AN ILLUSTRATED COLOUR TEXT

ORTHOPAEDICS AND TRAUMA

AN ILLUSTRATED COLOUR TEXT

ORTHOPAEDICS AND TRAUMA

RONALD McRAE MB FRCS(Eng) FRCS(Glas) FChS(Hon) AIMBI
Consultant Orthopaedic Surgeon, Ross Hall Hospital
Formerly Consultant Orthopaedic Surgeon,
Southern General Hospital, Glasgow, UK

ANDREW W. G. KINNINMONTH MB FRCS(Ed.)(Orth.)
Consultant Orthopaedic Surgeon and Honorary Senior Lecturer,
Glasgow Royal Infirmary University NHS Trust and
Stobhill NHS Trust, Glasgow, UK

With original drawings by RONALD McRAE

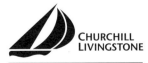
CHURCHILL
LIVINGSTONE

EDINBURGH LONDON NEW YORK PHILADELPHIA SYDNEY TORONTO 1997

CHURCHILL LIVINGSTONE
A Medical Division of Harcourt Brace and Company Limited

© Pearson Professional Limited 1997
© Harcourt Brace and Company Limited

◩ is a registered trademark of Harcourt Brace and
Company Limited

First published 1997
Reprinted 1998

ISBN 0 443-05135-6

British Library Cataloguing in Publication Data
A catalogue record for this book is available from the British Library.

Library of Congress Cataloguing in Publication Data
A catalog record for this book is available from the Library of Congress.

For Churchill Livingstone

Publisher Timothy Home
Project editor Jim Killgore
Design Sarah Cape
Page layout Kate Walshaw
Project controller Kay Hunston

The
publisher's
policy is to use
**paper manufactured
from sustainable forests**

Printed in China
GCC/02

PREFACE

Although orthopaedics and trauma are separate subjects, they both involve the study of bones and joints. Because of this, in most study courses, they are dealt with together. To conform with this common arrangement we have included both and, by doing so, hope that apart from convenience there will be gains in terms of consistency.

The contents of the book are loosely divided into two sections. At the beginning there is a description of fractures and dislocations in general, along with a number of orthopaedic conditions whose effects may often be widespread; later, and on a regional basis, specific fractures and orthopaedic problems are dealt with in more detail.

The layout of the book has been planned to avoid the daunting effect which a wordy text (often unrelieved by illustrations) may sometimes engender in the student. To this end it has been arranged that each topic is contained within a manageable double page spread, and is generously illustrated with representative radiographs, colour photographs and numerous line drawings (again in colour). To aid the assimilation of the information contained in each spread, there is a 'key points' summary box. This is consistently placed at the bottom right of the spread so that it may also be used to facilitate rapid revision.

Both subjects are large and expanding rapidly, and a comparatively small work cannot be fully comprehensive. Nevertheless, every effort has been made by careful planning and the elimination of superfluous text to include all that is considered to be essential for those at whom the book is aimed. (While it has been planned primarily for the use of medical students, physiotherapists, occupational therapists and nursing staff specialising in orthopaedics, there is sufficient detail for it to be of interest to family practitioners.) We hope that it will prove interesting, attractive and helpful.

Glasgow
1997

Ronald McRae
Andrew Kinninmonth

CONTENTS

GENERAL TOPICS IN ORTHOPAEDICS AND TRAUMA

REGIONAL ORTHOPAEDICS AND TRAUMA

DEVELOPMENTAL DISORDERS

There are many inherited disorders of bone, and most are uncommon. Some may not be evident at birth but only manifest themselves as growth occurs.

OSTEOGENESIS IMPERFECTA (BRITTLE BONE DISEASE)

This is an uncommon disorder with a variable pattern of inheritance. It is characterised by osteopaenia with a fracture diathesis, blue sclerae (Fig. 1), and deafness due to osteosclerosis. It has two main forms, namely the congenita and tarda: these are related to the age of presentation. The *congenita* form tends to be more severe and can lead to intra-uterine fractures and even stillbirth — either as a result of fractures or from intracranial haemorrhage during delivery. The survivors often develop abnormally: growth, particularly of the limbs, is retarded and the skull disproportionately large. Bone softening may lead to deformities of the limbs (Fig. 2), spine (Fig. 3) and of the rib-cage.

The *tarda* variety usually presents in the older child with fractures resulting from bone fragility. This form is generally inherited in an autosomal dominant pattern. Multiple fractures are common and may result from relatively minor trauma. As a child suffering from osteogenesis imperfecta nears adulthood, the tendency to fracture lessens; later, in females it rises again after the menopause. The radiographs show porotic, deformed bone, usually with evidence of healed fractures.

Treatment

There is no treatment other than for the specific fractures as they occur. Healing is usually rapid with appropriate immobilisation in a cast. In a few cases, prophylactic internal fixation with intramedullary rods is employed to reduce the frequency of fractures.

ACHONDROPLASIA

This is the most common of the family of skeletal dysplasias which produce abnormalities of chondrogenesis and osteogenesis. Most of these conditions result in shortness of stature, abnormal body proportions and skeletal malformations; they require specialist assessment.

Achondroplasia is of autosomal dominant inheritance, causes dwarfism, and is usually apparent at birth. Achondroplastics have disproportionately short limbs (the arms are especially affected), but the muscles are strong. Although the forehead is prominent, with a large vault and depressed nasal bridge, achondroplastics are generally of normal intelligence. On radiographs the tubular bones are short and wide with abnormal metaphyses (Fig. 4), but normal epiphyses.

The skull is large, although the base is usually underdeveloped. Although the spine is not usually short, the standing posture is abnormal in that there is a marked lumbar lordosis, a prominent abdomen, and usually flexion contractures of the hips. Spinal deformities are not uncommon, with narrowing of the spinal canal being the most important as it can cause a slowly progressive cord compression. In the lower limbs, genu varum is the most common deformity.

Treatment

Although the treatment is very protracted, leg lengthening procedures are often advocated and can lead to a significant improvement in the lower limb disproportion. The ability of the limb bones to produce new bone during leg lengthening procedures is excellent. Where there is narrowing of the spinal canal causing neurological symptoms, surgical decompression may be required. Genu varum may require realignment osteotomies.

DIAPHYSEAL ACLASIS (METAPHYSEAL ACLASIS, MULTIPLE EXOSTOSES)

Inherited as an autosomal dominant, this condition produces multiple exostoses which arise from the growth plates of long bones and occasionally from the scapulae and pelvis. The cause is a failure of remodelling during growth, with excess metaphyseal bone not being resorbed. Typically, the exostoses are bony with a cartilage covering and are usually easily palpable near the joints.

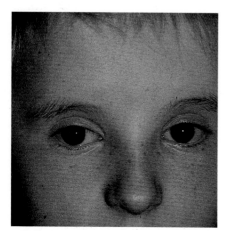

Fig. 1 **Child with blue sclerotics and osteogenesis imperfecta.**

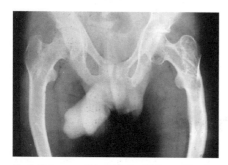

Fig. 2 **Osteogenesis imperfecta with femoral bowing and narrowing of the pelvis from bone softening.**

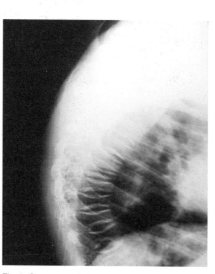

Fig. 3 **Osteogenesis imperfecta with multiple vertebral body deformities and a kyphosis.**

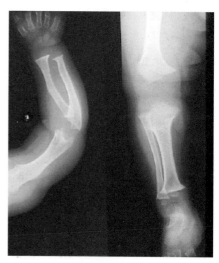

Fig. 4 **Achondroplasia with relative shortening of the long bones.**

Growth is not usually significantly retarded, but malalignment of the bones may occur. The radiographs typically show multiple sessile or pedunculated metaphyseal exostoses which point away from the joint (Fig. 5). The exostoses cease growth at the time of skeletal maturity of the affected bone and require no treatment unless they become symptomatic (e.g. from soft tissue friction). Rarely malignant change can occur and this should be suspected if enlargement is noted after skeletal maturity.

FIBROUS DYSPLASIA

This is a developmental defect which can affect one bone (monostotic) or several (polyostotic). Areas of endosteal bone are replaced with a fibrous matrix, with resultant weakening of the bone. Cases

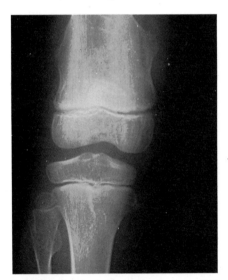

Fig. 5 **Diaphyseal aclasis affecting the femur, tibia and fibula.**

usually present with localised pain, gradually increasing deformity or fracture. The radiographs show a lucent area of disorganised bone with a 'ground glass' appearance. Unless there is a fracture, no breach occurs in the periosteum. In the polyostotic variety the long bones tend to be affected, sometimes in one limb only or scattered throughout the skeleton (Fig. 6). Sometimes the polyostotic variety is accompanied by skin pigmentation (and precocious puberty in girls), and this is known as Albright's syndrome.

Treatment
Intervention is confined to lesions which are painful, due to mechanical weakness or fracture, and those showing gradual deformity. In symptomatic lesions, curettage and bone grafting may be sufficient. If deformity accompanies the lesion, corrective osteotomy may also be required.

MARFAN'S SYNDROME

This is a disorder of autosomal dominant inheritance which produces a defect in collagen metabolism. Those affected are usually tall and thin, with long digits (arachnodactyly or 'spider bones') and generalised ligamentous laxity (leading to 'double jointedness', joint subluxations or dislocations). Skeletal deformity is common, in the form of scoliosis or rib anomalies such as pectus excavatum (funnel chest). Typically the patients have a highly arched palate and are prone to lens dislocations leading to myopia. Perhaps the most important potential complications are related to the heart and great vessels; aortic valvular disease

and dissection of the aorta are the most common problems, with the latter being the most frequent cause of death.

Treatment
Unfortunately, there is little that can be done to improve the orthopaedic deformities. Prompt treatment of any cardiac anomalies may reduce the risk of aortic dissection.

NEUROFIBROMATOSIS (VON RECKLINGHAUSEN'S DISEASE)

This disorder is inherited as an autosomal dominant condition. The skin manifestations are neurofibromas (which can be small subcutaneous nodules or more obvious cutaneous nodules) and café-au-lait spots which, if more than five are evident, are virtually diagnostic of the condition. The neuromas are usually innocent, but occasionally they are present on the peripheral nerves or cranial nerves (especially the 8th cranial nerve). Sometimes a patient with a neuroma in a spinal foramen will present with symptoms and signs identical to those found in a prolapsed intervertebral disc. Investigations such as a CAT or MRI scan should be able to differentiate between these two distinct pathologies (Fig. 7). Scoliosis develops in about 30–40% of affected children and frequently requires surgical stabilisation. In a few cases a neurofibroma may replace bone leading to fracture and a pseudoarthrosis; this is particularly important in the case of the tibia, where treatment may be extremely difficult. Neurofibromatosis itself does not require treatment.

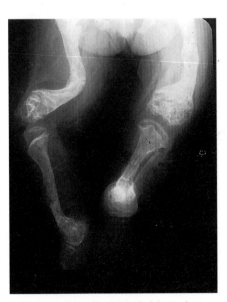

Fig. 6 **Gross deformities of the limb bones in polyostotic fibrous dysplasia.**

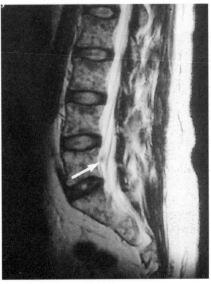

Fig. 7 **MRI scan showing the small dark shadow of a neurofibroma behind the body of L5.**

Developmental disorders

- Osteogenesis imperfecta only requires treatment if a fracture occurs or if others are anticipated.
- Achondroplastics can be improved by limb lengthening procedures, although this treatment is often protracted.
- Diaphyseal aclasis needs to be treated only if it causes local symptoms, but any increase in a lesion after skeletal maturity should arouse suspicion of malignant change.
- The most common cause of death from Marfan's syndrome is dissection of the aorta.
- Five or more café-au-lait spots are diagnostic of neurofibromatosis.

BONE INFECTIONS

Established bone infections are now relatively uncommon in the UK. This is primarily due to the availability of effective antibiotics, which are often able to abort an infection at an early stage. In adults, in countries with well-developed health care sevices, the most common precipitant is a surgical procedure such as fixation of a fracture or a joint replacement. In less well-developed countries, bone infections all too commonly result from delays in the treatment of open fractures.

ACUTE OSTEOMYELITIS

In children, acute osteomyelitis most frequently involves the femur, tibia or humerus. In the majority of cases the causal organisms are blood borne from a septic focus elsewhere, and generally lodge in a metaphysis (this is considered to be due to the high vascularity of this region where there are 'venous lakes' which have a relatively slow blood flow). There is sometimes a history of a previous minor injury in the affected area. The inflammatory response leads to increased pressure in the unyielding vascular channels within the bone causing great pain, marked local tenderness and swelling, and general toxicity with high fever. If untreated, pus may escape into the medullary cavity (Fig. 1) or form a subperiosteal abscess; this may in turn rupture, present beneath the skin, and eventually form a sinus. The periosteum may be widely stripped, forming a shroud of new bone (*involucrum*) with numerous openings (*cloacae*) through which pus may escape. Increased intra-osseous pressure may lead to local thrombosis and bone necrosis. Then, if the area of dead bone becomes detached from its surroundings it forms a *sequestrum* (Fig. 2). Sinuses, an involucrum and sequestra are the features of *chronic osteomyelitis* which is usually accompanied by impaired growth. As an irretrievable situation can arise within a few days, an accurate assessment and prompt treatment are essential (note that in those cases where the organisms enter by other routes, e.g. penetrating injuries, the pathological features are similar, but in adults widespread periosteal stripping does not occur).

Bacteriology

The most common organism is *Staphylococcus aureus*, followed by *streptococcus* and *pneumococcus*. Haemolytic streptococci

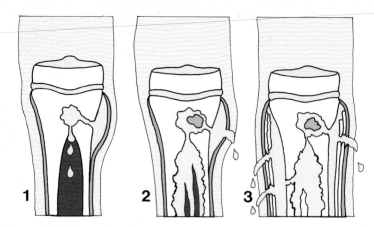

Fig. 1 **Osteomyelitis. (1)** A metaphyseal focus may spread to the medullary cavity, or subperiosteally. **(2)** Necrosis of bone and soft tissues may form an abscess cavity, a sequestrum (shown in grey) and a sinus; and the medullary cavity may become extensively infected. **(3)** Wide stripping of the periosteum (shown in green) may lead to the formation of a bony involucrum, cloacae, and multiple sinuses.

are now seldom involved. Gram negative organisms, especially *Escherichia coli* and *Pseudomonas pyocyanea*, account for about 10% of infections. Salmonella osteomyelitis is not uncommon in patients with sickle cell disease who are prone to the development of bone infarcts.

Diagnosis

The condition should be suspected in any child complaining of severe pain in a limb, especially where there is accompanying fever and toxicity. Clinically there is well-localised metaphyseal tenderness, usually with swelling and often redness, and the ESR and C-reactive protein (CRP) are elevated. The white count is generally raised, with an increased polymorph count (if it is not, this may indicate a poor defence response with toxic depression of marrow activity). Blood cultures should be carried out in an attempt to isolate a causal organism and establish bacterial sensitivities. Obtaining a specimen of pus by aspiration or surgical exposure may be desirable for the same reasons, but in view of the risks of introducing secondary infection this may be deferred until the results of initial treatment have been assessed. Radiographs are usually normal at presentation, but show periosteal reaction and rarefaction within 7–10 days.

Treatment

Bedrest and splintage of the limb is essential. Early use of high dose antibiotics may quickly abort an episode. Until sensitivities are obtained, two antibiotics can be given empirically, e.g. flucloxacillin and fusidic acid in high

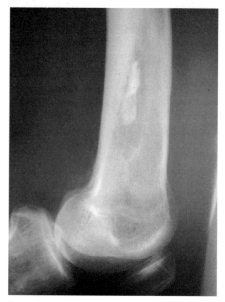

Fig. 2 **The radiograph shows a sequestrum in an abscess cavity in the distal femur.**

dosage. It is generally agreed that if the systemic upset is not controlled within 48 hours, surgical drainage and decompression of the metaphysis should be undertaken. This is often the case by the time the patient enters hospital, so that surgical drainage may be the first line of treatment. Once an antibiotic specific to the infection has been found, it should be continued for 4–6 weeks.

CHRONIC OSTEOMYELITIS

Once there is bone necrosis with sequestrum formation the scene is set for recurrent attacks of osteomyelitis. Bacteria and necrotic bone often become

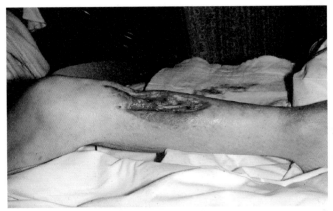

Fig. 3 **Chronic discharging osteomyelitis of the tibia secondary to the internal fixation of a fracture.**

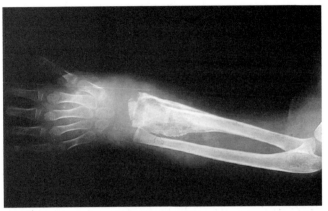

Fig. 5 **Tuberculosis of the distal radius in a child.**

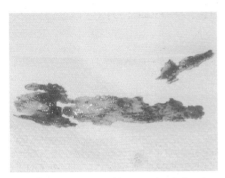

Fig. 4 **Sequestra removed from a case of chronic osteomyelitis.**

trapped in fibrous tissue in the area, and sometimes lie dormant for years. The radiographs in chronic cases show disorganised, thickened and sclerotic bone, sometimes with abscess cavities containing sequestra. The skin is often scarred and adherent to underlying bone, and there may be a chronic sinus which discharges continuously or intermittently (Fig. 3).

Treatment
In some cases, treatment by simple dressing of a chronic discharge may suffice. When there are recurrent exacerbations of the infection, with pain (especially likely if drainage is blocked) and the formation of abscesses, more active treatment will be required; it should also be noted that where there is a sequestrum a sinus is unlikely to dry up for any length of time. While temporary improvement may follow a course of an appropriate antibiotic, the only hope of a more lasting solution is by surgery. Then, as a minimum, drainage should be established, sequestra removed (Fig. 4), and infective granulation tissue excised. In some cases it may be possible to carry out a more radical excision of the diseased area and replace the defect with a vascularised bone graft; in others, amputation may be the only solution.

SUBACUTE OSTEOMYELITIS
In this condition, the onset is insidious with no history of a previous acute episode, injury or likely bacterial inoculation. The distal tibia and os calcis are most frequently affected, although any bone can be involved. The causative organism is usually a staphylococcus aureus, although Gram negative organisms may sometimes be isolated. The complaint is of low grade bone pain. Clinically, there may be little to find and the symptoms can easily be dismissed (it is not clear why these infections do not present acutely, especially as there is usually no history of previous antibiotic ingestion). The typical lesion on X-ray is a small rounded lucency surrounded by a rim of sclerotic bone (Brodie's abscess). It can be confused with an osteoid osteoma as there is often little systemic upset. In its other form, subacute osteomyelitis produces sclerosis (usually of a long bone) without pus formation (sclerosing non-suppurative osteomyelitis). The whole medullary cavity can be obliterated with new bone leading to sequestrum and sinus formation.

Treatment
This is similar to that employed in other forms of osteomyelitis, with surgical excision being the preferred method in Brodie's abscess.

SKELETAL TUBERCULOSIS
Tuberculosis (TB) can affect any part of the skeleton and is the result of haematogenous spread from an active focus in the lungs or lymphatic system. The infection tends to be chronic, with slow destruction of bone, and it may present as a relatively painless swelling containing tuberculous pus. It is common in the bodies of the vertebrae where the growth plates and the intervertebral discs are destroyed at an early stage. Large

tuberculous abscesses often form and there is sometimes neurological involvement (see p. 24). Elsewhere the causal organisms tend to lodge close to a joint (e.g. in the hip, the second most common area affected, the infection commences in the acetabular floor, the epiphysis, or the metaphysis, all within the joint capsule); the joint is then rapidly invaded so that the case becomes predominantly one of tuberculous arthritis. The diaphyses of the metacarpals or metatarsals may also be affected (tuberculous dactylitis), otherwise involvement of the shafts of the major long bones is quite rare (Fig. 5).

Treatment
This is the same as for joint TB, although surgical debridement may occasionally be required.

OSTEOMYELITIS SECONDARY TO FRACTURE FIXATION
This occurs when fixation is complicated by an early uncontrolled wound infection. The stability of the fracture must be maintained to ensure healing, and this may be achieved by the use of an external fixator or sometimes by leaving the metalwork in situ. In combination with radical surgical debridement and appropriate antibiotic cover, healing can be obtained in a high proportion of cases.

Bone infections
- Prompt diagnosis and early treatment are essential in any case of acute osteomyelitis.
- Chronic osteomyelitis is often very disabling, and in extreme cases amputation may be required.
- Tuberculosis of long bones is rare compared with tuberculosis of joints.

INFECTIVE ARTHRITIS

Without prompt diagnosis and treatment, infective arthritis can cause irreparable damage to the articular surfaces of a joint leading to rapidly advancing degenerative changes and permanent stiffness. Infection can result from the direct inoculation of organisms in penetrating injuries, from haematogenous spread, or by extension from an adjacent area of osteomyelitis. Predisposing factors include diabetes, rheumatoid arthritis, steroid therapy or leukaemia.

Pathology

The changes which occur in the joint are mainly due to the effects of the causal organism on the synovial membrane and articular surfaces. On reaching the joint, the infective agent causes an acute inflammatory synovitis. This reactive effusion is rich in leucocytes and fibrin. Chondral injury results from the action of proteases derived from the leucocytes, plasmin (a powerful chondrolytic agent released in the inflammatory exudate) and bacterial toxins which act directly on the chondrocytes (Fig. 1). In addition, normal synovial fluid production is inhibited, causing poor lubrication and further joint damage. If untreated, a fibrotic reaction occurs, leading to the formation of intra-articular adhesions and severe joint stiffness.

Bacteriology

Any pathogen, be it bacterial, viral or fungal, can cause a septic arthritis. Staphylococci, streptococci and Gram negative organisms are probably the most common in the UK, but other infections (such as brucella, typhoid, measles, mumps and many venereal infections) can cause an arthropathy.

Joint aspiration before antibiotics are commenced is highly desirable in all cases where infection is suspected so that any organism and its antibiotic sensitivities can be established.

ACUTE SEPTIC ARTHRITIS IN CHILDREN

In an unwell baby with a high fever, an infected joint can easily be missed unless the possibility is kept in mind and a careful examination is made; the consequences of overlooking a septic arthritis can be disastrous. The signs are usually obvious in the superficial joints (swelling, tenderness and pain on movement) but

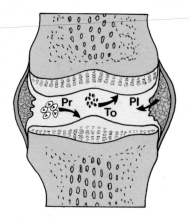

Fig. 1 **Chondral injury in joint infections results from plasmins (Pl), proteases (Pr) and bacterial toxins (To).**

are less so in the hip: there the joint is usually held in abduction, flexion and external rotation, and there is pain when any attempt is made to straighten it. In the older child, the diagnosis may be easier as a more detailed history may be forthcoming. In some cases antibiotics may have been started empirically, suppressing the signs (but not necessarily the outcome for the affected joint). At the start the radiographs may be normal or show some signs of joint distension. Later, narrowing or distortion of the joint, delayed development, or asymmetrical growth may become evident.

ACUTE SEPTIC ARTHRITIS IN ADULTS

This may have an acute or insidious onset; it is important to exclude predisposing features such as diabetes. Patients with rheumatoid arthritis have a particularly high incidence of joint sepsis which can be mistaken for a flare-up of their underlying disease. Intravenous drug abusers frequently present with a late septic arthritis as a result of injecting their hips when attempting to find their femoral vessels. As a group they suffer from bacteraemic episodes and may be significantly immunosuppressed; other joints can also be affected by haematogenous spread.

Clinically an infected joint is red, swollen, painful and resistant to attempted motion; associated pyrexia and leucocytosis leave little doubt about the diagnosis. Radiographs may be normal at the onset, but may show early narrowing of the joint space, a poor prognostic sign (Fig. 2).

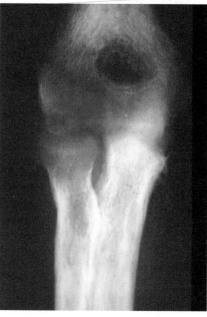

Fig. 2 **Infective arthritis of the elbow with narrowing of the joint space between the humerus and the ulna, and blurring of the articular margins.**

Vertebral involvement is not uncommon, with the end plates and disc spaces being affected first. This leads to necrosis of the disc and adjacent bone, typically producing a narrowed disc space and often bone sclerosis (this may help differentiate it from malignancies which destroy the vertebral bodies in the first instance). The infection often originates in the genitourinary tract, communicating via Batson's plexus (the anastomosis between the pelvic veins and the vertebral venous complex).

Investigations

Regardless of age a prompt diagnosis is essential. Joint aspiration, with an urgent Gram stain and aerobic and anaerobic cultures, should be carried out. Baseline haematological indices including haemoglobin, ESR and C-reactive protein (CRP) are useful for the purpose of monitoring progress.

Treatment

Early treatment is essential to avoid irretrievable damage to the articular cartilage; this follows along the lines described for osteomyelitis. In the hip, many advocate early surgical decompression, either by repeated aspirations or surgical lavage as an open procedure or arthroscopically. In all cases, high doses of appropriate antibiotics should be given and continued until the CRP settles.

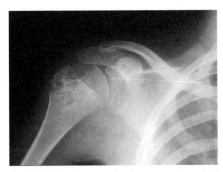

Fig. 3 **TB of the shoulder, with involvement of the metaphysis and epiphysis.**

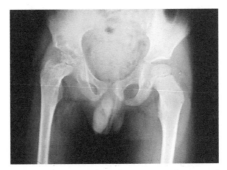

Fig. 4 **Advanced TB of the hip, with involvement of the acetabulum as well as the femoral epiphysis and metaphysis.**

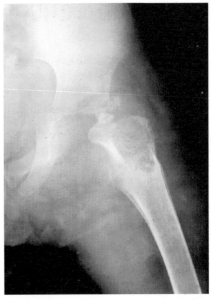

Fig. 5 **TB hip with disturbed epiphyseal growth and dislocation of the hip.**

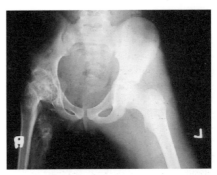

Fig. 6 **Gross destruction of the hip, with a calcified TB abscess in the thigh.**

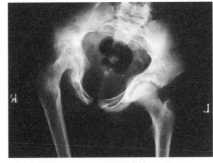

Fig. 7 **TB hip with spontaneous fusion in adduction.** There is associated true and apparent shortening of the limb, and compensatory tilting of the pelvis.

TUBERCULOUS ARTHRITIS

The destruction of the affected joint surface is slower than in other forms of infective arthritis, and it tends to be secondary to a synovial reaction (although marginal erosions may occur). The resultant tuberculous granulation tissue forms a pannus, producing softening and erosion of the articular surface; in combination with extensive fibrosis, this leads to a very stiff degenerate joint. Unlike the majority of pyogenic infections of bone, the growth plate may be penetrated (Fig. 3). The most common peripheral joints to be affected are the hip (Fig. 4) and knee. Clinically, the joint may be relatively painless in the first instance, with the patient complaining of a limp or altered function. Later the signs become more florid, and abscess formation within the joint may lead to its dislocation (Fig. 5); rupture of the joint capsule may lead to tracking abscesses (Fig. 6).

Investigations

Aspiration and synovial biopsy are necessary to establish the diagnosis, although it should be remembered that joint TB is usually a sequel to generalised disease; thus a full clinical assessment is required, including tuberculin testing, urine and sputum cultures, and an X-ray of the chest. Joint radiographs may show rarefaction and erosions of bone, and increased soft tissue density (indicating likely abscess formation). Changes which involve both an epiphysis and a metaphysis without sclerotic margins are typical of TB.

Treatment

The mainstay of treatment is antituberculous triple chemotherapy. In the early phase before joint damage has occurred, synovectomy may be helpful in retaining motion; but once joint damage has occurred little can be done to salvage the joint. Then the aim is to obtain fusion of the joint, either spontaneously (Fig. 7) or by means of surgery.

SEPSIS AFTER TOTAL JOINT REPLACEMENT

Prosthetic infections occur in acute and chronic forms, and it can be argued that the longer the prosthesis is implanted the more likely it is to become infected. The *acute form* occurs in the first week and results from the perioperative inoculation of organisms. The *chronic form* is more insidious, and the only feature may be X-ray evidence of loosening of the prosthesis; this may or may not be accompanied by pain. Clinically, there may be little else to find, but the ESR and CRP may be raised. Radioisotope scanning may show characteristic 'hot' areas around the prosthesis. Although there is a wide spectrum of potential pathogens, the most common are *Staphylococcus aureus* or *albus* (previously thought not to be a pathogen) and *Escherichia coli*.

Treatment

An acute infection may sometimes be aborted by antibiotics. If there is a major systemic upset in the presence of a markedly inflamed wound, antibiotics along with surgical lavage (or a more radical debridement) may salvage the situation, although regular review thereafter is necessary. In the chronic form the prosthesis usually has to be removed; if the infection can be eradicated, re-implantation of a further prosthesis may be possible. If this is not feasible, excision arthroplasty (e.g. of the hip) or joint fusion (e.g. at the knee) are the best options.

Infective arthritis

- Septic arthritis requires prompt diagnosis and treatment to minimise complications.
- Tuberculosis should always be regarded as a possible cause of septic arthritis.
- Regular ESR and CRP estimations are useful for monitoring treatment of joint infections.
- Pain in a prosthetic implant in the absence of X-ray evidence of loosening should raise suspicions about possible infection.

OSTEOARTHRITIS

Osteoarthritis is an extremely common degenerative process which is responsible for considerable disability in the form of pain, stiffness and restricted mobility. Two forms are recognised: primary and secondary osteoarthritis. In *primary osteoarthritis* the aetiology is uncertain, although it is likely that it is the end result of a number of pathological processes which lead to 'joint failure'. In *secondary osteoarthritis*, one or more of many well recognised predisposing factors are seen to be present (Table 1). With increasing knowledge, secondary osteoarthritis is now diagnosed more frequently than primary, e.g. in osteoarthritis of the hip, a predisposing abnormality can be found in 90% of patients.

Pathological features

The two fundamental features are *cartilage damage* and *mechanical failure*. Cartilage damage occurs in stages, and starts with a breakdown of the normal collagen fibre network and a reduction in proteoglycan concentration. This results in a loss of cartilage resilience, setting up a worsening spiral of events; the exposed collagen fibres have an affinity for water, which causes further swelling and proteoglycan depletion leading finally to loss of the mechanical integrity of the articular cartilage. Inflammatory responses to this process can result, and these exacerbate the course of events by releasing proteolytic enzymes which further degrade the joint surface. Conditions such as gout cause degeneration in a similar way, and hydroxyapatite crystals have been incriminated as a mediator in this particular disease. Mechanical factors play a significant role in the degenerative process. The forces crossing a joint may be either excessive or applied over an abnormally small area, or there may be a combination of both these factors. In congenital dysplasia of the hip or in genu varum, for example, the area of load transmission is not only small, but the actual force is increased because the deformity is associated with abnormal leverage between the surfaces.

Macroscopic appearances

Cartilage: At first there is fibrillation of the superficial layers giving a frayed appearance to the surface. Subsequently, the cartilage develops deep fissures with fragmentation and detachment of cartilage fragments, leading to exposure of

Table 1 **Aetiological factors in secondary osteoarthritis.**

- Congenital: e.g. acetabular dysplasia, congenital dislocation of the hip
- Developmental: e.g. Perthes' disease, slipped upper femoral epiphysis
- Metabolic: e.g. gout, pseudogout
- Infective: e.g. staphylococcal, tuberculosis, brucellosis
- Sexually transmitted: e.g. Reiter's syndrome, gonococcal
- Post-traumatic: e.g. from fractures involving the articular surfaces
- Genetic: e.g. haemophilia (and related diseases), Gaucher's disease, mucopolysaccharidoses, sickle cell anaemia
- Autoimmune diseases: e.g. rheumatoid arthritis, ankylosing spondylitis, psoriatic arthritis and other seronegative arthritides
- Avascular necrosis: e.g. idiopathic, or secondary to fracture, caisson disease, alcohol abuse or steroids

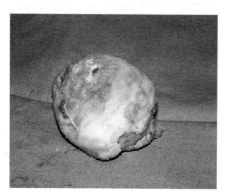

Fig. 1 **Femoral head (removed during the course of a joint replacement) showing loss of most of the articular cartilage.**

subchondral bone (Fig. 1) and the formation of loose bodies.

Subchondral bone: An abrasive mechanism is probably responsible for eburnation (polishing) of the exposed bone which may develop a smooth, ivory-like appearance. Areas of segmental necrosis and microfractures appear in the subchondral layers, resulting in increased osteoblastic activity which is responsible for increased uptake in isotopic bone scans. There is thickening of the subchondral plate and adjacent bony trabeculae leading to **sclerosis**, one of the cardinal radiological features of osteoarthritis.

Subchondral pseudocysts: These are seen both histologically and in radiographs and represent areas of bone which have been replaced by myxomatous fibrous tissue. The lesions are thought to be the result of high intra-articular pressure forcing synovial fluid through defects in the joint surface into the marrow spaces. Although almost invariably present in osteoarthritis, they are by no means exclusive to this condition.

Remodelling: This is a striking feature which leads to an alteration of the joint contours. It is commonly seen in the hip joint where the normal spherical shape of

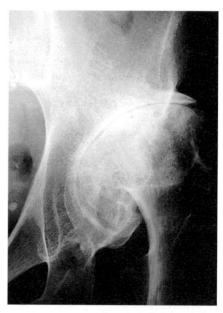

Fig. 2 **Osteoarthritis of the hip with remodelling the femoral head which is no longer spherical.**

the femoral head becomes flattened and marginal osteophytes (new bone) appear (Fig. 2). This process can lead to further restriction of joint mobility by acting as a physical block to motion.

Clinical Features

Symptoms

Pain is the cardinal and usual presenting symptom. It is often worsened by immobility, when the joint tends to stiffen up, or if there is any subsequent activity to gain relief. Pain at rest and nocturnal pain coupled with severely restricted mobility are the main indications for surgical intervention. *Stiffness*, particularly in the morning, is a variable phenomenon and usually reflects capsular fibrosis and/or protective muscle spasm. *Swelling*, often due to an effusion, is a common symptom but is only evident in superficial joints such as the knee or wrist. *Functional disability* in the upper limb or a limp in the lower limb (antalgic gait) are common reasons for referral.

Signs

Commonly only one joint is affected, usually a weight-bearing one (the knee or hip). There may be muscle wasting in the area, and in the palpable joints tenderness is almost universal. Palpable osteophytes or joint effusion may be responsible for swelling. Synovial thickening is not a major feature in osteoarthritis. In the case of the knee there may be obvious deformity (e.g. genu valgum or varum, or one of fixed flexion), while in the hip the joint may be flexed, adducted and internally rotated.

Investigations

It is important to exclude other causes of joint destruction such as gout or rheumatoid arthritis, whose course may be modified by specific treatments. In view of this a full haematological, biochemical and serological profile should be undertaken; in particular the ESR and rheumatoid factor (which are invariably negative in osteoarthritis) should be assessed. An X-ray examination of the affected joint should be carried out. The cardinal radiographic features are joint space narrowing, subchondral bone sclerosis, the formation of cysts and marginal osteophytes and sometimes loose bodies (Fig. 3). There may be joint subluxations which in the hands are associated with conspicuous local swellings of the DIP joints (Heberden's nodes, Fig. 4) or the PIP joints (Bouchard's nodes).

Treatment

Conservative measures

Weight reduction is important in the obese patient whose weight-bearing joints are affected. This not only reduces joint stresses, but may facilitate any surgical intervention should this become necessary. Physiotherapy is useful in maintaining a functional range of motion. Splintage can be useful in the acute arthritic joint but should be used for brief periods only to avoid producing stiffness. In the lower limb, a walking stick will help to reduce the loading on the affected joint. Modification of activities may help to relieve pain, although exercising within the limits of pain should be encouraged.

Medical treatment

Where the pain is mild, simple analgesics like aspirin or paracetamol can be used. In patients with more severe pain, non-steroidal anti-inflammatory agents such as ibuprofen or indomethacin, taken on a regular basis, can produce satisfactory relief. It is important to use these drugs

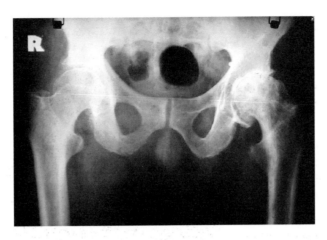

Fig. 3 **Early OA right hip, with slight joint space narrowing and early lipping.** Advanced OA on the left, with gross narrowing of joint space, marginal sclerosis of the acetabulum, and cystic changes in the femoral head.

with care if there is a history of gastro-intestinal pathology.

Surgical treatment

The primary aim of surgical intervention is the relief of pain. Before any operation is planned, the patient's general condition must be assessed to exclude severe concurrent medical conditions. There are four main surgical options:

Arthrodesis or joint fusion is the only certain way of rendering a joint pain-free. This procedure, however, has the tendency to increase the stresses in the related joints, and the effects of the absolute loss of movements on function must be carefully considered. It is sometimes advocated in a patient who is considered to be too young (because of long-term uncertainties) to have a joint replacement, and is a useful salvage procedure for a failed arthroplasty.

Arthroplasty (usually in the form of total joint replacement) is the most commonly performed operation in orthopaedics and is most effective at the hip and knee. By relieving pain and preserving or restoring joint movement it leads to restoration of function. Although the success rate is high, the risks of complications such as infection, loosening, mechanical failure and ultimate component wear must be kept in mind.

Osteotomy can be utilised to realign deformities and spread the transmitted loads more evenly (e.g. in genu varum where there are degenerative changes in the medial joint compartment). Even when performed in cases where deformity is minimal, pain relief may be achieved; this is thought to be due to painful subchondral venous hypertension being reduced by the bone division.

Excision arthroplasty has occasional use as a salvage procedure in infected hip arthroplasties, where by removing all foreign material (prostheses and cement)

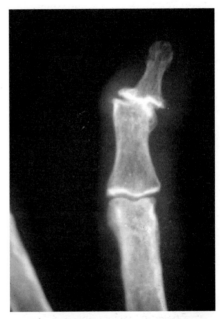

Fig. 4 **Subluxation of the DIP joint of a finger with prominence of the distal end of middle phalanx (Heberden's node).**

the infection may be allowed to settle. A fibrous joint is produced: this has some stability but mobility is restricted.

Osteoarthritis

- The incidence of osteoarthritis increases with age.
- It commonly affects a single joint.
- The pathology primarily involves the articular cartilage.
- Medical treatment should always be tried first.
- There are several surgical options but in the hip and knee, total joint arthroplasty is the treatment of choice for advanced disease.

DIETARY AND METABOLIC DISORDERS

These conditions are common in the general population, frequently passing unnoticed until a fracture or an acute inflammatory episode leads to a medical assessment.

OSTEOPOROSIS

Osteoporosis is specifically defined as osteopaenia with a parallel reduction in bone mineral and matrix below the range found in normal subjects of similar age and sex. Osteoporosis can to some extent be physiological in the sense that with age all our bones become relatively porotic, mainly due to a reduction in our activity; but if this is more extreme, pathological fractures may result from trivial incidents. After the age of 25 years the process affects everyone, but it is more rapid in women, particularly after the menopause. Caucasians seem more vulnerable than other races, so there may be a genetic predisposition. There are many other factors which may be implicated (Table 1).

Table 1 **Causes of osteoporosis**

1. Age-related and postmenopausal (the most common)
2. Endocrine
   - thyrotoxicosis
   - acromegaly
   - Cushing's syndrome
3. Disuse porosis, e.g. after injury or prolonged bedrest
4. Rheumatoid arthritis
5. Prolonged corticosteroid administration

Clinically osteoporosis is symptomless and may go unobserved until a fracture occurs (in the UK fractures have now reached epidemic proportions, with the distal radius (Colles) and the neck of femur being most common). If the spine is involved, there may be a progressive kyphosis and loss of stature, often from multiple vertebral compression fractures (Fig. 1).

Investigations

In essence, the biochemical and haematological indices are normal, but as osteoporosis often coexists with osteomalacia, care must be taken in interpreting the results. Apart from detecting fractures in the classical sites, plain radiographs are often unreliable in diagnosing osteoporosis as variations in exposure may give false impressions of osteopaenia or normality. Dual photon absorption densitometry on the other hand can now quantify bone mineralisa-

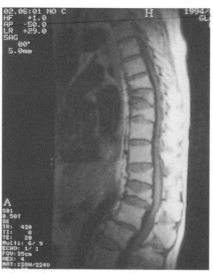

Fig. 1 **MRI scan showing multiple osteoporotic wedge fractures of the spine.**

tion and also allow an assessment of the effects of treatment.

Treatment

There is much debate about the best therapy. Maintaining bone stock by activity and hormone replacement therapy in perimenopausal women may be the most effective measures, although there is as yet no single remedy which can be recommended.

DISORDERS OF VITAMIN D METABOLISM

Vitamin D is a fat-soluble vitamin which is either absorbed from food or is synthesised in the skin by the action of sunlight on 7-dihydrocholesterol, producing cholecalciferol. This then requires further metabolism in the liver, and then the kidney, to produce the most active metabolite, 1, 25 dihydroxycholecalciferol. It is responsible for the absorption of calcium from the intestine and for normal bone mineralisation. Any of the steps in this process can be blocked.

RICKETS

This is a childhood disease which is caused by vitamin D deficiency and lack of sunlight. It leads to a failure of skeletal calcification, which is most evident at the sites of rapid growth, e.g. the metaphyses of long bones. In babies, little abnormality may be evident apart from some mild swelling of the bone ends and of the ribs (ricket rosary). Bone softening may lead to some deformity of the skull. Once

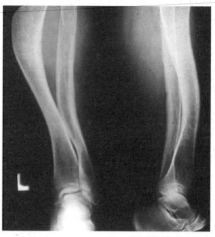

Fig. 2 **Rachitic deformities of the tibia persisting in adulthood.**

the child starts to walk, progressive bony deformity becomes more obvious, with the tibiae becoming bowed and rotated (Fig. 2). As vitamin D also influences muscle function a profound and disabling myopathy may occur.

Investigations

The serum calcium and phosphate levels are reduced and the alkaline phosphatase is raised. In the growing child, care must be taken in interpreting the latter; it should be compared with the normal range found in children in the same age group. The radiographs have a typical appearance, with widening and 'cupping' of the metaphyses.

OSTEOMALACIA

This is the adult equivalent of rickets, although the aetiology of the deficiency is more varied. It is often difficult to diagnose, presenting only as a fracture in an elderly patient. Clinically, patients may complain of generalised muscle and bone pain, made worse by activity or when pressure is applied to the subcutaneous surfaces of affected bones.

Several aetiological factors and patterns are recognised:

1. *Nutritional.* Up to 30% of elderly patients presenting with a fracture of the neck of femur have osteomalacia. Whilst the cause may be multifactorial, many have inadequate diets and, being frail and housebound, are never exposed to sunlight.
2. *Malabsorption.* Any form of malabsorption will inevitably cause a

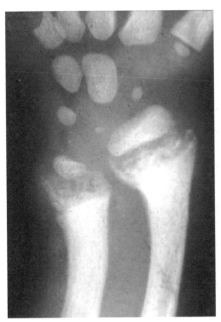

Fig. 3 **Metaphyseal cupping of radius and ulna due to renal rickets.**

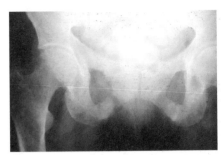

Fig. 4 **Osteomalacia: pseudofractures of ischial rami.**

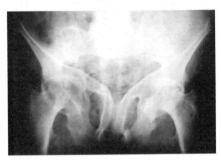

Fig. 5 **Osteomalacia: triradiate deformity of the pelvis.**

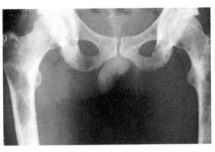

Fig. 6 **Hyperparathyroidism with multiple femoral cysts.**

degree of osteomalacia, e.g. after partial gastrectomy or in the presence of gluten enteropathy.
3. *Renal osteodystrophy* (renal rickets). This occurs secondary to chronic renal failure, which produces phosphate retention and a failure of 1, 25-dihydroxycholecalciferol production. This in turn leads to calcium malabsorption, secondary hyperparathyroidism, and defective osteoid maturation (Fig. 3).
4. *Drug-induced.* The most important drugs which may lead to osteomalacia are anticonvulsants such as phenytoin and phenobarbitone.

Investigations
In the absence of renal failure the biochemical abnormalities may not be as clear cut as in rickets. The calcium and phosphate may be normal or low, although the bone isoenzyme alkaline phosphatase is invariably raised. Osteomalacia is sometimes diagnosed empirically if the serum levels of calcium and phosphate, when multiplied together, give a figure lower than 2.25 (SI units) or 28 (mgms/100cc). Vitamin D estimations or an iliac crest biopsy can be carried out where there is still difficulty in making a diagnosis. Radiographs of osteomalacia typically show pseudofractures (Looser's zones, Fig. 4). These are areas of demineralisation usually situated in the concavity of long bones (in Paget's disease the convexity is involved), the pelvic rami and the lateral edge of the scapulae. They are probably traumatic in origin. In the spine, the vertebral bodies may collapse,

becoming biconcave in shape (so-called 'codfish' vertebrae); bone softening may lead to bowing of the long bones and deformity of the pelvis (Fig. 5).

Treatment
Therapy is directed to the cause. Dietary advice, exposure to sunlight, and calcium with vitamin D supplements (orally or by injection) are usually enough to resolve the condition within a short time. In some cases long-term treatment may be required.

HYPERPARATHYROIDISM
This is a relatively rare condition. Primary hyperparathyroidism in most cases is caused by an adenoma which classically leads to an elevation of serum calcium and depression of serum phosphate. Renal calculi may form and be painfully excreted. Bone changes are seen radiographically as subperiosteal erosions, particularly in the hands, and cystic changes (osteitis fibrosa cystica, Fig. 6) in the long bones (so-called brown tumours as they have a high concentration of haemosiderin). Symptoms are often mild and dismissed by the patient, but lethargy, general malaise and nausea may become prominent. Secondary hyperparathyroidism (more common than primary) results from calcium malabsorption and vitamin D deficiency associated with renal failure.

Treatment
Where symptoms are present, primary hyperparathyroidism is treated by excision of the adenoma. In secondary cases, careful supplementation of calcium and vitamin D may help to control the symptoms.

HYPERCALCAEMIA IN MALIGNANCY
This is a problem which occurs commonly in malignant disease and must not be confused with hyperparathyroidism. It is probably caused by a combination of bone destruction and a humoral agent secreted by the malignancy. The clinical features are diverse, to some extent depending on the rapidity of onset. Drowsiness, headaches and hallucinations with intractable vomiting in the late stages are all features of the hypercalcaemia.

Treatment
If severe and life threatening, careful rehydration and attention to fluid balance is essential. Drugs such as Mithracin are useful, but require to be used with great care.

Dietary and metabolic disorders

- Osteoporotic fractures are common in the ageing population.
- Maintaining bone stock with exercise and hormone replacement therapy may help prevent osteoporosis.
- Osteomalacia is present in up to 30% of elderly patients presenting with fractures.
- Once detected, osteomalacia is eminently treatable with calcium and vitamin D supplements.

GOUT AND PSEUDOGOUT (CRYSTAL SYNOVITIS)

These two disorders commonly affect the general population and present in very similar ways. They can be difficult to differentiate, but with care this should be possible.

GOUT

This is a disease which has been recognised for centuries and is characterised by attacks of acute arthritis secondary to the release of the crystals of monosodium urate monohydrate into the joint cavity. In addition, deposits of sodium urate can be found in all tissues but particularly around the joints and kidneys; if found on the skin they are known as tophi (Fig. 1). (The disease is now so eminently treatable that the massive cutaneous tophi seen in the past are now relatively rare.) Some 20% of urinary tract calculi consist of uric acid; these form in affected individuals as a result of the high renal excretion of uric acid. Uric acid is produced at the end stage of purine metabolism in the breakdown of nucleic acids (Fig. 2.)

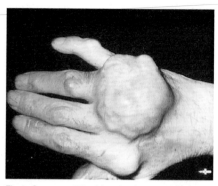
Fig. 1 Gross gouty tophi on the dorsum of the hand.

Hyperuricaemia is the primary cause of gout, but there are people with an increased level of uric acid in the blood who never manifest the disease. Urate concentration is variable in all of us, and is a combination of genetic predisposition and environmental factors. Fifty per cent of gout sufferers are overweight and there is a strong connection with excessive intake of alcohol (which blocks the renal secretion of uric acid). Foods that are high in purines (i.e. those which are protein rich) may raise the urate level. Diuretics, such as frusemide and the thiazides, alter the renal excretion of uric acid and may precipitate an attack.

It should be remembered that an attack of gout may be promoted by conditions or situations which produce rapid cellular turnover, e.g. myeloproliferative disease, multiple myeloma and, importantly, chemotherapy treatment. The stress of surgery is also a common precipitant.

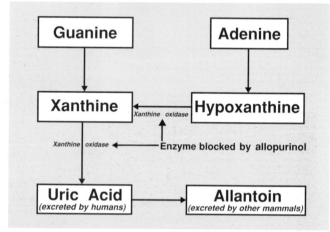
Fig. 2 The key stages in purine metabolism.

Clinical features

Gout is the most common form of inflammatory disease seen in men over 40 years, accounting for 85% of the total; about 25% have a strong family history. In the absence of a precipitating cause it is rare in patients below this age. The initial episode tends to affect the lower limbs, with the first metatarsophalangeal joint being the favourite (and classical) site. With recurrent attacks more joints may be recruited, although the axial skeleton is rarely affected. Typically the onset is abrupt, unlike in other inflammatory conditions, producing a painful, swollen and inflamed joint (Fig. 3).

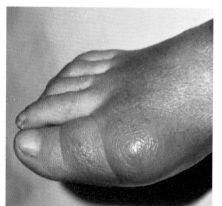
Fig. 3 Acute gout affecting the MP joint of the great toe.

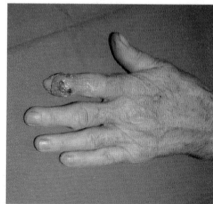
Fig. 4 Ulceration of the skin over digital tophi.

Surrounding desquamation may occur. In some cases gout may be mistaken for a septic arthritis as there may be a low grade fever and leucocytosis.

If the process is allowed to become chronic, tophi form, most commonly in the synovium, subchondral bone, the lobes of the ear, the olecranon bursa and achilles tendon. They may lead to ulceration of the overlying skin (Fig. 4). Tophus production is related to the urate level and reflects the severity and uncontrolled course of the disorder. Secondary renal disease may intervene, and there is a higher incidence of hypertension in affected individuals. (Beware the 'infection', particularly of the digits, which fails to settle on antibiotics as this may be an atypical gout.)

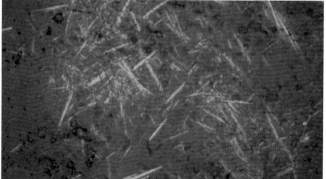
Fig. 5 Urate crystals in gout.

Investigations

During an acute attack the level of urate should be raised at some stage, but absence of a raised urate does not exclude the diagnosis. The presence of uric acid crystals in the synovial fluid is diagnostic; aspiration also allows a specimen to be taken for bacteriological culture to exclude infection. The crystals show negative birefringence under polarised light microscopy (Fig. 5).

Radiographs in the early stages are invariably normal, but with progression of the disease, punched-out lytic lesions appear at the joint margins; the joint space becomes narrowed and is ultimately lost (Fig. 6).

Treatment

There are two aspects of treatment: firstly to control an acute attack and, secondly, to avoid recurrent episodes in those identified as being vulnerable. The latter is of particular importance in suppressing the formation of tophi and calculi, and in avoiding joint destruction. The patient is first advised about diet, alcohol intake and the avoidance of drugs such as aspirin and thiazide diuretics. Then, in the acute attack, non-steroidal anti-inflammatory agents should be used promptly and in maximum dosage. (Note, however, that none of these drugs has any effect on the concentration of uric acid.) Treatment of hyperuricaemia in the absence of gouty attacks is controversial and should probably be avoided unless the level is very high. (When it is, those affected almost invariably go on to have repeated attacks.)

Long-term treatment is usually reserved for susceptible individuals who have recurrent attacks. The best agent is probably allopurinol, which inhibits xanthine oxidase (Fig. 2) thus reducing the concentration of uric acid. Patients are required to take this medication on a lifelong basis; failure to continue is a common cause of relapse.

PSEUDOGOUT (CALCIUM PYROPHOSPHATE DEPOSITION DISEASE)

This disorder closely mimics gout and the two conditions can be difficult to differentiate. Both can be responsible for acute and chronic arthropathies. The main difference is that pseudogout is secondary to the deposition of calcium pyrophosphate dihydrate crystals (CPPD). This typically produces a characteristic pattern of calcification in the articular cartilage of the affected joints — so-called chondrocalcinosis (Fig. 7). It is notable that as in gout the deposits can be found in tendons, synovium, and ligaments.

There is an increasing prevalence of chondrocalcinosis with age, but overall acute attacks are less common than in gout. Men are affected more often than women (1.4 : 1) and it is rare before the age of 50 years. Large joints such as the knee, shoulder and wrist are frequently involved, with the metatarsophalangeal joint of the great toe being rarely affected.

Clinically, the attacks are more prolonged than in gout, but severe pain is usually absent. Like gout, the onset may be acute, although the systemic effects are generally (although not invariably) less marked. The knee is affected in the majority of acute cases (60%), with about 5% having multiple joint involvement. As a direct result of the condition degenerative changes gradually ensue in the affected joints.

Investigations

There is no biochemical test for this condition. The main diagnostic criterion is the finding of CPPD crystals in synovial fluid following joint aspiration. These show positive birefringence in polarised light (this is negative in gout) and is diagnostic. Remember however that crystals are not always found, and the diagnosis should not be excluded if the clinical picture otherwise fits.

Radiographs show chondrocalcinosis most frequently in the knee and radio-ulnar joint of the wrist. Remembering that the incidence of chondrocalcinosis increases with age may help prevent a case being treated inappropriately as one of gout or septic arthritis.

Treatment

The acute attack is best treated with non-steroidal anti-inflammatory agents which usually lead to resolution. Repeated aspirations to reduce the concentration of CPPD may help in resistant cases, although this regime runs the risk of introducing infection. There is no known method of suppressing the crystal deposition as in gout, and therefore the measures described above should be employed without delay.

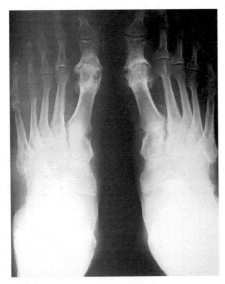

Fig. 6 **Advanced changes in both first metatarsophalangeal joints due to gout.**

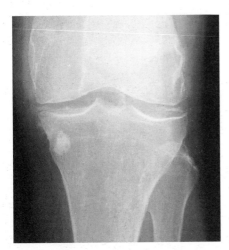

Fig. 7 **Chondrocalcinosis of the knee with involvement of the menisci.**

Gout and pseudogout

- Gout is more common than pseudogout, and both affect men more frequently than women.
- Both are rare under the age of 40 unless there is a predisposing factor.
- Uric acid is raised at some time in an attack of gout, but a normal level does not exclude the diagnosis.
- Microscopic examination of a joint aspirate, with the use of polarised light, can confirm the diagnosis in cases of both gout and pseudogout.
- Non-steroidal anti-inflammatory agents can be used effectively to treat both conditions.

RHEUMATOID ARTHRITIS

This is a chronic, systemic inflammatory disorder of unknown aetiology, characterised by joint involvement. The inflammatory process is often intermittent, and frequently leads to progressive joint destruction, deformity, and incapacity.

Pathology
It starts in the synovial membrane of the joints or tendon sheaths. The swollen synovium produces exudate which contains many agents which are destructive (e.g. proteolytic enzymes, collagenases, proteases) and others which are regulatory (hyaluronic acid, prostaglandins and lymphokines). In addition, plasma cells and lymphocytes are present in varying quantities. The latter in particular play a major role in the production of polyclonal immunoglobulin (some of which is rheumatoid factor). Within the synovial fluid, immune complexes are frequently found, and these can activate complement, cause release of chemotactic agents, and encourage further ingress of inflammatory cells. The synovial proliferation (pannus) spreads over the surface to form marginal erosions and later gradual destruction of the articular cartilage.

The main form of rheumatoid factor is the IgM antibody type (IgM RF). Its presence is a consequence of the disease process, and it is used to group cases into those which are seropositive and those which are seronegative. It is an autoantibody against gamma-globulin and may be responsible for aggravating the inflammatory process. The serological titre is related to the virulence of the disease, but it should be remembered that a low titre can be found in a proportion of the normal population. Rheumatoid nodules on extensor surfaces occur in patients who have a positive rheumatoid factor.

Clinical features
The peak presentation is between 35 and 45, with a higher incidence in females. This, along with the remissions which often occur during pregnancy, may reflect hormonal influences. It can occur at any age, even in children (Still's disease or juvenile chronic arthritis). Most frequently it starts as a symmetrical polyarthritis affecting the small joints of the hands and feet, but its presentation may be protean. It may be slowly progressive (and this tends to have the worst prognosis), episodic or fulminating.

Symptoms
General symptoms include early morning stiffness, weight loss, fever, malaise and fatigue; local symptoms include joint swelling and pain.

Signs
The affected joints or tendon sheaths may show signs of inflammation, with tenderness, redness, increased local heat and swelling. Other evidence of joint involvement varies with the location.

Hands. Bilateral, symmetrical involvement is common, often commencing in the PIP joints before affecting the MP joints. As it progresses, laxity of the collateral ligaments of the MP joints leads to ulnar deviation of the fingers (Fig. 1), and joint subluxations may occur. Swanneck (hyperextension of the PIP joints and flexion of the DIP joints, Fig. 2), or boutonnière (fixed flexion of the PIP joint and hyperextension of the DIP joint) deformities lead to significant reduction of grip strength and manual dexterity. Instability of the joints of the thumbs can reduce pinch strength and lead to the typical Z-deformity (fixed flexion deformity of the IP joint and hyperextension of the MP joint, Fig. 3). Sudden loss of function of a finger may follow an acute tendon rupture. In the case of an extensor tendon under the retinaculum there may be an associated 'dropped' finger.

Wrists. Synovial swelling can lead to compression of the median nerve. As the disease progresses, destruction of the radiocarpal joint produces a volar subluxation, and involvement of the inferior radioulnar joint leads to loss of pronation and supination; both may cause considerable disability (Fig. 4).

Shoulder and elbow. These are commonly affected leading to restriction of motion. In the shoulder, rupture of the rotator cuff may occur as the disease progresses. Pain will lead to further compromise of upper limb function.

Knee. Chronic effusions and synovial hypertrophy can lead to rapid destruction of the joint (Fig. 5). Fixed flexion and valgus deformities may develop (note that in osteoarthritis of the knee varus deformity is more usual). Large, and often asymptomatic popliteal cysts are common. Unlike solid tumours they typically fluctuate in size. If they rupture,

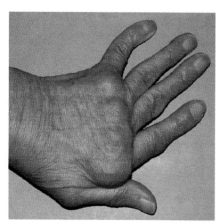

Fig. 1 **Ulnar deviation of the fingers.**

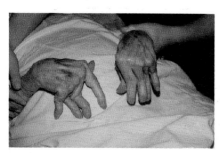

Fig. 2 **Swan-neck deformities of all the fingers but the right index.**

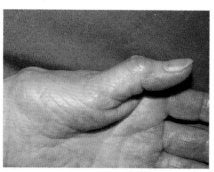

Fig. 3 **Z-deformity of the thumb.**

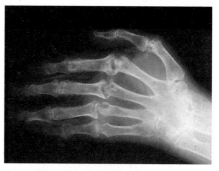

Fig. 4 **Destruction of inferior radioulnar, radiocarpal, carpal and MP joints.**

they can cause severe pain and swelling in the calf, commonly mistaken for a deep venous thrombosis.

Hips. Disability here may be marked, even when radiological changes are minor. It should always be remembered that rheumatoid patients often take high doses of steroids, with the risk of avascular necrosis.

Spine. The cervical region of the spine is most commonly affected. Instability, especially at the atlantoaxial joint, must be excluded by flexion and extension views. This is most relevant where general anaesthesia is being contemplated. Extra care to correctly support the neck, particularly during intubation, is mandatory.

Feet. Flattening of the medial longitudinal arches, MP joint subluxations and other toe deformities are common, leading to complaints of metatarsalgia and difficulty in getting shoes to fit. Painful calluses develop, and walking may be seriously impaired.

Extra-articular manifestations.
Although basically a joint disease, other organs may be involved, often in an insidious way. In the eyes, scleritis can cause blindness if neglected; keratoconjunctivitis sicca occurs in about 10% of patients and may be associated with dry mouth (Sjögren syndrome). In the chest, pulmonary effusions are often small and only seen on routine chest X-ray, but can be severe. At the worst extreme is severe pulmonary fibrosis, which is associated with a high titre of rheumatoid factor. Involvement of the cardiovascular system may lead to pericardial effusions and pericarditis, and rheumatoid vasculitis can cause pathology in any system: in the skin it manifests as ulcers, haemorrhages, or in severe cases even gangrene. In the

urinary tract, amyloidosis of the kidneys is not uncommon and may prove fatal. In the nervous system, primary neuropathy is relatively uncommon, although cervical myelopathy due to subluxation of the cervical spine is not. Anaemia is a universal finding and is commonly multifactorial in origin; often it is secondary to gastrointestinal loss following ingestion of anti-inflammatory drugs. In Felty's syndrome there is a combination of anaemia and splenomegaly.

Investigations
Few investigations are specific, although a high titre of RF is highly suggestive and indicative of a poor prognosis. Other helpful tests include a full blood count and an ESR or C-reactive protein. Biopsy is useful to exclude other conditions affecting the synovium (e.g. tuberculosis and pigmented villonodular synovitis). In doubtful cases a table of diagnostic criteria may be employed (Table 1).

Radiological features
The principal changes include soft tissue swellings, juxta-articular osteoporosis, marginal erosions, joint space narrowing, and deformity. The hands are often affected earliest.

Table 1 **Criteria for diagnosis of rheumatoid arthritis (American Rheumatism Association).**

1. Morning stiffness
2. Pain on motion, or tenderness in a joint
3. Swelling of a joint due to fluid or soft tissue
4. Swelling of a second joint
5. Symmetrical joint swelling
6. Typical rheumatoid nodules
7. Typical X-ray changes
8. Positive test for serum rheumatoid factor
9. Synovial fluid forming poor mucin clot with dilute acetic acid
10. Characteristic synovial histology
11. Characteristic histology of rheumatoid nodule

Criteria 1–5 must be present for at least 6 weeks. If 7 of these criteria are present, the diagnosis is of classical rheumatoid arthritis.

Treatment
Medical
Aspirin in high doses was the most common treatment, but its use has been largely superseded by newer agents such as naproxen (Naprosyn) or piroxicam (Feldene). They reduce stiffness and synovitis, and improve mobility. Where the disease is poorly controlled, *second line treatment* may be employed: this may involve the use of gold salts, penicillamine, antimalarials (chloroquine), or immunosuppressants (e.g. azathioprine). None are free from complications, and careful monitoring of urine and haematological indices is required. *Third line treatment* is the use of steroids (e.g. prednisolone). The dose should be prescribed at the lowest level compatible with disease control to minimise the side-effects. Intra-articular steroids may be utilised in the accessible joints.

Surgical treatment
Synovectomy used to be the mainstay of treatment, but with better medical treatment it has become less frequently required. It is used before there are significant radiographic changes, or perhaps in younger patients. In the bigger joints, such as the hip and shoulder, it can be performed arthroscopically. It is particularly rewarding in the MP joints of the hand, where it may be combined with a realignment procedure to correct ulnar drift of the fingers. In areas of tenosynovitis, such as on the dorsum of the wrist or in the digital flexor sheaths, it may prevent tendon ruptures.

In the late stages, joint replacement is often used, particularly in the hip and knee. It can often restore pain-free function. Excision arthroplasty may be used in the MP joints of the feet, or as a salvage procedure in infected joint replacements. Arthrodesis is now confined to the digital joints, the ankle and the wrist, and as a salvage procedure, e.g. for failed knee replacements.

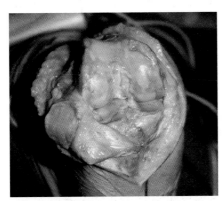

Fig. 5 **Synovial thickening and destruction of articular cartilage seen at time of joint replacement.**

Rheumatoid arthritis
- Rheumatoid arthritis is a systemic disease, with a peak onset between the ages of 35 and 45.
- Women are affected more frequently than men, in the ratio 2.5:1.
- A high titre of rheumatoid factor is usually diagnostic.
- Synovitis is the main pathology.
- Severe joint destruction can occur early in the disease.
- 50% of patients are controlled by medical treatment.
- Surgery may be helpful in restoring function.

PAGET'S DISEASE (OSTEITIS DEFORMANS)

This condition was first described by Sir James Paget in 1877 and is a chronic focal bone disease of unknown aetiology. It is characterised by an increase in the activity of osteoclasts (bone resorption cells) and a secondary increase in the activity of osteoblasts (bone forming cells). The incidence is high in the UK, New Zealand and parts of Australia, but is relatively uncommon in other parts of the world, and this is especially so in South-East Asia and Norway. Both familial and environmental factors may be involved. No clear precipitating factors have been identified, but a possible viral infective aetiology has been suggested.

Incidence

Paget's disease affects men and women equally, and usually presents in the over-50 age group; frequency increases with age. Diagnosis in the young, where it is rare, should be avoided unless there is histological confirmation.

Pathology

Histologically the bone looks markedly abnormal; it shows disorganised areas of lamellar and woven bone (containing abundant osteoclasts) laid down in a random fashion (Fig. 1). Bone resorption is closely coupled to bone formation, and it seems that the pathology lies with the osteoclast, and that the osteoblastic activity is a reactive response to the pathological process.

Clinical features

Many patients are asymptomatic, and diagnosed as a result of radiographs being taken for other purposes (e.g. pelvic X-rays to exclude a fracture after a fall). The disease can affect any bone but favours the long bones: e.g. femur (49%), tibia (25%), pelvis (71%), and lumbar spine (51%). Other common areas are the skull, thoracic spine and the scapulae. It can affect one bone (monostotic form) or several (polyostotic). The condition may start many years before presenting clinically; the bone involved becomes progressively affected, and as it is stressed it may become deformed and painful, or it may fracture. Pain is common, and tends to be mild and boring in character; it is not well controlled with analgesics. Deformity develops slowly and is dependent on the stresses applied and the bone involved.

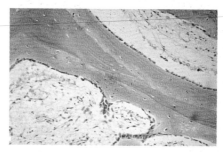
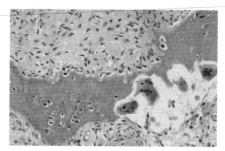

Fig. 1 **Right, microscopic appearance of Paget's disease, with disorganised areas of lamellar and woven bone which have been laid down in random fashion. Left, normal bone for comparison.**

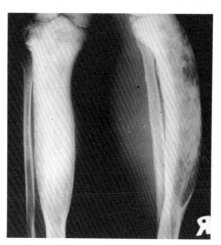

Fig. 2 **Paget's disease of the tibia, with striking alteration of bone texture and anterior bowing.**

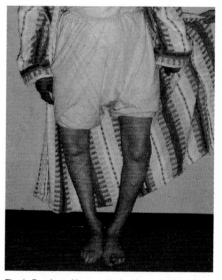

Fig. 3 **Bowing of legs typical of Paget's disease; the tibiae and femora are involved.**

In the *tibia*, which is easily palpable, the bone is thickened with a sharp anterior edge and anterior bowing (Fig. 2). Lateral bowing of the *femur* and tibia may be obvious clinically (Fig. 3). The *skull* may enlarge (requiring an increase in hat size), and can produce deafness or even optic nerve compression. *Backache* and *nerve root impingement* are not uncommon. In its active phase, the disease can be responsible for a non-specific malaise or headaches, and in its extreme form there may be high output cardiac failure due to the high vascular demands of the affected bone.

Diagnosis

The plasma alkaline phosphatase is elevated, particularly during the active phase, and there is an increase in the urinary excretion of hydroxyproline. In advanced cases, the radiographic appearances are distinct and of reliable diagnostic value. They show typical expansion and deformity of the bone; the pattern of the trabeculae is coarse, and they are widely separated with a 'streaky' appearance (Fig. 4). In its vascular phase there may be areas of porotic bone adjacent to areas of relatively sclerotic bone, reflecting differences in vascularity; while the tibia is most commonly affected, bone softening may lead to deformity of the pelvis and femur (Fig. 5). With increasing deformity, single or multiple stress fractures may develop; these cause local pain and may be forerunners of complete fractures. The skull can display an odd 'geographical' distribution of disease (osteoporosis circumscripta), not to be confused with the 'pepper-pot' appearance of hyperparathyroidism or the punched out lesions of myeloma.

Isotope bone scans using Technetium labelled biphosphonates can clearly display the affected bones at an early stage, even prior to changes appearing on plain X-rays. Multiple X-rays (so-called

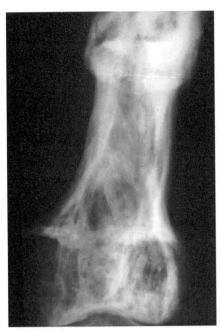

Fig. 4 **Typical 'streaky' appearance of distal femur where there are two healing fractures.**

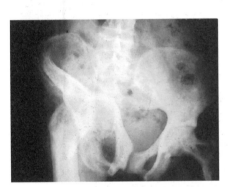

Fig. 5 **Distortion of the pelvis and femoral neck (coxa vara) as a result of Paget's disease.**

skeletal surveys) should be avoided if possible; the areas to be X-rayed should be determined by the results of the isotope scan.

Complications

Generally these are minor, but some patients may develop deafness or visual disturbance. The main problems are two-fold, namely *fracture* and *secondary sarcoma*.

Fractures are most common in the long bones, especially the femur and tibia, and may require internal fixation. They generally heal satisfactorily, although at a slower rate than normal.

The incidence of sarcomatous change is uncertain, but thought to be about 5–10%. In a patient with known Paget's disease, malignant change should be suspected if there is increased pain, swelling and tenderness in the affected bone.

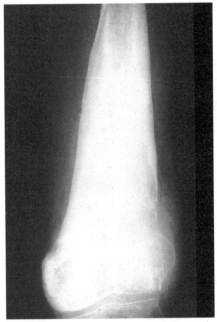

Fig. 6 **Paget's sarcoma, with areas of bone destruction just proximal to the femoral condyles on both sides, and early formation of extra-osseous masses.**

Although the diagnosis may be confirmed by the radiographs, a confirmatory biopsy is usually required.

Treatment

This is only necessary in the face of symptoms. The usual indication is pain, with or without recurrent stress fractures. Apart from analgesics, there are numerous more specific medical treatments, of which the most common and most effective group of drugs appear to be the Biphosphonates, e.g. etidronate and pamidronate. They act by inhibiting the osteoclasts on the advancing layer of absorption, thus halting the progression of the disease; they also inhibit bone mineralisation and ectopic calcification, the former being a risk of treatment. Such therapy may produce clinical

remission in about 90% of cases, although 6 months may elapse before this is reflected in the biochemistry.

Surgical treatment is confined largely to fracture management. As many of the patients presenting with fractures tend to be elderly, and as healing tends to be slow, internal fixation is usually advised. Bone vascularity or great hardness can pose technical problems. Where there are recurrent stress fractures with severe deformities, correction may be attempted with multiple osteotomies and intramedullary nail fixation (the so-called 'shish kebab' operation).

PAGET'S SARCOMA

This is sarcomatous change occurring in a bone affected by Paget's disease. It is relatively rare and said to have an annual incidence of 1.7 per 100 000 population. It becomes increasingly common with age, and has a peak incidence in the 60–80 age group. Men are twice as likely as women to develop it. The bones most frequently involved are the femur, pelvis, humerus, scapula and skull. There is usually increasing pain and tenderness in the site of established Paget's disease, which may not even have been previously diagnosed. About 30% present with a pathological fracture. Radiographs may not be diagnostic, but previous films, if available for comparison, are often helpful. Areas of bone destruction should be viewed with suspicion (Fig. 6). Any extra-osseous mass is almost diagnostic.

Treatment

This is often palliative as the prognosis is poor. Amputation in peripheral lesions may give the best results as the tumours are not usually susceptible to radiotherapy or chemotherapy. The average survival from the time of diagnosis is 1 year, and may be worse if the patient presents with a pathological fracture.

Paget's disease (osteitis deformans)

- The primary cause of Paget's disease is excessive osteoclastic activity.
- Pain is the most common presenting complaint, with or without an associated fracture.
- Plasma alkaline phosphatase is elevated in active disease.
- Radiographs are usually diagnostic when the disease is advanced.
- Biphosphonates offer the best treatment at present.
- Beware of the possibility of malignant change.

NEUROMUSCULAR DISORDERS

In assessing any condition in this group, a carefully taken history is essential. It is particularly important to record the pattern of progression, whether worsening, static or improving, and whether it was evident at birth. Some are inherited, and a family history (and possibly examination of other members of the family) is essential in confirming a pattern of inheritance.

CEREBRAL PALSY

This is defined as a non-progressive motor disorder resulting from an irreparable injury to the central nervous system. This usually occurs during foetal development or in the perinatal period; the most common causes are anoxia, cerebral trauma or haemorrhage, infections or severe postnatal jaundice (kernicterus). Although the injury to the brain is static, the muscle imbalance which results from it produces a dynamic state which leads to a situation which changes continually during growth. The motor deficit has a very variable pattern which depends on the extent and site of the lesion. Some patients are severely spastic, while others may have a flaccid paralysis or have athetoid or ataxic movements. A careful assessment is necessary of the child's mental abilities as this has a bearing on how the child cooperates with treatment. While mental retardation is common, it must be remembered that many are of normal intelligence. Some have communication or learning difficulties which result from their physical impairment.

Clinically, there may be few signs at birth, the condition manifesting itself with delays in reaching the normal developmental milestones; or motor imbalance and incoordination, with upper motor neurone signs, may appear. The motor problems can produce various deformities, but the most common are related to spasticity. In *the lower limbs* there may be fixed flexion/adduction of the hips, flexion of knees, and equinus of the ankles. In *the upper limbs* there may be internal rotation of the shoulders, fixed flexion of the elbows, and flexion of the wrists. The disorder can affect one side (hemiplegia), both sides (diplegia, with the legs more frequently involved than the arms), or all four limbs (quadriplegia).

Treatment

All therapies are dependent on the ability of the child (and parents) to cooperate.

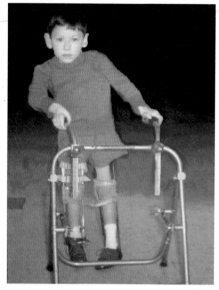

Fig. 1 **Polio which has affected both legs and the spine; mobilisation with leg calipers and a frame.**

Although the brain injury is non-progressive, the treatment must continue until growth has stopped as the muscle imbalance invariably tends to cause recurrent and often progressive problems. Attention must be paid to avoiding contractures by regular splintage and physiotherapy, and wherever possible to maintain postural control and mobility. Surgery is reserved for intractable joint contractures, or for restoration of muscle balance by tendon release or transfer. It is important to maintain an educational programme to maximise the child's potential and to remember that many of the patients are of normal intelligence.

ACUTE ANTERIOR POLIOMYELITIS

While still a serious problem in many Third World countries, polio has become rare in the UK since the introduction of an effective vaccine. It is caused by the poliovirus which enters via the gut or nasopharynx and settles in the anterior horn (motor) cells of the cord or in the brain stem. After a 2 week symptomless incubation period the patient develops flu-like symptoms, often with muscle pains and neck rigidity; this lasts for 48 hours and is followed by paralysis of rapid onset. The extent of the paralysis is variable. The lower limbs are most commonly affected, but at higher levels the spinal or respiratory muscles (including the diaphragm) may be

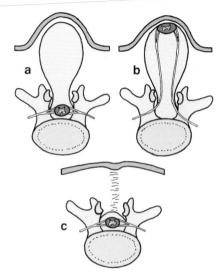

Fig. 2 **Spina bifida. (a)** Meningocoele; **(b)** meningomyelocoele; **(c)** occulta.

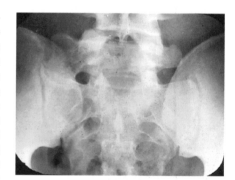

Fig. 3 **Spina bifida occulta L5 with partial sacralisation.**

involved: then respiratory support is necessary for survival. After a period of 1–2 months a period of recovery sets in, continuing for 1–2 years. Muscle power charting may help in assessing progress and establishing a prognosis. Any residual paralysis is flaccid, and if extensive may be seriously disabling. In the absence of muscle stimulation, growth of the affected limb(s) will be retarded and the limb bones become atrophic. Note that sensation is not materially affected in polio.

Treatment

Deformity due to muscle wasting and imbalance may be inevitable, and there may be joint instability and limb shortening. In the lower limb, splinting with calipers (Fig. 1) or other devices may be required, along with shoe raises to compensate for growth inequality. Surgery (in the form of tendon transfers or joint fusions) may occasionally be required to maximise function.

SPINA BIFIDA

This is caused by an intrauterine failure of fusion of the neural arches, although some argue that it may be secondary to a segmental rupture after fusion has occurred. The incidence is about 2–3 per 1000 births, with a prevalence in first-born children and socially deprived families. Over 60% of the defects are in the lumbar or lumbosacral region; more proximal lesions have a poorer prognosis. Associated conditions such as hydrocephalus and cardiac, genitourinary or gastrointestinal anomalies are not uncommon, and must be identified early to avoid complications.

In closed lesions the skin is intact but rarely normal. There may be a dimple or patch of hair to alert the examiner's suspicions. In the open variety there is an obvious saccular herniation of the meninges. The neural structures may lie in their normal position relative to the spinal canal (meningocoele, Fig. 2), or

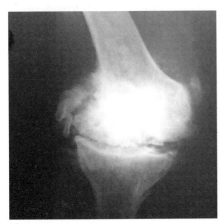

Fig. 4 **Advanced muscular dystrophy.**

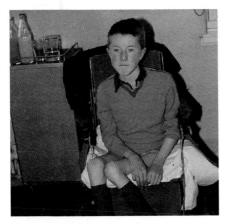

Fig. 5 **Charcot's disease of the knee.**

be displaced into the sac (meningomyelocoele). In the extreme form, a dysplastic spinal cord may be visible at the bottom of the defect (myelocoele). Elevation of alpha-fetoprotein during pregnancy may indicate spina bifida (although it is also elevated in multiple pregnancies). Further investigation by ultrasound or fetoscopy can readily confirm the diagnosis. After birth, radiographs show a complete loss of the posterior elements at the site of the lesion. (Note that spina bifida occulta (Fig. 3) may be discovered accidentally. It may be symptom-free or associated with pes cavus.)

Treatment

If the alpha-fetaprotein is elevated, termination of pregnancy can be considered, although not without full counselling of the parents.

If the pregnancy is continued, the subsequent treatment of these children requires a multidisciplinary team including neurosurgeons, orthopaedic surgeons, urologists, paediatricians, physiotherapists, orthotists and social workers. Early surgical closure is indicated if the baby is strong enough to withstand this procedure. In addition, a ventricular shunt may be required to drain an associated hydrocephalus, and a urinary diversion may become necessary (as 90% of affected children have some involvement of the urinary system).

Orthopaedic care is largely related to splintage to enhance mobility and to avoid ulceration in skin deprived of sensation. Charting of the neurological defect should be attempted as soon as possible as this may allow the necessity for early splintage to be predicted. Surgical intervention is aimed at the restoration of muscle balance and the correction of bony deformities such as scoliosis. Much time and effort is put into the treatment of affected children to try to allow them to walk, but many are ultimately confined to a wheelchair.

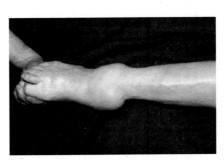

Fig. 6 **Charcot's disease of the ankle (tertiary syphilis).**

MUSCULAR DYSTROPHIES

This is a family of inherited diseases which characteristically produce progressive muscle wasting. They are all rare, but the most common are the Duchenne and Becker types; these are X-linked (boys being affected), with the Becker type being a more benign form. (There are other rarer forms of muscular dystrophy with variable inheritance patterns.) In the Duchenne type, children become progressively weaker and are usually wheelchair-bound by their early teens (Fig. 4). Death results from respiratory muscle weakness. In both types, cardiac conduction anomalies may exist, and these have a bearing on any surgical procedures which may be required.

Investigations

These include estimation of creatine phosphokinase levels (which are invariably raised in muscular dystrophy), EMG studies, and muscle biopsies.

Treatment

The principal aim of treatment is to maintain mobility and avoid contractures. This can often be effected by the use of splints and physiotherapy. Surgery is reserved for resistant cases.

CHARCOT'S DISEASE OF JOINTS

These may follow any local or systemic disorder which causes sensory loss, e.g. diabetes, syphilis and spina bifida. It is characterised by gross joint destruction (Figs 5 & 6) and instability, generally unaccompanied by pain. It is important that the condition is clearly recognised as any attempt at joint replacement is doomed to failure, and even fusion can be difficult to achieve. Splintage to stabilise the affected joint and allow ambulation is usually the main form of treatment.

Neuromuscular disorders

- Cerebral palsy is a non-progressive brain injury which can lead to progressive dynamic muscle imbalance during growth.
- Poliomyelitis produces a motor deficit but no sensory loss.
- If the maternal alpha-fetaprotein levels are elevated, it is likely that the foetus has a neural tube defect.
- Charcot joints can occur in any condition which produces a sensory deficit.

NERVE COMPRESSION SYNDROMES IN THE UPPER LIMB

Mechanical compression of a nerve within a nerve tunnel may occur when there is a discrepancy between the size of the tunnel and what passes through it. The *tunnel itself* may be reduced in size, e.g. by a local fracture or arthritic lipping, or *the contents* may increase in volume as a result, for example, of synovitis, oedema, ganglions or other tumours. Patients with diabetes are particularly susceptible to nerve compression.

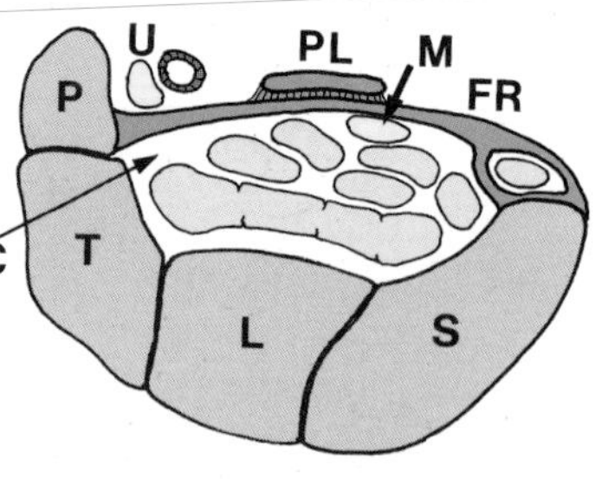

Pathomechanism

Direct compression is the main component but traction and pressure may compromise the blood supply. Transient pressure may produce dysfunction which recovers if the compression is quickly relieved. Prolonged pressure leads to Wallerian degeneration and ultimately intraneural fibrosis with permanent loss of function.

Clinical assessment

A firm diagnosis can often be made on the examination findings alone. It is important to ensure that the motor or sensory changes coincide with the distribution of a specific nerve. If the deficit extends beyond the normal territory of a nerve, it is likely that the compression lies proximal to the suspected tunnel. If there is doubt about the level, nerve conduction tests may be required.

CARPAL TUNNEL SYNDROME

This is the most common syndrome, affecting the median nerve as it passes below the transverse carpal ligament at the wrist (Fig. 1). It may arise from distortion of the tunnel after a distal radial fracture, but more commonly it is seen as a result of conditions affecting the contents: these include rheumatoid synovitis (and related diseases), diabetes (which increases the vulnerability of the nerve to compression) and pregnancy (secondary to fluid retention, with recovery normally occurring after childbirth). Less commonly it may occur in hypothyroidism, amyloid disease, acromegaly, gout (with uric acid deposits in the canal), ganglions, lipomas and neuromas. Patients with renal failure, who have arteriovenous shunts in the forearm, are prone to this condition, although the mechanism is not clear.

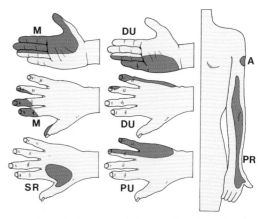

Fig. 1 **The carpal tunnel (C), formed by the scaphoid (S), lunate (L) and the triquetral (T), roofed over by the flexor retinaculum (FR).** It contains the flexor tendons and the median nerve (M). U=ulnar nerve and artery; PL=palmaris longus; P=pisiform.

Fig. 2 **Sensory distribution in the upper limb.** M=median; SR=superficial (distal) radial; DU=distal ulnar; PU=proximal ulnar; A=axillary; PR=proximal radial.

Clinical features

It is four times more common in women than men, peaking in the 4th and 5th decades. The typical history is of paraesthesia in the distribution of the median nerve (Fig. 2). At night, the patient often wakens after 3–4 hours sleep and frequently gives a history of obtaining relief from her paraesthesia by shaking the hand. Symptoms may also be precipitated by direct pressure on the volar aspect of the wrist, but generally they occur spontaneously. The motor deficit typically affects the thenar muscles and the lateral two lumbricals. Once wasting is evident, urgent treatment is required. Unfortunately many patients have atypical symptoms, often with sensory changes involving the whole hand or forearm.

Diagnosis

The main clinical tests, if positive, reproduce the sensory symptoms. In the Tinel test the nerve is firmly and repeatedly tapped over the carpal tunnel; in the Phalen test the wrist is held in a flexed position for 30 seconds (this reduces the

room within the carpal tunnel); in the sphygmomanometer test, which must be interpreted with caution, the cuff is inflated to just above the systolic pressure for 1–2 minutes. Where surgery is contemplated the diagnosis should be confirmed by nerve conduction tests.

Treatment

A resting night splint or an injection of hydrocortisone can be tried in mild cases. Diuretics can be helpful when fluid retention is a factor (e.g. in pregnancy). The mainstay of treatment in persistent cases is surgical decompression. This usually leads to an early improvement in the sensory symptoms, but motor deficits have a more variable recovery.

PROXIMAL COMPRESSION OF THE MEDIAN NERVE

This is rare, but includes the following:

- Just above the elbow, a supracondylar spur with an anomalous ligament

(Struthers) bridging the medial epicondyle can compress both the brachial artery and the nerve as they pass beneath (Fig. 3).
- Just distal to the elbow, compression may occur at the origin of the pronator teres (pronator syndrome) leading to both motor and sensory symptoms. It may be precipitated by repetitive and strong muscular contractions.
- In the upper forearm, compression may occur secondary to an anomalous band at the origin of the sublimis muscle (anterior interosseous syndrome), causing weakness of the flexor pollicis longus and the lateral half of the flexor digitorum profundus. The distal joints of the index and thumb hyperextend when a pinch grip is attempted; the thenar muscles innervated by the median nerve are unaffected.

ULNAR NERVE COMPRESSION

This is much less common than carpal tunnel syndrome, but if it occurs in the cubital tunnel at the elbow, and leads to intrinsic muscle motor deficit, recovery is the exception rather than the rule. Fortunately, most patients seek help before the syndrome reaches this stage. The local anatomy may be abnormal (e.g. there may be an aponeurotic band proximal to the elbow joint or an anomalous band as the nerve enters the flexor carpi ulnaris) and these must be dealt with at any surgical exploration. Less commonly the nerve may be compressed in the hand, either in its canal adjacent to the carpal tunnel (canal of Guyon) or more distally in the tunnel which carries the deep palmar branch. Each has a distinctive clinical presentation and diagnosis is dependent on a sound knowledge of the local anatomy.

The nerve is vulnerable to external pressure at the elbow in the anaesthetised or unconscious patient and particular care must be taken to protect it in these circumstances. Fractures of the medial epicondyle can lead to distortion of the cubital tunnel and subsequent neural symptoms. Supracondylar fractures in the child may lead to acute kinking of the nerve due to the deformity. Ununited fractures of the lateral humeral condyle or supracondylar fractures with disturbance of the carrying angle (generally cubitus valgus) can lead to an ulnar neuritis of delayed onset (tardy ulnar palsy). If the nerve is excessively mobile it may be damaged by friction against the medial epicondyle.

Clinical features
The onset is often insidious, but unfortunately a delay of more than 6 months in seeking help may result in a poor prognosis. The sensory and motor characteristics depend on the site of compression. In proximal lesions, the sensory loss is more extensive due to involvement of the dorsal cutaneous branch. Motor loss affects the flexor carpi ulnaris, the ulnar innervated half of the flexor digitorum profundus and the intrinsic muscles of the hand (excluding those innervated by the median nerve). While intrinsic muscle wasting of the hand is usually obvious, forearm muscle wasting is often less pronounced. Where weakness is severe the muscle imbalance results in an ulnar claw hand, with hyperextension of the metacarpophalangeal joints and acute flexion of the interphalangeal joints of the ring and little fingers. Compression in the canal of Guyon leads to some intrinsic motor loss, with sensory changes confined to the volar surface of the hand. Deep palmar branch compression produces purely motor signs in the hand but tends to spare the branch to the abductor digiti minimi, leading to an abducted posture of the little finger. Beware, however, of the patient with wasting of all the intrinsics (i.e. including the thenar muscles), when other causes must be suspected. These include motor neurone disease, peroneal muscular atrophy (an inherited, chronic, slowly progressive peripheral neuropathy), syringomyelia (where typically there is a cystic lesion in the central region of the cervical cord) and a T1 lesion (e.g. from malignant infiltration from an apical lung tumour). In all but the latter, the wasting is bilateral and symmetrical (Fig. 4).

Treatment
In most cases surgical exploration at the defined site of compression is necessary. At the elbow, anterior transposition in combination with decompression of the nerve is usually necessary to avoid recurrence.

RADIAL NERVE COMPRESSION

Entrapment of the nerve is relatively rare, although direct acute compression is relatively common. In the so-called 'Saturday night palsy', a patient under the influence of alcohol or drugs falls asleep with the arm over the back of a chair, leading to prolonged direct compression of the nerve at mid-humeral level; this site is also vulnerable in humeral shaft fractures. The typical clinical presentation is of weakness of the extensor muscles of the wrist (drop wrist), fingers, and thumb, with sensory changes in the 1st dorsal web space. There is usually complete spontaneous recovery in about 3 months (during which time an appropriate splint is usually worn), and in most cases it is safe to adopt an expectant policy.

POSTERIOR INTEROSSEOUS NERVE COMPRESSION

Compression of this nerve is rare. It may occur as it passes through the fibrotendinous band at the supinator origin (arcade of Frohse). The onset is usually insidious and there is no sensory upset. There is weakness of the finger and thumb extensors and abductor pollicis longus. The absence of a wrist drop and sensory change distinguishes it from radial nerve palsy (note that the nerve is vulnerable to injury during surgical explorations of the forearm).

SUPERFICIAL RADIAL NERVE INJURY

This is relatively common after a direct blow to the radial aspect of the wrist, where the nerve is superficial and vulnerable. It is often misdiagnosed as a sprain or even a fracture but, characteristically, produces a painful dysaesthesia. The altered sensation is across the dorso-radial aspect of the hand and often involves the ulnar aspect of the thumb and radial aspect of the index finger, leading to altered pinch sensation. The treatment is expectant, but the patient must be warned that the recovery may be protracted.

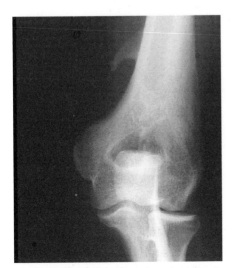

Fig. 3 **Supracondylar spur sometimes associated with median nerve (and brachial artery) compression.**

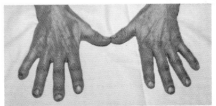

Fig. 4 **Bilateral interosseous muscle wasting.**

> **Nerve compression syndromes in the upper limb**
> - A clear knowledge of anatomy is essential in diagnosing nerve compression syndromes.
> - Carpal tunnel syndrome is by far the most common compression syndrome.
> - Major motor and sensory deficits indicate a proximal lesion.
> - Neurophysiological tests can clarify the site of pathology.
> - Beware the T1 lesion with a complete intrinsic palsy.

NERVE COMPRESSION SYNDROMES IN THE LOWER LIMB

These are less common than those of the upper limb, but early recognition is important to avoid long-term disability. As in the upper limb, a sound knowledge of the regional anatomy is essential to avoid delay in diagnosis. Neurophysiological tests, such as nerve conduction studies, may be required.

SCIATIC NERVE

The nerve is made up of the 4th and 5th lumbar and the 1st, 2nd and 3rd sacral nerve roots. While the 4th and 5th roots are most commonly compressed as a result of a lumbar disc prolapse (see Prolapsed intervertebral disc), involvement of the sciatic nerve itself may occur under a number of circumstances. Patients who are *bedridden*, *comatose* or *under prolonged anaesthesia* may lie for prolonged periods in one position, causing proximal compression of the nerve. *Haematoma formation* or *late scarring* in the buttock region after surgery or local fracture can cause distortion and subsequent compression. When giving an injection into the buttock, it should always be given in the 'safe area' to avoid potential damage to the nerve (Fig. 1). The nerve may be *directly injured in posterior dislocation* of the hip.

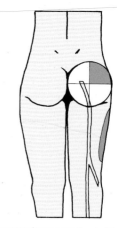

Fig. 1 **The upper and outer quadrant of the buttock (and the lateral aspect of the thigh) are comparatively safe areas for injections.**

Clinical features

The presentation is dependent on the severity and level of compression. In severe cases there may be weakness or paralysis of the posterior thigh muscles and all the muscles below the knee level in association with a complete sensory loss in the cutaneous distribution of the nerve (Fig. 2). This distinguishes it from the sciatica of disc prolapse which has a specific root distribution for both the motor and sensory deficits. As with any other nerve compression injuries it must be treated expeditiously to avoid permanent neurological deficits.

Piriformis syndrome is a rare form of sciatic nerve compression which is difficult to diagnose because of its variable presentation. The most common pathology is a fibrous band deep to the piriformis which kinks or compresses the nerve as it leaves the pelvis via the sciatic notch. Clinically it presents with sciatica-like pain which (unlike sciatica from other causes) is aggravated by resisted abduction/external rotation of the hip and/or internal rotation of the extended thigh. It is worsened by walking or stooping and there may be a local palpable and tender swelling. The straight leg raising test may be positive. The diagnosis can be confirmed by nerve conduction tests and treatment is usually by surgical decompression.

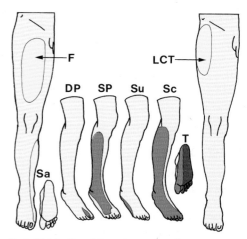

Fig. 2 **Distribution of the main cutaneous nerves in the lower limb.** F=femoral; Sa=saphenous; DP=deep peroneal; SP=superficial peroneal; Su=sural; Sc=sciatic; T=tibial (with medial and lateral plantar divisions); LCT=lateral cutaneous nerve of thigh.

COMMON PERONEAL NERVE

The sciatic nerve splits into the tibial and the common peroneal nerves proximal to the knee. The common peroneal nerve is most at risk as it winds around the fibular neck where it is susceptible to pressure from tight bandaging, ill-fitting plaster cast or poorly supervised treatment in a Thomas splint. Ganglions or synovial thickening (e.g. from rheumatoid arthritis) in the proximal tibiofibular joint or local tumours (Fig. 3) may also cause local compression of the nerve; the nerve may also be injured in fractures of the medial tibial table.

Clinical features

Whilst the presentation can be acute or chronic, mild or severe, the features are characteristic. Tenderness at the head of the fibula indicates the site of pathology, especially if local pressure produces pain in the sensory distribution of the nerve (Fig. 2). Motor weakness involves all the muscles of the anterior and peroneal compartments (ankle and toe dorsiflexors, foot invertors and evertors) producing a 'drop foot' which can make walking difficult (note that in a disc prolapse affecting the 5th lumbar nerve root the tibialis anterior muscle may be spared).

Treatment

Where a traumatic origin is likely, a watching policy can be adopted as the condition usually shows signs of spontaneous recovery within three months. However, where local pathology is responsible (e.g. a ganglion) surgical exploration is mandatory.

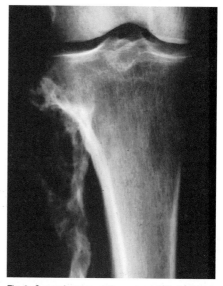

Fig. 3 **Osteoclastoma of the proximal fibula with an associated common peroneal nerve palsy.**

LATERAL CUTANEOUS NERVE OF THIGH (MERALGIA PARAESTHETICA)

The nerve originates from the 2nd and 3rd lumbar roots and runs under the inguinal ligament near the anterior superior iliac spine. Its course is very variable and it sometimes crosses the inguinal ligament, where it is particularly vulnerable. In many cases no obvious cause of injury may be found, but damage sometimes results from wearing tight fitting corsets, direct pressure during pregnancy or local trauma. The nerve may also be accidentally injured during surgical approaches to the hip. Beware the patient who has unremitting pain in the distribution of the nerve as this may be due to infiltration by an abdominal malignancy.

Clinical features and treatment

The patient complains of either pain or dysaesthesia in the distinct distribution of the nerve which is entirely sensory. If a careful history can identify a cause, treatment is directed towards eradicating it. If the cause is obscure, a conservative policy is usually adopted as most cases tend to resolve with time. The results of surgical exploration are rather unpredictable.

SAPHENOUS NERVE

The saphenous nerve is the entirely cutaneous terminal part of the femoral nerve. It may be injured (as distinct from being compressed) during surgical stripping of the long saphenous vein for varicosities or to obtain grafts. It is most commonly injured on the medial side of the ankle. The typical sensory loss is along the medial side of the foot. If the nerve is injured at or above the knee, the loss will also involve part of the thigh. It can cause a severe dysaesthesia which is difficult to treat. Physiotherapy in the form of a desensitisation programme can sometimes help, although the disturbed sensation is rarely abolished.

FEMORAL NERVE

Femoral nerve palsy is relatively rare as the nerve is normally well protected within the pelvis as it lies on the iliacus muscle (on leaving the pelvis it rapidly splits into its many branches). A haematoma in the iliacus muscle deep to its overlying fascia is the usual cause; this may result from hyperextension injuries of the hip (e.g. in karate), from pelvic fractures or in patients with a bleeding diathesis. The striking feature is paralysis of the quadriceps muscle, with instability of the knee and difficulty in walking. More distally the nerve may be injured in anterior surgical approaches to the hip joint or from the exothermic reaction of acrylic cement which has accidentally extruded anteriorly while being used to secure the acetabular component of a hip replacement. Proximal root compression from a high disc prolapse may be differentiated from a femoral nerve palsy (which it can mimic) by the history and examination and the usual absence of pain in the latter.

Treatment

Iliacus haematoma injuries often resolve over a 3–6 month period and a watching policy is generally adopted. Unfortunately, the effects of thermal injuries tend to be more permanent and no specific treatment is of benefit.

TIBIAL NERVE

The tibial nerve runs behind the medial malleolus to the sole of the foot, splitting into the medial and lateral plantar nerves. En route it may become compressed, giving rise to paraesthesia in the sole of the foot and sometimes intrinsic muscle wasting (tarsal tunnel syndrome, Fig. 4). This may be caused by a ganglion, a bony prominence or local trauma (note that the tibial nerve may also be injured in the region of the soleal arch in proximal tibial fractures).

Treatment

Surgical exploration is necessary to decompress the nerve and remove the offending pathology.

DEEP PERONEAL NERVE

The nerve is vulnerable to compression as it passes under the extensor retinaculum on the dorsum of the foot (anterior tarsal tunnel syndrome, Fig. 4). This may be due to a ganglion or a local bony protuberance, often secondary to osteoarthritis, and results in paraesthesia radiating over the dorsum of the foot to the hallux and 2nd toe. There may be weakness of the extensor hallucis brevis and extensor digitorum brevis, although this is often difficult to confirm clinically. The symptoms may be aggravated by high-heeled or tightly laced shoes and by plantar flexion. Treatment is usually by surgical exploration. More proximally, the deep peroneal nerve is sometimes affected by rising pressure within the anterior compartment of the leg (anterior compartment syndrome). This may be due to oedema resulting from excessive exercise or tibial shaft fractures (where haemorrhage is an additional factor). There is often severe pain, loss of sensation in the first web space and, later, with impending muscle necrosis, paralysis of the dorsiflexors of the ankle and toes. In this situation, surgical decompression of the compartment is essential to avoid permanent soft tissue damage.

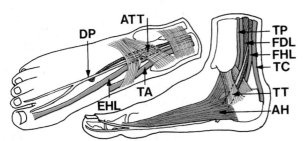

Fig. 4 **The tarsal tunnel (TT) runs between the two layers of the flexor retinaculum, leading the tibial nerve and vessels deep to abductor hallucis (AH).** TP=tibialis posterior; FDL=flexor digitorum longus; FHL=flexor hallucis longus; TC=tendo calcaneus. The anterior tarsal tunnel (ATT) contains the deep peroneal nerve (DP) and dorsalis pedis artery. Its roof is formed by the extensor retinaculum. EHL=extensor hallucis longus; TA=tibialis anterior.

Nerve compression syndromes in the lower limb

- A clear knowledge of lower limb anatomy is essential in establishing a diagnosis.
- The most common compression syndrome in the lower limbs is one secondary to a disc prolapse.
- Major motor and sensory deficit suggests a proximal lesion.
- Neurophysiological tests may aid diagnosis.
- Beware unremitting pain; this may be related to malignant infiltration.

KYPHOSIS

The thoracic spine (as seen from the side) is curved, with the convexity lying posteriorly. When this curve is increased to more than 40 degrees, kyphosis is said to be present (it may be measured by the Cobb method used for scoliosis). There are two main patterns: regular and angular. A *regular curve* is spread over an appreciable length of the spine and involves several or many vertebrae; the cause is usually benign and often secondary to a generalised disease process. In *angular kyphosis* the alteration in contour is abrupt, often resulting in the marked prominence of a single vertebral spine (gibbus). It results from localised vertebral collapse and the underlying cause is usually acute and significant (such as fracture, tumour or infection).

Kyphosis often results in back pain and the deformity may cause problems from the cosmetic point of view. Kyphosis does not itself tend to compromise respiratory function, but may do so if associated with a scoliosis (kyphoscoliosis). Lateral radiographs, the most important part of any investigation, allow measurement of the deformity and the assessment of any local abnormalities; they will also determine whether the kyphosis is congenital or acquired.

CONGENITAL KYPHOSIS

There are several congenital abnormalities which may lead to kyphosis. There may be a *failure of development* of the anterior part of one or more vertebral bodies, leading to anterior wedging. There may be a *failure of segmentation*, where the vertebrae fail to split into their component parts (Fig. 1). Regular follow-up is essential in both these cases as with growth either may lead to progressive deformity. Surgery is usually advised if the deformity worsens beyond 50 degrees or is predicted to do so. Generally a fusion of the affected segment is carried out using internal fixation (e.g. Harrington rods). Where a neurological deficit is evident, spinal decompression may also be required. In some types of *spina bifida*, kyphotic (and scoliotic) deformities may occur as a result of vertebral body deformities, paralysis, or both. Deterioration can be extremely rapid. The goal in treatment is to produce a spine of normal height centred over a level pelvis. Methodology is specialised, although in most cases extensive spinal fusion will be needed at

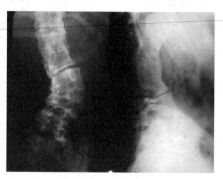

Fig. 1 **Congenital failure of segmentation leading to kyphoscoliosis.**

some stage. Orthotic treatment may in some cases allow this to be delayed until puberty.

ACQUIRED KYPHOSIS

This deformity may occur as a consequence of any disease process other than a congenital anomaly. There are many causes which include the following.

SPINAL FRACTURE

This is the most common cause of acquired kyphosis in adults and children. Longitudinal (axial) loading of the spine may result in acute compression with wedging of one or more vertebral bodies. In the adult the deformity is immediate and often stable (see p. 64), but in children (where fracture is in fact rather uncommon) the deformity can worsen with growth. In all these cases the kyphosis is angulatory.

In the elderly suffering from osteoporosis, spinal fracture may occur as a result of minimal trauma (even coughing or sneezing). There is usually (but not always) pain at the time of any fresh fracture, although this generally settles within a matter of weeks. In many cases the fractures involve several vertebrae, with the result that the kyphotic curve is often *regular*. Over a period, with repeated fractures, the deformity gradually worsens. The sufferer may not even appreciate that there is a major deformity, although she (osteoporosis is commoner in women) may have noticed a loss of height or some difficulty in the fit of clothing. Compensatory extension occurs in the lumbar area of the spine (increased lordosis); this often becomes the source of pain rather than the area of the thoracic fractures. Note that in the related condition of *senile kyphosis* there

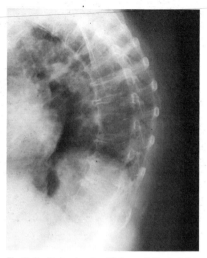

Fig. 2 **Senile kyphosis with loss of disc height anteriorly and regular kyphosis.**

may be a marked regular kyphosis secondary to anterior disc degeneration, with or without osteoporotic fractures (Fig. 2).

INFECTION

Spinal infection is relatively rare, but can present as a pyrexia of unknown origin. It is sometimes not diagnosed until extensive investigations have been made but, on the other hand, it may present with severe backache, systemic upset and spinal deformity. Worldwide the most common infection is tuberculosis; in the UK and other European countries its incidence is on the increase, but pyogenic bacterial infections (such as coagulase positive *Staphylococcus*, *E. Coli* or *Pseudomonas pyocyanea*) are more common.

TUBERCULOSIS OF THE SPINE

This accounts for 50% of cases of bone and joint tuberculosis. It is most common in children and the onset is often slow and insidious, with aching pain and gross spinal stiffness. Radiographs at the earliest stages show narrowing of a single disc space; later the vertebral bodies are involved, leading to anterior and sometimes lateral wedging (Fig. 3). Local abscesses may expand and track distally (Fig. 4). The spinal cord may be involved (as a result of abscess pressure, sequestra, angulation or spinal artery thrombosis) leading to paraplegia. Renal spread is not uncommon. The initial investigations, apart from local radiographs, should include X-rays of the chest, a Mantoux test and, in the case of the lumbar region,

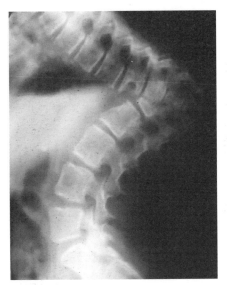

Fig. 3 **TB spine, with gross vertebral destruction, a gibbus and an endangered spinal cord.**

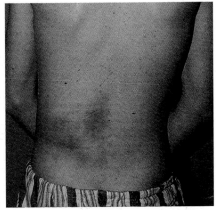

Fig. 4 **Lumbar abscess (left) secondary to spinal tuberculosis.**

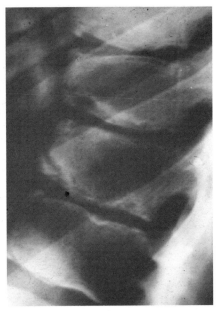

Fig. 5 **Disturbance of the epiphyseal plates and anterior wedging typical of Scheuermann's disease.**

an IVP. In the early stages it may mimic other infections (and vice versa) and generally the only way of establishing a firm diagnosis is by obtaining specimens for histological and bacterial examination. As the abscess is small at first, and the early removal of necrotic bone and pus is to be desired, many surgeons like to perform this with a local debridement. Later, when there is gross bone destruction with little new bone formation and large abscesses, the diagnosis is seldom in doubt.

The mainstay of treatment is the prolonged use of antituberculous drugs. These include rifampicin, isoniazid and ethambutol, and are always used in combination. Drug resistance is becoming a serious problem and sensitivities should always be obtained. Abscesses should be evacuated surgically. Fusion may occur spontaneously, but there is now a tendency to aggressive surgery, with removal of all infected material and extensive grafting of the affected areas. When the cord is involved, decompression may lead to recovery in the early stages, but is less successful in well established cases.

PYOGENIC OSTEITIS OF THE SPINE

This is more common in the adult and is blood borne, sometimes from the urinary tract (via Batson's plexus). About 70% of pyogenic infections are in the lumbar spine. The vertebral end plates are affected first; later the discs may be destroyed by proteolytic enzymes and bacterial toxins. The infection usually spares the posterior elements and typically the radiographs show a narrowed disc space with destruction of the end plates. This in turn can lead to a kyphosis

secondary to anterior wedging of the vertebral bodies. New bone can form and adjacent vertebrae tend to fuse spontaneously.

Clinically, the onset may be acute or insidious. In the former, the patient will have local pain, high fever and major systemic upset. Muscle spasm is present and nerve root irritation may be evident. In the latter, a long history of mild backache may be obtained and the patient can present with a deformity or neurological symptoms. Laboratory investigations are commonly unhelpful and non-specific, although the ESR is usually raised. In the radiographs of the affected area, new bone formation and the absence of extensive spinal abscesses are more suggestive of pyogenic infection than tuberculosis. Where the findings favour the former, aspiration or needle biopsy of the abscess or disc space under X-ray control is often diagnostic and can exclude malignancy. CT or MRI scans will clarify the extent of the disease.

Bedrest, splintage to control pain, and appropriate antibiotic therapy are mandatory and usually result in spontaneous fusion.

SCHEUERMANN'S DISEASE

Also known as vertebral epiphysitis this affects adolescents, and there may be a familial predisposition. The aetiology remains obscure, but it may be that the vertebral end plates sustain microfractures as a result of recurrent minor trauma which result in growth disturbance with progressive kyphosis. For the diagnosis to be made at least three vertebral bodies must be involved. The case may present with backache or deformity. Stiffness is often a feature and a neurological assessment should be made. The radiographic appearances are usually diagnostic (Fig. 5). In mild cases the

treatment is symptomatic, but where the deformity is severe, bracing during growth or even surgical stabilisation may be considered.

TUMOUR

It should always be remembered that a neoplasm in the body of a vertebra can cause a local kyphus as destruction progresses. The anterior elements and pedicles are commonly affected, but usually the disc space is spared until the condition is advanced: this may help to differentiate it from an infection. The most common spinal tumour is a metastasis (e.g. from breast, lung, prostate and kidney). Primary tumours (e.g. myeloma) are rare. Treatment of the uncomplicated case is dependent on the nature of the primary. Where there is impending or recent paraplegia, decompression should be undertaken unless the case is terminal.

Kyphosis

- The most common cause of kyphosis is osteoporotic fracture in the elderly.
- In congenital kyphosis the deformity is likely to get worse with growth.
- Spinal infections, although rare, are important and may be impossible to diagnose without bacteriological or histological confirmation.
- Scheuermann's disease is the most common cause of kyphosis in the adolescent.

LOW BACK PAIN

Back pain is a very common problem which is responsible for almost half of all the work days lost due to musculoskeletal disorders in the UK. The average episode of low back pain lasts about 4–6 weeks. The cause is generally benign, but careful evaluation is necessary in order to recognise a potentially serious condition or one where surgical treatment may be required.

The *degree of disability* is very variable and not necessarily closely related to any mechanical problem in the back. It may vary according to the personality, occupation and recreational activities of the patient; symptoms can be 'conditioned' by relatives and friends or exacerbated by the patient's personal problems. Conversely, many patients carry on stoically, not allowing their backache to be any more than an inconvenience to them.

It is important to establish a diagnosis, and in some cases this may be suggested by the history of how the condition started and progressed. In addition, the symptoms, the clinical examination (based on sound anatomical knowledge) and the results of any radiographs or other investigations should be in agreement.

SYMPTOMS

Pain. The site of pain and any reference to the lower limbs needs to be identified. Pain radiating into the leg down to the ankle and foot is known as 'sciatica'; depending on its distribution, it indicates irritation of the L4, L5 or S1 nerve roots. The term is much abused: pain radiating into the thigh (but not below the knee) is a very common symptom in mechanical back pain, but this is NOT a sciatic distribution. Note also the daily pattern of pain: mechanical back pain usually varies with posture and activity; unremitting pain is a feature of both malignant infiltration, psychogenic pain and malingering, requiring careful assessment.

Paraesthesia. While pain of varying intensity is the main symptom resulting from nerve root compression, paraesthesia in the affected nerve root distribution is common. It may be very disturbing and at times the only symptom.

Stiffness. This is usually secondary to pain and muscular spasm but, if prolonged, may lead to fixed deformities which become difficult to rectify. It tends to vary with activity and posture.

Urinary symptoms. Difficulties with micturition may indicate significant neurological compression of the cauda equina, often from a central disc prolapse, and should be treated as a surgical emergency.

Bowel disorders. Constipation may also result from caudal compression or from rectal tumours, but more frequently follows the use of analgesics such as codeine. Careful assessment is necessary.

EXAMINATION

General mobility. The assessment should begin as soon as the patient enters the examination room. The way he moves, dresses and undresses, or climbs onto the examination couch should be observed. Be wary if there is a disparity between the history and examination findings, e.g. the patient who undresses and dresses freely when unaware of being observed yet later appears to be in great pain during the formal examination.

Muscular spasm. This is a good indicator of pathology and may produce a shift (or lean) to the affected side; this is very common in disc prolapse.

Movements. Flexion can be assessed visually or by direct measurement. The latter (Fig. 1) may be repeated with the patient sitting forward on the examination couch. Less than 5 cm is indicative of a significant limitation of lumbar flexion (be aware that in touching the toes the greater part of the movement occurs in the hips). Assess the degree of lateral flexion

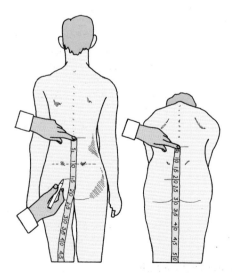

Fig. 1 **Assessing flexion in the lumbar spine.** Mark the ends of a 15 cm length of spine (with the 10 cm mark level with the dimples of Venus); holding the upper end of the tape, ask the patient to bend forwards as far as possible. Note the increase in the measurement.

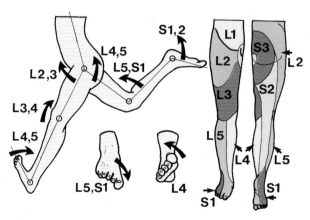

Fig. 2 **Root (segmental) distributions.** Note that motion in each joint is controlled by four nerve roots running in sequence. Hip – flexion L2, 3; extension, L4, 5. Knee – extension (and the knee jerk) L3, 4; flexion L5, S1. Ankle – dorsiflexion L4, 5, plantarflexion (and the ankle jerk) S1, 2. (Inversion involves L4 and eversion L5, S1.) A useful mnemonic for the lower limb dermatomes is that we kneel on L3, stand on S1 and sit on S3.

and whether it is the same on both sides (note that no rotation occurs in the lumbar spine).

Muscle strength and sensation. These should be carefully assessed as they will indicate which nerve roots are affected (Fig. 2). Test the tendon reflexes and plantar responses.

Where the pattern does not fit a nerve root(s) distribution, suspect other neurological conditions (e.g. multiple sclerosis, Vitamin B_{12} deficiency (causing 'glove and stocking' paraesthesia) or motor neurone disease causing a proximal myopathy); or that the patient is malingering.

Nerve root tension. This can be demonstrated with the *straight leg raising (SLR)* or *bowstring* tests which tension the sciatic nerve and thereby its roots; both are performed with the patient supine. In the SLR test the knee is kept extended and the hip gradually flexed by raising the heel from the couch until pain restricts the motion (Fig. 3). The pain should be in the sciatic distribution below the knee if a lateral disc prolapse is

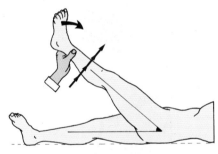

Fig. 3 **The straight leg raising test.** When performing this, note the angle at which the patient first complains of pain, the site of the pain and whether it is aggravated by dorsiflexion of the foot.

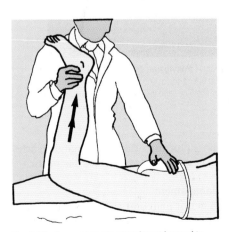

Fig. 4 **The femoral nerve stretch test is used to assess L2, 3, 4.** Tension on these roots is produced by flexion of the knee, and may be increased by extension of the hip.

compressing the L4, L5 or S1 nerve roots (the most common involvement). In the bowstring test, both the hip and knee are flexed to 90 degrees; this puts no tension on the nerve. The knee is then slowly extended until there is complaint of pain. Pressure applied to the tibial nerve behind the knee in a positive test will cause pain in the distribution of the sciatic nerve.

The *'flip' test* can be used to catch out malingerers. On the pretext of examining their back, the patient is asked to sit upright with the knees extended. The malingerer will sit happily, whilst the genuine patient will rise until the affected nerve root is placed under tension and then suddenly collapse or 'flip' back onto the couch because of pain.

The *femoral nerve stretch test* may be used to assess tension in the roots of the femoral nerve (L2, 3, 4), particularly where disc prolapses affecting the proximal part of the lumbar spine are suspected (Fig. 4). The patient lies prone (or in the lateral position) with the hip extended. The knee is slowly flexed; if no reaction is produced, the hip is hyperextended. A positive test produces pain down the anterior thigh.

Rectal examination. This is necessary in any patient who complains of any urinary or bowel symptoms. Anal tone, the state of the prostate and the presence of any rectal masses and other abnormalities should be noted.

INVESTIGATIONS

Blood tests. These are not absolutely necessary in the typical back pain patient, but where some doubt exists about the diagnosis, haematological and biochemical screens are indicated. These should include a full blood count, ESR, bone biochemistry and protein electrophoresis (the latter to exclude myeloma). If an inflammatory polyarthropathy is suspected, an additional autoantibody screen may be required.

X-rays. A-P and lateral radiographs of the lumbar spine, usually with an additional localised lateral projection of the lumbosacral junction, are standard. These would be expected to exclude fracture or neoplasia and confirm the presence of degenerative changes and most other significant pathologies.

SPECIAL INVESTIGATIONS

Computerised axial tomography (CAT or CT scans). These allow clear definition of many of the common pathologies, e.g. disc protrusion, tumour, spinal stenosis.

Magnetic resonance imaging (MRI). The indications are similar to those for CAT scanning, but it is better for infective or neoplastic problems and disc protrusions. It is considered safe to use in pregnancy.

Isotopic bone scans. These involve the injection of a radioisotope, usually Technetium, which is taken up by the bone in areas of increased activity. It is especially useful in illustrating metastatic deposits, fractures and infective foci.

DIAGNOSIS

Having followed the above procedure you should be able to decide whether the patient's condition falls into one of the following four categories:

- The backache does not arise from the spine, e.g. it is prostatic, renal, gynaecological or rectal in origin, and will require appropriate investigation and treatment.
- It is due to a prolapsed intervertebral disc.
- It is due to some other distinct (and usually radiologically proven) spinal pathology such as osteoarthritis, spondylolisthesis, etc.
- By a process of elimination, the backache arises from mechanical causes or is psychogenic in origin.

Low back pain

- A careful history and examination are essential in diagnosing any case of low back pain.
- Pain in the sciatic distribution is referred below the knee and is caused by nerve root irritation or compression.
- Loss of urinary or bowel control requires emergency assessment.
- Plain X-rays can exclude most simple pathologies, but special investigations may be necessary where the pathology is more complex.

SERONEGATIVE SPONDYLOARTHROPATHIES

This group of inter-related conditions includes ankylosing spondylitis, psoriatic arthropathy, Reiter's disease, intestinal arthropathies and some forms of juvenile chronic arthritis. All are associated with the human lymphocytic antigen complexes (HLA-B27), absence of rheumatoid factor in the serum and lack of rheumatoid nodules (Table 1). They affect the insertions of tendons and ligaments (entheses) leading to severe stiffening of the affected joints.

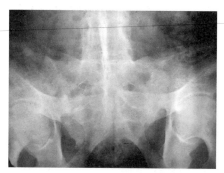
Fig. 1 **Advanced ankylosing spondylitis with fused sacroiliac joints.** The distal lumbar spine is also ankylosed, with ossification in the interspinous ligaments.

Table 1 **Common clinical features in seronegative polyarthropathies.**

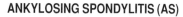

- Peripheral arthritis — usually lower limbs, and asymmetrical
- Radiological sacroiliitis
- Rheumatoid factor negative
- Association with HLA-B27
- Absence of characteristics of rheumatoid arthritis (nodules and extra-articular features)

ANKYLOSING SPONDYLITIS (AS)

This is a chronic inflammatory disease which mainly affects the axial skeleton. The synovial joints and tendon and ligament attachments to bone are involved. There is almost invariably X-ray evidence of sacroiliitis which generally confirms the clinical diagnosis (Fig. 1). About 20% of HLA-B27 positive patients ultimately develop the disease and the prevalent age of onset is in the 2nd and 3rd decades. Males are affected more often than women.

Clinical features

In many the symptoms are mild, with a minor degree of low back pain or morning stiffness. In others the disease is rapidly progressive and disabling. It typically presents in a young adult male with back pain and stiffness of insidious onset. Sacroiliac disease produces pain in the buttocks. There may be pain at the insertions of the Achilles tendons or the plantar fascia. As the condition progresses, it may involve any or all of the spine (Figs 2 and 3), and the major limb joints (particularly the hips, knees, shoulders and elbows). Bony or fibrous ankylosis occurs in the articulations which have been affected; when this occurs, pain tends to improve but at the expense of mobility. Chest expansion is often reduced, leading to impaired pulmonary function.

In the lumbar region the spine flattens, with loss of the lordotic curve; in

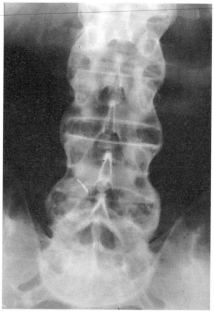
Fig. 3 **Ankylosing spondylitis with typical 'bamboo spine' appearance.**

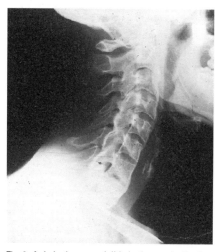
Fig. 2 **Ankylosing spondylitis in the cervical spine with interbody and facet joint fusions.**

the thoracic and cervical spine there is usually a progressive kyphosis (Fig. 4) which in extreme cases may prevent forward vision as the chin comes into permanent contact with the chest. Extra-articular features of AS include fatigue, weight loss, low grade fever, uveitis and conjunctivitis. Fibrotic lung disease, pulmonary tuberculosis and cardiac pathology (e.g. aortic incompetence and conduction defects) are less common but important.

Investigations

Routine blood tests can be normal, although a high ESR is usual. Alkaline phosphatase and creatinine phosphokinase are often raised. Estimation of the HLA-B 27 is not routinely undertaken, unless the diagnosis is in doubt (remember that 8% of the normal population are positive). The sacroiliac joints are almost invariably involved in ankylosing spondylitis, and radiographs which

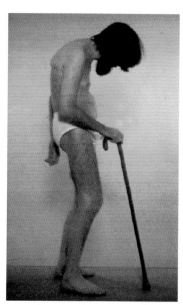
Fig. 4 **Ankylosing spondylitis.** Note the loss of lumbar lordosis, and the fixed flexion deformities (of the hips, and the thoracic and cervical spine).

show blurring of the joint margins, sclerosis, erosions or fusion are diagnostic.

Management

Relief of pain and stiffness and maintenance of posture are the main objectives of treatment. Non-steroidal anti-inflammatory agents are the mainstay of medical treatment as second line drugs, such as methotrexate or steroids, have limited use. Physiotherapy, including extension exercises, may be advised in an attempt to preserve spinal alignment. Surgery is sometimes required, either in the form of joint replacement (particularly in the case of the hip) or spinal osteotomy, where a kyphotic deformity is particularly gross.

PSORIATIC ARTHRITIS

There is an association between psoriasis and arthritis: 7% of those suffering from psoriasis will develop arthritis.

Clinical features

Commonly, the skin, nails and distal interphalangeal joints of the fingers are involved, but there is a wide spectrum of presentation (Fig. 5); this may be asymmetrical in pattern or symmetrical like rheumatoid arthritis. There is a close association between the involvement of the nails and joints, but skin and joint disease have a variable temporal relationship: indeed, there are patients who have an arthropathy for many years before skin lesions appear, making diagnosis difficult. The small joints of the fingers and toes are often very stiff at an early stage unlike in other arthropathies. The major joints can also be involved, but to a much lesser degree than in rheumatoid arthritis. Stiffness of the spine is, however, seen not infrequently and can be mistaken for AS. It is similarly disabling, although the spinal deformities seen in psoriasis are less severe.

Investigations

There is no specific test for psoriasis, although anaemia is common and the ESR and C-reactive protein may be raised. Radiological changes are seen in the small joints of the hands and feet and these are often very severe. Ultimately, the joints may ankylose. In the spine, osteophytes are non-marginal, but nonetheless can cause stiffness and pain.

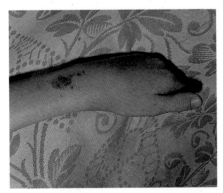

Fig. 5 **Psoriatic arthritis with some puffy swelling of the wrist and a psoriatic patch in the distal forearm.**

Treatment

The majority of patients need only symptomatic treatment with simple analgesics or non-steroidal inflammatory agents. As in rheumatoid disease some patients require second line treatment and in extreme cases steroids may be necessary. Surgical treatment in the form of joint reconstructions or fusions may be required to maintain mobility and relieve pain.

REITER'S DISEASE

This is characterised by urethritis, conjunctivitis and arthritis. In the UK it is invariably a consequence of venereal exposure, but in some parts of Africa and in the Middle and Far East it can follow an attack of dysentery. There has been some controversy about its aetiology, but it is clear that there is an association with Chlamydia Trachomatis infection in the venereal form and Shigella Flexneri in the dysenteric form. Patients who develop the disease are invariably HLA-B27 positive and there is thought to be a genetic predisposition to developing the syndrome following infection with Chlamydia.

Clinical features

It presents with urethritis (often in a patient attending a genitourinary clinic). This is followed shortly afterwards by conjunctivitis and arthritis. These can be of varying severity, with the arthritis tending to manifest itself about 1–3 weeks after the onset of the urethritis. There can be accompanying systemic upset such as fever and weight loss. Other associated problems are moist erosions with raised edges on the penis (circinate balanitis) and, in about 30% of cases, pigmented lesions on the soles of the feet which may ultimately erupt into areas of thickened skin (keratoderma blennorrhagicum). Painless ulcers on any of the buccal surfaces is a problem which is often overlooked.

The arthritis tends to affect the main weight-bearing joints, especially the knees and ankles. Whilst there is a natural tendency to resolution, the syndrome can be recurrent and ultimately cause joint destruction. An asymmetrical sacroiliitis is common and such a finding should arouse suspicion. Areas of periostitis with fluffy new bone formation are sometimes seen, particularly around the calcaneus ('lover's heels').

Treatment

Bedrest during the acute phase is helpful and tense effusions may have to be aspirated. Otherwise the treatment is largely symptomatic, using non-steroidal anti-inflammatory agents. Tetracyclines have been used, although their efficacy is unsubstantiated. Steroids do not seem to have a role to play in Reiter's, apart from intra-articular injections which may help to relieve swelling and pain. Surgical intervention is rarely required, except in severe and persistent cases.

ENTEROPATHIC ARTHRITIS

This is relatively uncommon, but should always be borne in mind in a patient with an atypical presentation. It occurs in association with a number of inflammatory bowel conditions: ulcerative colitis, Crohn's disease, bacillary dysentery, Whipple's disease and Behçet's disease. The first two are the most common and the arthropathy can be of varying type and severity. It tends to affect the peripheral joints and the pattern usually follows that of the underlying condition. It affects 15–20% of patients suffering from the underlying enteric disease which may have its associated systemic and cutaneous manifestations (e.g. perianal lesions, erythema nodosum and uveitis). The arthropathy tends to be self-limiting and, in most cases, non-deforming. In making a diagnosis, reliance must be placed on the clinical picture as investigations tend to be non-specific. Treatment is centred on control of inflammatory bowel disease. If remission can be achieved the arthritis is not usually a problem and surgery is seldom required.

Seronegative spondyloarthropathies

- The seronegative spondyloarthropathies share common clinical features.
- They are usually HLA-B27 positive.
- Ankylosing spondylitis is the most common of these conditions.
- In psoriatic arthritis the arthropathy can appear before the skin lesions.
- Surgical intervention is seldom required in psoriatic arthritis and is usually confined to the weight-bearing joints.

BENIGN BONE TUMOURS

These are relatively common, but require careful assessment to establish a diagnosis and exclude malignancy, so that a decision may be made quickly regarding treatment. Many are easily recognised by their position and appearance on plain radiographs, but where doubt exists, radioisotope, CAT or MRI scanning and bone biopsy may be necessary. The majority of benign bone tumours occur in the adolescent or young adult and cease growth when skeletal maturity is established.

OSTEOID OSTEOMA

This typically affects males more commonly than females, and usually presents between the ages of 10 and 25. The history is of severe and persistent pain which is typically abolished by aspirin. The femur and tibia are most commonly affected, although the spine (usually a pedicle), can be involved. The lesion is usually found in the cortex of the bone, and there is reactive sclerosis around a radiolucent central nidus (Fig. 1). The nidus consists of immature osteoid tissue and highly vascular cellular tissue; it is rarely larger than 1 cm in diameter and may be difficult to spot. Where doubt exists, tomography or CAT scanning can be helpful. A radioisotope scan always shows an intense 'hot spot' in the affected area. (Note that the simple bone

tumour known as an osteoblastoma is similar in character and histology, and many argue may be the same entity.)

Treatment
Surgical excision, if complete, is curative.

CHONDROMA

This is probably the most common of all bone tumours, and is often first seen in a fracture clinic where it presents as a pathological fracture. There are two varieties of the tumour, the enchondroma and the ecchondroma. The *enchondroma* is confined within the intact cortex, although it may cause it to balloon and become structurally thin. The *ecchondroma* (Fig. 2) protrudes beyond the cortex of the bone. Both most commonly occur in the tubular bones of the hands and feet, and less frequently in the larger tubular or flat bones. (This is in contrast to chondrosarcoma.) Malignant transformation is rare in solitary chondromas, but it can occur in up to 25% of cases of multiple enchondromatosis (Ollier's disease).

Treatment
Excision and curettage are usually curative, although larger lesions may require supplementary bone grafting. Small lesions discovered incidentally rarely give trouble but should be watched.

OSTEOCHONDROMA

This is also a comparatively common tumour, and it typically occurs on the external surface of a metaphysis (usually

the distal femur, proximal humerus or proximal tibia). It is thought that it results from a failure of remodelling during growth. This leads to a typical pedunculated (Fig. 3) or sessile growth arising from the metaphysis. It is not uncommon for an osteochondroma to remain unnoticed for years and only be identified after a minor injury. The patient may vehemently deny its pre-existence, although the radiographs confirm its typical appearance and long standing nature. These tumours always stop growing at skeletal maturity and any enlargement thereafter should be treated with suspicion. (Note that multiple tumours of this pattern are a feature of diaphyseal aclasis.)

Treatment
The tumour can cause local irritation of tendons or other soft tissues as they override the swelling during movement. Excision may be indicated because of this, or to alleviate any anxiety. The tumours typically have a cartilage 'cap' which makes them larger than their X-ray appearances would suggest.

SOLITARY BONE CYST (UNICAMERAL BONE CYST)

This tumour occurs predominantly in boys close to adolescence; the most common sites are the proximal humerus and femur. It often presents in a fracture clinic as a pathological fracture (Fig. 4). On X-ray it appears as an ovoid radiolucent area with thinning of the overlying cortex (which may be slightly expanded). Although it may tend to abut the growth plate, it never penetrates it.

Treatment
Where the tumour is found in association with a fracture, it may resolve

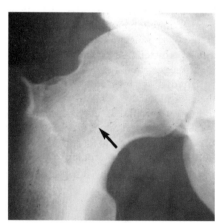

Fig. 1 **The pointer indicates an osteoid osteoma in the femoral neck.**

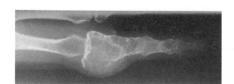

Fig. 2 **Ecchondroma of a proximal phalanx.**

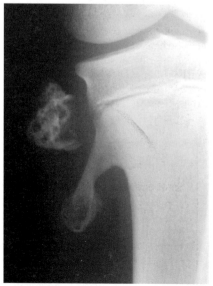

Fig. 3 **Pedunculated metaphyseal osteochondroma.**

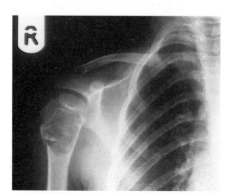

Fig. 4 **Bone cyst with pathological fracture.**

spontaneously as union proceeds (which it usually does at the normal rate). If this does not occur, or in other circumstances, excision and curettage is normally advised; this may be supplemented by packing the cavity with bone grafts. There is some evidence that intracystic injection with methylprednisolone may be as effective as surgery.

ANEURYSMAL BONE CYST

This tumour is characterised by having blood-filled cavities separated by fibrous septa and areas of new bone formation. It affects adolescents and young adults, with the metaphyseal regions of long bones and the vertebral column being most frequently involved. The X-rays usually show an eccentric radiolucent lesion expanding beyond the margins of the thinned cortex (Fig. 5). Growth may be extremely rapid, giving the mistaken impression of malignancy.

Treatment

Complete surgical removal of the lesion is usually curative. Some advocate radiotherapy alone or in combination with surgery.

JUXTA-ARTICULAR BONE CYSTS (INTRAOSSEOUS GANGLIONS)

These occur in mature adults, and their frequency increases with age. They are common in the distal tibia, acetabulum (Fig. 6) and carpus. The typical radiographic appearance is of a well defined, radiolucent cystic space with a sclerotic

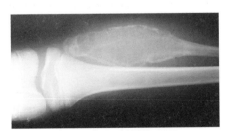

Fig. 5 **Aneurysmal bone cyst of the fibula.**

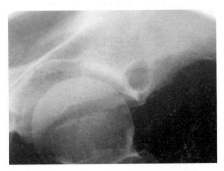

Fig. 6 **Intraosseous ganglion of the acetabulum.**

margin. They are similar to the cysts of osteoarthritis. Their cause remains obscure, but they may be due to fibrous metaplasia with superimposed mucoid degeneration.

Treatment

Deroofing and curettage of the lesion is usually curative, but if it is large, bone grafting of the defect may be necessary to maintain bony integrity.

FIBROUS CORTICAL DEFECT

This tumour occurs in the metaphysis during growth, and if incorporated within bone is known as a non-ossifying fibroma. Most are found as incidental X-ray anomalies or may present with fractures. They appear as well circumscribed lesions and can be difficult to differentiate from simple cysts.

Treatment

No specific treatment is necessary unless it is a cause of recurrent fracture. Then curettage and bone grafting are usually curative.

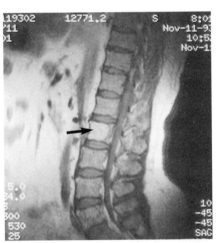

Fig. 7 **MRI scan showing haemangioma of a vertebral body.**

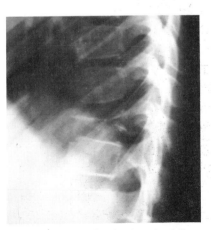

Fig. 8 **Flattened vertebra due to eosinophilic granuloma.**

HAEMANGIOMA

A few occur in the skull and long bones, the latter being more likely to produce symptoms and pathological fracture. The majority, however, affect a vertebral body and are an incidental finding. Radiographs show increased density and striations in the vertebral body, which in spite of the absence of bone destruction or expansion may be mistaken for malignancy. An MRI scan may be helpful in clarifying the diagnosis (Fig. 7).

Treatment

This is conservative where a symptomless tumour is found in a vertebral body. Where there is a pathological fracture of a long bone, stabilisation with or without fixation is necessary. Radiotherapy can be used in inaccessible areas, but should be reserved for symptomatic lesions only.

EOSINOPHILIC GRANULOMA (HISTIOCYTOSIS 'X')

This is one of a family of conditions which includes Hand–Schüller–Christian and Letterer–Siwe disease. All have eosinophilic granulomas as part of the syndrome, but the only one the orthopaedic surgeon is likely to see is the solitary eosinophilic granuloma of bone. This is usually discovered in adolescence, most frequently in the skull, jaw, vertebral bodies, ribs or the metaphyseal regions of long bones. Pain is the presenting feature, and any systemic effects suggest the more complex family members of this condition. Radiographs show a lucent area with thinning of the cortex and, on occasions, rapid expansion. Vertebral body lesions have a typical flattened and dense appearance, with no alteration of the intervertebral discs (Fig. 8).

Treatment

Biopsy is essential, but curettage usually succeeds in eradicating it. Multiple lesions suggest other forms of the disease, and this must be clarified by investigation.

Benign bone tumours

- Benign tumours are relatively common.
- Plain radiographs are usually sufficient to establish a diagnosis.
- Increased size of a tumour after skeletal maturity should arouse suspicion of malignant change.

MALIGNANT BONE TUMOURS

Primary malignant bone tumours are rare, and account for less than 0.05% of all deaths from malignant disease. Advances have been made in the treatment of these tumours, although the prognosis still remains poor in many of them.

Before any therapeutic decisions can be made, the precise classification of a tumour is essential. This requires a multidisciplinary team to carefully assess its clinical, radiological and pathological features. Non-invasive investigations which give information about the extent and dissemination of the lesion should be performed before any biopsy is done so that the tissue planes are not disturbed. These can include radioisotopic scanning, angiography, and CAT and MRI scanning. Open biopsy can be a reliable method of diagnosis, but needle biopsy is becoming the method of choice. The opinion of one or more pathologists specialising in bone tumours is always highly desirable as interpretation of the specimens is often difficult. Definitive treatment should be embarked upon only after a clear diagnosis has been made by the multidisciplinary team and the merits of each case discussed.

GIANT CELL TUMOUR (OSTEOCLASTOMA)

This occurs predominantly in males in the 20–40 year age group after skeletal maturity has been reached. Although this tumour is usually benign, it can cause much local destruction, sometimes being described as locally malignant. When first seen however it may be found to be of low grade malignancy, or at a later stage it may undergo malignant change. The most common sites are in the distal femur, proximal tibia and the distal end of the radius. These tumours are found in the epiphyses lying close to the joint surfaces and are often eccentrically placed. They may transgress the old growth plate and spread into the metaphysis and shaft. Microscopic examination shows that they consist of masses of giant cells of the osteoclast type. The histology may however vary within a specimen and make the diagnosis of malignancy and its grading very difficult. Radiologically, the lesion is radiolucent with indistinct margins and thinning of the adjacent cortex (Fig. 1).

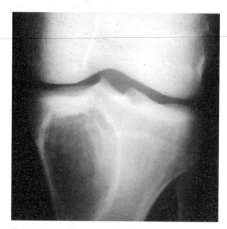

Fig. 1 **Giant cell tumour of proximal tibia.**

Treatment

This depends on the grading. Simple tumours may be treated by curettage (sometimes with chemical cauterisation of the cavity) and bone grafting or cement augmentation of the defect. As the more aggressive tumours have a tendency to recur, en-bloc resection with the use of a replacement allograft may give a better result.

OSTEOSARCOMA (OSTEOGENIC SARCOMA)

This is the most common of the primary bone tumours, affecting males predominantly in the second decade. It is rare after the age of 40 years unless associated with Paget's disease. It usually presents as a painful swelling, and there is often a history of previous trauma (the trauma simply draws the patient's attention to the lesion, and has no aetiological significance). Clinically, the mass may be fixed to the overlying tissues, and in a young person this sign must always be presumed to be evidence of malignancy until proven otherwise.

Radiographs can be very variable, but usually show disorganised areas of bone, with lytic and sclerotic regions. The edge of the lesion is usually poorly defined, and the cortex may be locally destroyed (Fig. 2). The tumour also gives rise to new bone formation (as its correct etymology indicates). There are typically raised periosteal reactions at the tumour margins (Codman's triangles), and spiculated new bone formation ('sun-burst spiculation'). This is very characteristic, but not invariably diagnostic. Osteogenic sarcoma tends to metastasise to the lungs and pleura; with better imaging

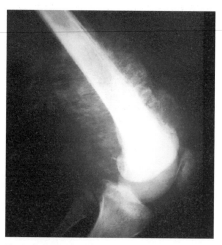

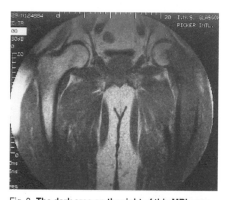

Fig. 2 **Osteosarcoma of distal femur with sun-burst spiculation.**

Fig. 3 **The dark area on the right of this MRI scan shows a chondrosarcoma which has replaced the major portion of the (L) femur up to the level of the epiphyseal plate.**

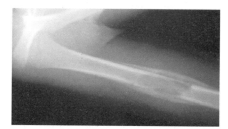

Fig. 4 **Ewing's sarcoma with bone destruction and periosteal reaction.**

(such as by CAT scanning) it now seems likely that metastases are already often present at the time of presentation.

Treatment

Advances in treatment in recent years have tended to lead to a more hopeful prognosis. This relates to several factors. Firstly, there is better understanding of the tumour, and improved imaging has made efforts at staging more reliable. Secondly, both pre- and post-operative chemotherapy regimes have led to eradication of micrometastases. Thirdly, advanced surgical techniques may often allow salvage of a limb when in the past amputation was the standard procedure.

CHONDROSARCOMA

This is a tumour which is usually found in adults between the ages of 25 and 65. It is rare under the age of 20. The tumour may arise without there being any obvious local abnormality, or it may occur secondary to an osteochondroma or other pre-existing pathology. There is a wide variation of behaviour. The most common sites are in the proximal femur (Fig. 3), pelvis and humerus. This tumour tends to favour the metaphyseal areas, but may extend into the diaphyses. Histologically it can sometimes be difficult to separate low-grade malignancies from benign lesions, and it requires an experienced pathologist to interpret the sections. No such doubt exists with the highly malignant variety. In radiographs chondrosarcomas are seen to be destructive, and contain within them areas of spotty calcification. If the cortex of the bone is breached, then the tumour may form lobulations which can be detected by palpation. This may follow secondary change in a pre-existing lesion.

Treatment

These tumours are usually unresponsive to chemotherapy or radiotherapy, and surgery is therefore the mainstay of therapy. Radical excision and prosthetic replacement is the treatment of choice, but where extensive infiltration is present, amputation is the better option.

EWING'S SARCOMA

This is a tumour which causes confusion and remains somewhat controversial as its origin has not been clearly defined. It is a round cell sarcoma, but can be difficult to differentiate from malignant lymphoma and metastatic adrenal neuroblastoma.

It occurs in the 5–20 age group, predominantly affecting boys. It may involve the diaphysis or metaphysis of the long bones, or occasionally the pelvis. Unlike other tumours systemic effects are common, with fever, anaemia, lymphocytosis and an increased ESR. Radiographically, the appearances vary widely, but usually show bone destruction (Fig. 4), associated with a layered periosteal reaction ('onion skinning'). Taken in isolation however this feature is not diagnostic.

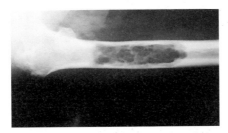

Fig. 5 **Myeloma of the proximal femur.**

Treatment

Aggressive chemotherapy in combination with radiotherapy have been responsible for improving the prognosis. Radical surgical resection has become more popular, and this may ultimately reduce the role of radiotherapy.

MYELOMA

This is a tumour of plasma cells which can produce a single lesion (plasmacytoma) or multiple lesions. It favours those bones which have an abundant red marrow (such as the vertebrae, skull, ribs, pelvis and the metaphyseal regions of the long bones). It affects males predominantly in the 45–65 age group. They present with unremitting pain or a pathological fracture. There may be a systemic upset such as anaemia, weight loss and renal complications (e.g. calcinosis, amyloidosis and pyelonephritis).

The ESR is typically highly raised to a figure which is often in excess of 100 mm/hour; this alone should alert suspicion. Investigation must also include protein electrophoresis (as an abnormal immunoglobulin band is present), urinalysis for Bence–Jones protein (present in 50% of cases), and if doubt exists, a marrow puncture. Radiographs show lytic lesions (Fig. 5). These may be multiple, and indistinguishable from secondary deposits.

Treatment

Chemotherapy is the mainstay of treatment, but radiotherapy is useful for rapid relief of pain as the tumours are radio sensitive. Internal fixation is necessary for pathological fractures. Rarely spinal lesions may cause neurological symptoms and require decompression.

METASTATIC BONE TUMOURS

In adults, these are much more common than primary malignant tumours. The likeliest sources of the primaries are lung, breast, prostate (Fig. 6), kidney and thyroid, although any tumour can metastasise to bone. The favoured sites are those

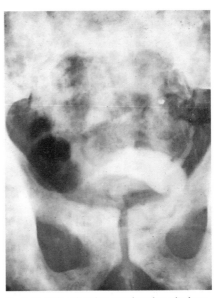

Fig. 6 **Multiple sclerotic secondary deposits from a carcinoma of the prostate.**

bones which have a rich blood supply (such as the vertebrae and proximal femora). The features are pain, swelling and pathological fracture. It should always be remembered that although deposits can be painful because of the infiltration, if the pain is only present on weight-bearing then the bone is mechanically unsound and will ultimately fracture.

Investigations are dependent on the site of the primary if this is known. Radioisotope scanning may allow clarification of the extent of spread.

Treatment

This is aimed at the primary lesion or towards palliation, and usually takes the form of radiotherapy or chemotherapy. Internal fixation is reserved for the treatment of fractures or bones which are mechanically suspect.

Malignant bone tumours

- Careful assessment of any malignant bone tumour is necessary before any treatment can be planned.
- CAT and MRI scanning may clarify the extent of local spread; and radioisotope scanning metastatic spread.
- Chemotherapy has been responsible for an improved prognosis in osteosarcoma.
- In chondrosarcoma, if complete excision is possible, radical excision with prosthetic or allograft reconstruction is the treatment of choice.

COMPLICATIONS OF JOINT REPLACEMENTS

Joint replacement can produce rapid relief of pain and stiffness, giving freedom of motion and an impressive improvement in limb function. There is however a widely held popular belief that replacement solves all joint problems, that it is always successful, and that its effects are permanent. Unfortunately this is not the case. All joint replacements ultimately tend to fail, either by fracture, loosening, infection or wear. The longer the time that has elapsed since the replacement, the greater the chances of failure; whether a problem occurs is in many cases dependent on the longevity of the patient. The most common implants are for the hip and knee, although replacements at other sites are being performed with increasing regularity.

INTRA-OPERATIVE COMPLICATIONS

Haemorrhage. Whilst many joint replacements are performed under a tourniquet (e.g. knees and elbows), some such as hips and shoulders are not. The periarticular tissues are very vascular, and the haemostatic mechanisms in bone can be slowed by the surgical manipulation during implantation of the prosthesis. Even with a tourniquet, care must be taken to avoid vascular injury — this will become evident on its release!

Nerve injury. The nerves most commonly injured are the ulnar nerve at the elbow, the sciatic (and occasionally the femoral) at the hip, and the common peroneal nerve at the knee. (The latter is particularly vulnerable during correction of a valgus deformity; then the nerve is usually subjected to tension and, if this persists, recovery is unlikely.) Nerves may be injured directly, necessitating surgical repair, or they may be injured indirectly by a tense postoperative haematoma; if this is suspected a watching policy can usually be adopted.

Fracture. This can be a disastrous complication as it can lead to the procedure having to be abandoned in order to deal with the fracture. The most common fracture (infrequent though it is) involves the femoral shaft and occurs during hip replacement procedures. It usually follows overzealous rotation to dislocate the hip preparatory to removal of the femoral head. The bone is particularly vulnerable in osteoporotic patients and in those suffering from rheumatoid arthritis. In some cases, the fracture can

be stabilised and the procedure continued (e.g. at the elbow and knee), but in others (e.g. at the hip) it may have to be abandoned until the fracture has healed.

Methylmethacrylate cement. This 'sets' by polymerisation, and the reaction is exothermic, producing temperatures up to 80 degrees centigrade (normal tissues are damaged at temperatures in excess of 43 degrees centigrade). Some of the heat may be dissipated by tissue irrigation and by the prosthesis itself (which acts as a heat sink) so that only occasionally is this reaction harmful. As the cement cures it can produce an acute hypotensive episode which is thought to be related to a hypersensitivity reaction. As a precaution the anaesthetist should be alerted and the patient well hydrated before the cement is inserted.

Tourniquet palsy. Many operations on the limbs are done under tourniquet to give a bloodless field. The generally agreed maximum ischaemia time for a pneumatic tourniquet is under 3 hours. As this level is approached, some patients may experience transient paraesthesia and some weakness distal to the site of the tourniquet following its release. A more common cause of palsy is over inflation of the cuff (or ill-advised use of a non-pneumatic tourniquet). Twice the systolic pressure in the lower limb and 50–70 mm Hg higher than systolic pressure in the upper limb is recommended for normotensive individuals.

EARLY POSTOPERATIVE COMPLICATIONS

Haematoma formation. Haemorrhage in the postoperative period can be excessive, and may sometimes require re-exploration to evacuate any haematoma and control bleeding points. Later, an insidious haematoma may become evident with swelling and external bruising. If a large haematoma persists there is an increased risk of wound infection, but as there is a risk attached to surgical evacuation, each case must be decided on its relative risks.

Deep venous thrombosis (DVT). There is a possibility of DVT in any operation, but this complication is particularly associated with joint replacement procedures in the lower limb. In hip replacements, the limb can be held in a rotated position for prolonged periods,

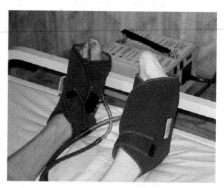

Fig. 1 **Mechanical compression boots with controller and antiembolism stocking for DVT prophylaxis.**

kinking the femoral vein and causing venous stasis. It is estimated that the incidence of DVT after hip and knee replacements is between 40% and 60% if no prophylactic measures are taken. With prophylaxis, such as graduated compression stockings, the administration of low molecular weight heparin or the use of mechanical compression boots (Fig. 1), the incidence of DVT can be significantly reduced. In half of those suffering from a DVT there are no obvious clinical signs apart from a low grade flickering pyrexia. In any swollen, painful leg a DVT should be considered, and the circulatory flow investigated by Doppler sound methods. If confirmed, full heparinisation should be instituted.

Pulmonary embolism (PE). The incidence in unprotected patients is between 5% and 15%. This can be reduced to less than 4% with the DVT prophylactic measures outlined above. Fatal pulmonary embolism is usually secondary to major pelvic thrombi, and often occurs without any previous signs of DVT. Its incidence is in the order of 0.5–1% of patients.

Urinary retention. This is common after lower limb surgery, particularly after hip replacements when the patient may lie postoperatively in the supine position for 48 hours. Spinal anaesthesia may play a part, although this complication is also common after general anaesthesia. It is more frequent in men, often being prostate related; any prostatic symptoms should be investigated and appropriately treated before replacement surgery. If retention occurs, catheterisation is necessary: this should be covered by antibiotics, as there is often a transient bacteraemia both during insertion and removal of the catheter, with the risk of hamatogenous

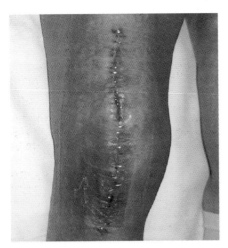

Fig. 2 **Early wound infection after total knee replacement.**

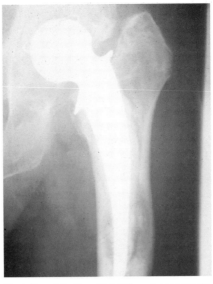

Fig. 4 **Deep infection of total hip replacement with loosening at the cement/bone interface.**

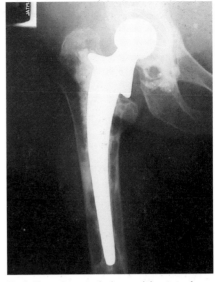

Fig. 5 **Extensive osteolysis round the stem of a total hip replacement.**

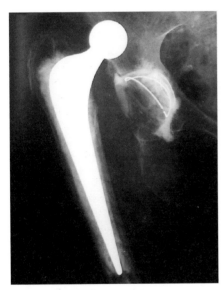

Fig. 3 **Dislocated total hip replacement.**

spread to any haematoma in the area of the prosthesis.

Early infection. This occurs within the first week, and is usually secondary to contamination during surgery or a transient bacteraemia following a postoperative chest or urinary infection (Fig. 2). Prophylactic perioperative antibiotics minimise the risk, but do not abolish it. If the infection is mild it may be aborted by antibiotic therapy, but if there is a major systemic upset in the presence of a markedly inflamed wound, surgical lavage or a more radical debridement may be necessary.

Dislocation. This can occur at any stage after any joint replacement, but is most common within the first 6 weeks in the hip (Fig. 3), shoulder and elbow. The hip is by far the most frequently dislocated, usually as a result of flexion and internal rotation. Prompt reduction under anaesthesia is required, followed if necessary by a period of splintage.

LATE POSTOPERATIVE COMPLICATIONS

Deep infection. Late infection occurs after 3 months and usually has an insidious onset. It is the result of haematogenous or direct contamination, and the causal organisms can lie dormant for many months. The first symptom may be pain at rest and during activity, and this may be alleviated by a course of antibiotics. X-rays may show loosening of the prosthesis (Fig. 4), but aspiration may be required to confirm infection. Treatment is complex, but removal of the prosthesis and cement is usually necessary; staged reinsertion may be possible if the infection is under control.

Aseptic mechanical loosening. The longer the prosthesis remains in situ, the higher the incidence. This is related to the mechanical stresses applied to the prosthesis during normal use. The symptoms are of pain on activity, with little at rest: this may distinguish it from infections, where pain tends to be constant. Revision surgery is frequently necessary to alleviate the symptoms.

Wear debris. The particulate debris produced as a result of polyethylene wear (e.g. from the acetabular component of a hip prosthesis) can cause a severe granulomatous reaction; this may lead to osteolysis and prosthetic loosening (Fig. 5). The resultant loss of bone stock can make revision surgery difficult, but specialised bone grafting techniques (such as 'impaction grafting') may allow the restoration of bone integrity.

Prosthetic failure. Fracture of a prosthesis generally requires its replacement.

As prostheses are manufactured to close tolerances, it is often possible to replace the broken part only, rather than all components of the joint replacement.

Fractures around prostheses. These are becoming increasingly common as the prosthetic population rises. In many cases the treatment is in line with standard fracture management. Unfortunately, some produce loosening of the prosthesis which may require revision.

Silicone synovitis. This is unique to the silastic prostheses used in the replacement of finger, toe and wrist joints. The pathology is secondary to wear of the silicone which causes a granulomatous reaction, leading to osteolysis and loosening. It is more common in osteoarthritics as they place more physical demands on their joints. Treatment is by removal of the prosthesis and curettage of the underlying bone; this creates a fibrous arthroplasty which often gives remarkably good function.

Complications of joint replacements

- All joint replacements tend to fail with time.
- DVT is very common after lower limb joint replacement procedures, and prophylaxis is essential.
- Urinary catheterisation after joint replacement must be covered by antibiotics.
- Late infection and aseptic mechanical loosening are difficult to differentiate.

FRACTURES: Basic definitions and concepts

A fracture is present when there is loss of continuity in the substance of a bone. There is a widespread misconception that a 'break' and a 'fracture' are somehow different. This is not so: the terms are synonymous.

GREENSTICK FRACTURE

Fractures of this type are confined to the more malleable bones of children (although not all children's fractures are of this pattern). Greenstick fractures are caused by indirect violence; there is minimal damage to the periosteum and the side of the bone away from where force is applied tends to buckle. The bone ends remain in apposition, although angulation is common (Fig. 1).

SIMPLE FRACTURE

This term has the potential for much confusion. It is preferable to reserve it to describe a fracture which has resulted in the formation of two bone fragments only. ('Simple' has also been used to describe any fracture which is closed, but this is probably best avoided.) To the lay mind the word 'simple' gives the impression that the injury and its treatment are straightforward; this is often not the case!

TRANSVERSE FRACTURE

The fracture runs across the bone roughly at right angles to its axis (Fig. 2). Fractures of this pattern may be caused by direct or indirect violence. They are often stable, with the tension of the surrounding muscles maintaining the bone end in contact. This advantage counteracts the effect of the smallness of the area of bone involved in the process of union.

OBLIQUE FRACTURE

When the line of a fracture is inclined at 30 degrees or more it is described as being oblique (Fig. 2). Fractures of this pattern may also result from direct or indirect violence. They are often unstable, with muscle tension leading to displacement and shortening.

SPIRAL FRACTURE

The fracture line spirals round the bone (Fig. 2). The cause is generally indirect violence in the form of a twisting force

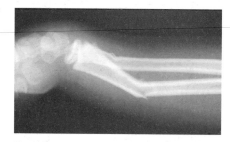

Fig. 1 **Greenstick fractures of the radius and ulna.**

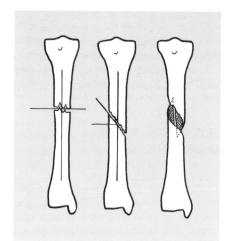

Fig. 2 **Transverse, oblique and spiral fractures.**

applied some distance away, e.g. a spiral fracture of the tibia may result from a twisting force applied to the foot. These fractures are usually unstable, but the large area of bone involved in the fracture can accelerate union.

MULTIFRAGMENTARY FRACTURE

When the violence causing the injury results in the formation of more than two bone fragments, the fracture can no longer be described as 'simple' (as in the preferred use of the term) but 'multifragmentary'. (Fractures of this pattern are also often referred to as comminuted fractures; the causal violence is usually severe (high energy) and may be direct or indirect (Fig. 3).) In some multifragmentary fractures there is a wedge of bone or 'butterfly' fragment (so-called from its shape) while at the same time there is still actual or potential contact between the main bone fragments (Fig. 4). If this is lost (in the multifragmentary complex fractures), gross instability is nearly always a problem. As the degree of violence which produces this pattern of fracture is generally great, there may be damage to other structures (e.g. skin, major vessels, nerves) as well.

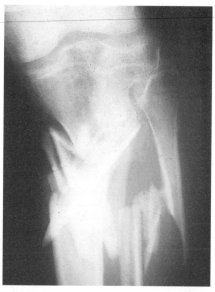

Fig. 3 **Highly comminuted fracture of the proximal tibia as a result of a high velocity injury.**

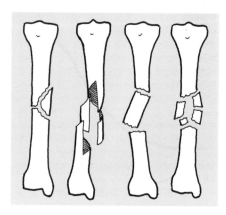

Fig. 4 **Comminuted fracture with butterfly fragment (far left); multifragmentary complex fractures of spiral, segmental and irregular pattern (right).**

Multifragmentary complex fractures may be spiral, segmental or irregular. In segmental fractures (often referred to as double fractures) there is often a problem with union at one of the distinct fracture levels.

IMPACTED FRACTURE

Impacted fractures occur in cancellous bone (e.g. in the heels, the vertebral bodies or the ends of the long bones) (Fig. 5). There is local crushing of the bone, with one fragment being driven into the other. They are often (but not always) stable and unite rapidly.

AVULSION FRACTURE

An avulsion fracture may result when the sudden contraction of a muscle causes it

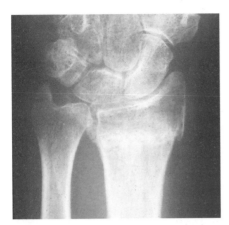

Fig. 5 **Impacted fracture of the distal radius (Colles' fracture).**

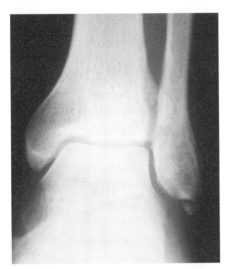

Fig. 6 **Avulsion of the bony attachment of the lateral ligament following an inversion injury of the ankle.**

to pull off the small area of bone into which it is inserted. Avulsion fractures may also arise in another set of circumstances: if a joint is stressed, one of the ligaments supporting it may either tear or pull off its bony attachment (Fig. 6). The discovery of a small fragment of bone in relation to a ligament insertion may indicate that a joint has been momentarily dislocated and may be potentially unstable.

ARTICULAR FRACTURE

A fracture may involve the articular surface of a joint (Fig. 7). In some cases this may only amount to a hair-line crack running through the bone to the articular surface, while in others there may be gross comminution with complete disruption of the joint surface. In all cases there is an increased risk of joint stiffness. If the disruption is severe, treatment may be technically difficult and disabling stiffness, pain and secondary osteo-arthritis may result. As a general rule

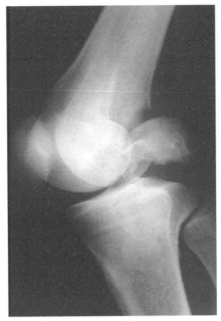

Fig. 7 **Displaced fracture of a femoral condyle involving the knee joint.**

mobilisation of the injured joint should be commenced as soon as it is safe to do so; the joint surfaces should be accurately reduced whenever this is feasible; in some cases the technical difficulties of open reduction and internal fixation, and the risk of the complications which may follow surgery, must be carefully weighed against the outcome which might be expected from the deployment of more conservative measures.

FRACTURE-DISLOCATION

A fracture-dislocation is present when a joint has dislocated and there is in addition a fracture of a related bony component (Fig. 8).

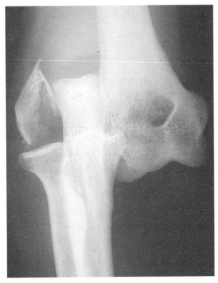

Fig. 8 **Dislocation of the elbow with fracture of the lateral condyle.**

OPEN FRACTURE

A fracture is classified as being open (old terminology 'compound') when the skin overlying the fracture is broken, with the establishment of a route through which organisms may pass in to the fracture site. The more extensive the damage to the skin, the greater the difficulty in treatment and the increased risk of infection. Open fractures may be classified into three groups of increasing severity, with the worst group being subdivided into three:

- *Type I open fractures*. The skin wound is less than 1cm in length and is clean.
- *Type II injuries*. The wound is greater than 1cm, but there is no extensive skin damage (such as skin loss or the formation of flaps (Fig. 9)).
- *Type IIIA open fractures*. These include fractures where in spite of extensive skin damage there is adequate soft tissue coverage of bone; also included in this group are multifragmentary fractures with the same or lesser degrees of skin damage.
- *Type IIIB injuries*. There is extensive soft tissue loss and exposure of bone (Fig. 10).
- *Type IIIC open fractures*. These are associated with an arterial injury which requires repair.

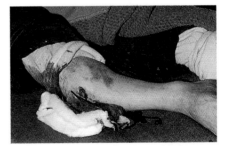

Fig. 9 **Type II open fracture.** The proximal tibia has fractured and a bone end has penetrated the skin. This pattern of fracture is often referred to as being 'open (or compound) from within out'.

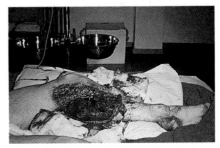

Fig. 10 **Type IIIB open fracture.** A severe crushing injury has damaged the skin and fractured the tibia. This is an 'open from without in' pattern of injury.

DISLOCATIONS, EPIPHYSEAL INJURIES, DEFORMITIES, HEALING

DISLOCATIONS

In a *dislocation* there is complete loss of congruity between the articulating surfaces of a joint. In a *subluxation*, loss of contact is incomplete. Joint subluxations may occur during the course of rheumatoid arthritis or pyogenic joint infections and may proceed to full dislocations.

EPIPHYSEAL INJURIES

Traction epiphyses are situated at principal muscle insertions and may be avulsed by violent muscle contraction. Unless the displacement is particularly severe, symptomatic treatment is all that is usually required. *Pressure epiphyses* are situated at bone ends and take part in an articulation. They are associated with longitudinal bone growth and have a specialised blood supply.

In some cases the blood supply to a pressure epiphysis may be disturbed by injury, leading to avascular necrosis. In others, the growth plate may be affected. The disturbance may be complete, leading to cessation of growth at that end of the bone and a degree of shortening, depending on the site and the age of the child (in relation to the time when epiphyseal union normally occurs). It may on the other hand be partial, leading to uneven growth with shortening and angulation (Fig. 1).

Five types of epiphyseal injuries are recognised (Salter and Harris Classification, Fig. 2):

- Type I. The whole epiphysis moves relative to the shaft (Fig. 3).
- Type II (the most common). The displacing epiphysis takes a small fragment of the metaphysis with it (Fig. 4).
- Type III. The epiphysis is fractured and part of it displaces.
- Type IV. These injuries are similar, but take a part of the metaphysis with them.
- Type V. Part or all of the epiphysis is crushed, usually with interference of growth.

FRACTURE DEFORMITY

Deformity occurs when the main fracture fragments move in relation to one another. This can have a great number of effects which may occur singly or in combination. If severe, the deformity may be conspicuous and the disturbance cosmetic. It may lead to shortening of the limb, which is of greater importance in

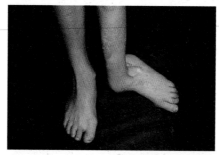

Fig. 1 **Old injury to distal tibial epiphysis leading to lateral cessation of growth.**

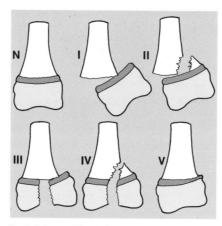

Fig. 2 **Salter and Harris Classification of epiphyseal injuries.** N=Normal.

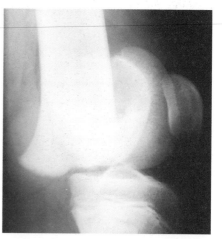

Fig. 3 **Type I injury distal femoral epiphysis.**

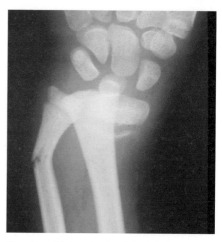

Fig. 4 **Type II injury distal radial epiphysis, with a greenstick fracture of the ulna (which is medially angulated).**

the lower limb where the gait may be affected. Angulatory deformity in the forearm bones may affect pronation and supination, while in the lower limb it throws abnormal stresses on the joints, leading perhaps to secondary osteoarthritis. If a fracture involves a joint, persisting deformity will interfere with the function of that joint and be a potential cause of pain, stiffness and degenerative changes.

There are three types of deformity: displacement, angulation and rotation.

Displacement (or translation). This is always described in terms of movement of the distal fragment. The distal fragment may be said to be medially, laterally, anteriorly, posteriorly, proximally or distally displaced. In the most severe cases there is total loss of bony contact (Fig. 5); more commonly some apposition remains and this may be described as a percentage of the whole, e.g. 'there is 50% bony apposition'.

Angulation. Here one fragment lies at an angle to the other. This may be described in terms of the direction in which the distal fragment is tilted or where the point of the angle lies, e.g. in a fracture of the

tibia where the distal fragment is tilted laterally the angulation is medial. This terminology is, unfortunately, confusing and must be used with great care.

Rotation. One fragment rotates in its long axis relative to the other; this rotational (or torsional) deformity may be one of external rotation or internal rotation (Fig. 6) or, in the case of the radius, pronation or supination. It may not be obvious in routine radiographs but is important to recognise, especially in the case of the upper limb: there, if undiscovered and untreated, it may lead to conspicuous loss of pronation, supination, or both.

Treatment

The treatment of deformity depends on its degree and site. In some cases an appreciable amount may be accepted (e.g. in the case of certain deformities occurring in young children where the powers of remodelling are great) but in

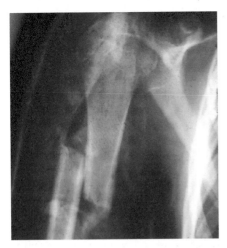

Fig. 5 **Lateral and proximal displacement, with complete loss of bony apposition, of a midshaft fracture of the humerus, in plaster at 8 weeks.** Note proximal and distal bridging callus.

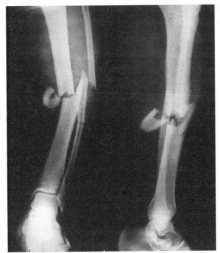

Fig. 6 **Comminuted, open (note gas shadows in calf), complex, midshaft fracture of tibia (with double fracture of the fibula), with lateral angulation (medial tilting of distal fragment), and external rotation.** Note on right that the upper tibia is pointing to the front while the foot is to the side.

the majority of cases reduction (by manipulation, traction or an open procedure) will be required.

FRACTURE HEALING

Stage 1. After any fracture under normal circumstances, bleeding from the bone ends and surrounding tissues leads to the production of a fracture haematoma. Into this there is an ingrowth of blood vessels from the periphery and the clot is replaced with fibrovascular tissue (Fig. 7). Collagen fibres are laid down and mineral salts deposited.

Stage 2. New woven bone is formed by cells derived from the periosteum and forms collars round the ends of each bone fragment (subperiosteal new bone formation). Bone is also formed to a lesser degree in the medullary cavity in the region of the fracture (medullary new bone). Under normal circumstances these exuberant formations of new bone blend together, creating bridging callus. In some cases fibrous tissue intervening between the bone ends may also be stimulated into the formation of new bone (tissue induction). As this process develops, the fracture becomes progressively less mobile as the fracture is splinted with new bone and the need for additional support declines.

Stage 3. Once rigidity in the fracture has been established, the process of cortical (or endosteal) bone union can proceed. If the bone ends are in close contact, osteoclasts tunnel across the fracture line; they are then followed by blood vessels and osteoblasts which form new Haversian systems. If there is fibrous tissue between the bone ends this must be removed before endosteal callus can be formed; this is generally achieved by the ingrowth of callus from the medullary cavity.

Stage 4. Once the cortical bone of the fracture has united, remodelling can commence. Haversian systems are laid down along the lines of stress and osteoclasts remove the bridging callus.

Complications

In Stage 1, if the blood supply to the area is poor or there is undue mobility at the fracture site, cartilage may form instead of new woven bone, interfering with the process of union.

In Stage 2, wide separation of the bone ends may prevent callus from bridging the bone ends.

The processes in Stage 3 are slow. If a fracture has been treated by rigid internal fixation, bridging callus does not appear; the internal fixation device, which gives significant local support, can seldom be safely removed until 18 months or so have elapsed since the fracture.

In Stage 4, the remodelling process is excellent in childhood. Gross displacements, including complete loss of bony contact, generally remodel well. Good, though less dramatic, corrections of angulation are usual. The correction of rotational deformities is, however, poor. These remodelling powers become less satisfactory after the age of 10, until at adolescence they become similar to those of adults.

TIMES TO UNION

Fractures involving cancellous (or woven) bone unite rapidly: usually by 6 weeks union is so far advanced that the bone can resist normal stresses, allowing mobilisation and resumption of normal function. Important cancellous bone fractures include Colles' fractures of the wrist, fractures of the proximal humerus (humeral neck fractures), fractures of the calcaneus and fractures of the vertebral bodies.

On the other hand fractures which involve cortical bone (such as the shafts of the main long bones) are slow to unite. A fracture of the tibia in an adult takes on average 16 weeks to unite and some femoral shaft fractures may take up to 6 months before union is sufficiently far advanced to allow unsupported weight bearing.

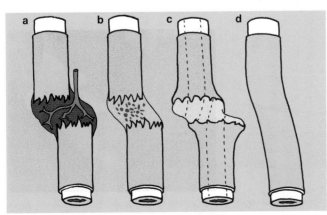

Fig. 7 **Some stages of union. (a) & (b)** Vascularisation and replacement of clot with fibrovascular tissue; **(c)** bridging callus derived from subperiosteal collars and medullary cavities; **(d)** re-modelled bone.

Dislocations, epiphyseal injuries, deformities, healing

- Traction and pressure epiphyses are quite distinct in terms of their situation, how they may be injured, their treatment and their possible complications.
- Angulation and rotation are the two most important fracture deformities.
- In the majority of cases, particularly in children, displaced fractures remodel very well.
- Fractures involving cancellous bone unite much more rapidly than fractures involving cortical bone.

FRACTURE COMPLICATIONS (I)

The many complications which occur in association with fractures may be classified into (i) those of a general nature, (ii) those involving other structures in the area of the fracture and (iii) complications which are particular to fractures as a whole.

GENERAL COMPLICATIONS OF FRACTURES

In common with many other injuries, fractures may be associated with internal haemorrhage, shock and the metabolic responses to trauma. In open fractures, there may be external haemorrhage and infection.

Prolonged recumbency may cause difficulties, particularly in cases of multiple injury and in lower limb fractures which by necessity or design are treated conservatively. Potential complications include hypostatic pneumonia and urinary tract infections, deep vein thrombosis, pressure sores, muscle wasting and demineralisation of the skeleton

Internal fixation of fractures, which is often performed in an attempt to minimise these risks, may in itself be complicated by blood loss, wound infection, mechanical failure of the internal fixation devices and the effects of anaesthesia.

LOCAL COMPLICATIONS

Involvement of arteries
A major limb artery may become kinked or stretched over an angled fracture, leading to impairment or loss of the distal circulation; this is most commonly seen in supracondylar fractures of the humerus in children (see p. 74). In the majority of cases the blood supply is restored by reduction of the fracture, but if not, exploration may be required.

In some cases the affected artery may be divided, and this is more common in open injuries. Where an arterial repair is required (and this is best performed by an experienced vascular surgeon) it is essential to fix the fracture first (usually by plating or the use of an external fixator).

Note that there can also be serious involvement of the circulation to skin and muscle in the region of the fracture by concurrent crushing, post-traumatic swelling (Fig. 1) or infection. The distal circulation may also be affected by rising pressure (from swelling or infection) within any of the closed compartments of a limb or from a cast that is too tight.

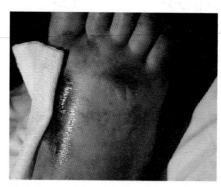

Fig. 1 **Run-over injury of the foot.** In spite of prompt elevation, bandaging and splintage some necrosis of skin is inevitable here.

Involvement of nerves

There may be an *immediate* neurological disturbance. This is seen most often after certain injuries (e.g. shoulder dislocations may be complicated by an axillary nerve palsy and fractures of the humeral shaft by radial nerve palsy) but any peripheral nerve may be vulnerable (Fig. 2). In many cases the affected nerve may have been stretched or locally compressed, leading to a lesion in continuity (neuropraxia), with recovery commencing after about 6 weeks. Less commonly the nerve may be divided; this is more frequent in open fractures. Where possible a nerve injury of this type should be treated by formal repair.

In some cases there is *delay* in the onset of symptoms. The period may be *short* (e.g. a few hours) when the nerve palsy is the result of rising pressure (from haemorrhage and oedema) in one of the muscle compartments of a limb (e.g. paralysis of the deep peroneal nerve in the anterior compartment of the leg following a tibial shaft fracture, which

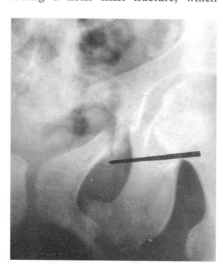

Fig. 2 **Obturator nerve palsy following a pelvic fracture.** The arrow points to the site of injury.

requires immediate treatment by decompression of the affected compartment).

The delay may be *moderate*: for example, a partial median nerve palsy may appear a few weeks after a Colles' fracture of the wrist. This fracture lies in the floor of the carpal tunnel. As it heals (particularly if there is residual deformity) it may lead to indirect pressure on the nerve. This may be treated by a carpal tunnel decompression.

The delay may be *long*, sometimes as great as several years after the initial injury. The most striking example of this is the so-called tardy ulnar nerve palsy which is often seen in adults a number of years after a childhood injury about the elbow. (This is often a supracondylar fracture of the distal humerus; some disturbance of epiphyseal growth may lead to a cubitus valgus deformity which may result in slow stretching of the nerve as it winds round the medial epicondyle.) Tardy ulnar nerve palsy may lead to paraesthesia in the ulnar distribution of the hand, with wasting of the intrinsic muscles; it is often treated by release and anterior transposition of the nerve at the elbow (Fig. 3).

Damage to nerve roots, the spinal cord or cauda equina may complicate spinal fractures or subluxations, and are the prime reason for the most careful handling of these injuries.

Involvement of tendons
Tendons may become bound down. This may occur when tendons which run close to a fracture adhere to local callus or fibrous tissue so that they lose their function. This can be a great problem in phalangeal fractures, when there is often a conflict between the need to immobilise the finger to allow the fracture to heal without deformity and the need for early mobilisation to avoid stiffness. This

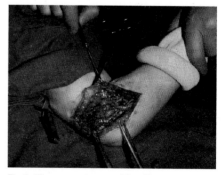

Fig. 3 **Ulnar nerve transposition.** The nerve has been brought forwards from behind the medial epicondyle; to bury it, a slit will be made in the forearm muscles over which it presently lies.

clash in the aims of treatment has an important bearing on the manner in which certain fractures are best treated.

Tendons may be compressed. This leads to functional impairment and pain (e.g. angulation of a calcaneal fracture may lead to the peroneal tendons being compressed between the lateral aspect of the calcaneus and the lateral malleolus; this may be treated by a decompression procedure).

Tendons may rupture. Some months after a Colles' fracture of the wrist (even when undisplaced) the long extensor tendon to the thumb may rupture, with loss of the ability to extend the distal phalanx. This may be due to the tendon becoming frayed by rubbing against the fracture, or it may result from some impairment of the blood supply of the tendon. This is usually treated by a tendon transposition procedure, using extensor indicis.

Involvement of viscera
A fractured rib may puncture a lung leading to a pneumothorax and the need for drainage. A pelvic fracture may damage the urethra, bladder or bowel and require appropriate surgery. Paralytic ileus may complicate fractures of the pelvis or lumbar spine, where the autonomic control of the bowel becomes affected by a retroperitoneal haematoma; nasogastric suction and fluid replacement will be required. Severe abdominal distension, vomiting and collapse sometimes occur shortly after the application of plaster jackets or other extensive body casts and may be due to compression of the duodenum by the superior mesenteric artery (cast syndrome). Removal of the cast, passage of a large bore gastric tube and fluid replacement may be required.

COMPLICATIONS PARTICULAR TO FRACTURES

Slow union
The processes of union occur in a normal manner and in sequence, but at a rate that is slower than would normally be expected.

Delayed union
Union is delayed, but as distinct from slow union there may be radiological signs of abnormality, such as absorption of bone at the fracture site, with the formation of a gap between the bone ends and poor bridging callus.

Hypertrophic non-union
There is complete failure of union: the bone ends appear sclerotic. They are also

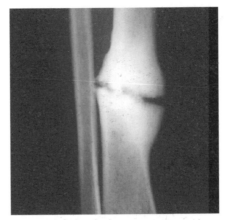

Fig. 4 **Hypertrophic non-union of the tibia.**

typically expanded at the level of the fracture — the so-called 'elephant's foot' appearance. The gap between the bone ends is filled with indolent cartilage and fibrous tissue, but the blood supply is undisturbed (Fig. 4).

Atrophic non-union
Again there is complete failure of union. The bone ends are usually osteoporotic and avascular and tend to become tapered and rounded off (Fig. 5).

CAUSES AND TREATMENT OF UNION DISTURBANCES

In many cases there may be little to explain why the process of bone healing has been impaired, but well-known factors include: (i) excessive mobility at the fracture site, particularly during the early stages, may prevent the formation of bridging callus (in some cases this may be due to inadequacy of fixation); (ii) inadequate bridging callus may in turn prevent the formation of endosteal callus; (iii) the presence of infection and (iv) disturbance of the blood supply to the fracture site may interfere with any of the stages of healing.

Established non-union is usually treated by rigid internal fixation of the fracture and the local application of bone grafts (generally pieces of cancellous bone obtained from between the inner and outer walls of the pelvis in the region

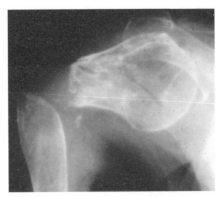

Fig. 5 **Atrophic non-union of a fracture of the proximal humerus.** Note the gross lateral angulation.

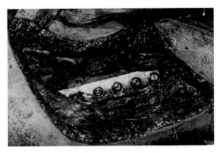

Fig. 6 **Non-union of a fracture of the humerus.** This has been treated by rigid internal fixation (with a plate and screws) and the application of cancellous bone grafts obtained from the pelvis.

of the iliac crest). In cases of atrophic non-union it is also advisable to remove any fibrous tissue between the bone ends, while in cases of hypertrophic non-union rigid internal fixation without bone grafting may suffice (Fig. 6).

Slow union requires no other treatment than patience, along with continued fixation of the fracture.

Delayed union may lead to problems with joint stiffness. As the period of fixation is extended, there is frequently some doubt as to whether the case may be progressing to non-union. Careful surveillance is required, with no delay in performing appropriate surgery should progress in union cease or the signs of non-union supervene. In some cases union may be stimulated by pulsed electromagnetic fields using suitable equipment.

Fracture complications (I)
- Both open and closed fractures may cause oligaemic shock.
- Always check the limb distal to a fracture to exclude a circulatory problem.
- The majority of cases of arterial circulatory problems respond to prompt reduction of the fracture.
- Increased pressure within a closed compartment leading to nerve compression must be dealt with promptly.
- Delays in fracture union may often lead to stiffness in the associated joints.
- Most cases of non-union are best treated by internal fixation and bone grafting.

FRACTURE COMPLICATIONS (II)

MALUNION AND SHORTENING

Malunion is said to be present when a fracture has united in a less than perfect position so that the resulting deformity interferes with function or is responsible for a displeasing appearance (Fig. 1). It may be due to persisting angulation, rotation or malalignment of joint surfaces. Many cases are preventable. If impending malunion is detected before the fracture has united, it may be avoided by forcible manipulation or wedging of a plaster; once united, correction can only be made by osteotomy, and the risks of this procedure must be carefully weighed against possible benefits.

Moderate limb shortening may occur in oblique and spiral fractures; more severe shortening may be seen in off-ended fractures. It is not a problem in the upper limb. In children, lower limb length discrepancies usually correct spontaneously in a year by epiphyseal overgrowth on the affected side. In adults, loss of 1–2cm in length is compensated by pelvic tilting and does not require treatment. Losses in excess of this may be treated by alteration to the footwear.

In children, injuries involving the epiphyses (especially Salter and Harris Groups III, IV and V) may be followed by **growth disturbance**. If the whole width of the epiphysis is affected, the bone may not grow to be as long as it should; if part only is affected, there will be uneven growth and deformity (Fig. 2). In some cases this may be avoided by skilled treatment of the initial injury or by later surgery (epiphyseolyis); in late cases shortening of an unaffected paired bone (e.g. of the ulna in fractures of the radius) or an osteotomy may be required.

AVASCULAR NECROSIS

A fracture may disrupt the blood supply to a bone fragment, leading to its death. When this occurs in the shaft of the bone there is seldom any problem; the living bone actually unites with the necrotic fragment which is then progressively revascularised. This same process occurs when the avascular segment involves the articular surfaces, but the inevitable bone softening and distortion may lead to early, painful, secondary osteoarthritis. This is seen most often in the hip joint after fractures of the femoral neck (Fig. 3), in the wrist after fractures of the scaphoid (Fig. 4), and in the ankle after fractures of the neck of the talus.

While avascular necrosis is itself untreatable, its effects in the lower limb may be reduced by avoiding weight bearing during the revascularisation period (to prevent deformity by pressure). Thereafter treatment is dictated by the severity of the secondary osteo-arthritis (e.g. avascular necrosis of the head of the femur causing marked pain and stiffness in the hip from secondary osteoarthritis may be treated by a total hip replacement).

LOSS OF JOINT MOVEMENT

Nearly every fracture carries the risk of some reduction of movement in the related joints and the loss of function that this may entail, so that this complication assumes great overall importance. Loss of movement may be the result of factors occurring within the joint, close to the joint or remote from the joint.

Intra-articular factors

Causes of a general nature include fibrous adhesions resulting from (i) organisation of a joint haematoma; (ii) articular cartilage damaged by trauma; (iii) articular cartilage which has undergone degenerative changes as a result of prolonged immobilisation.

Causes of a mechanical nature may occur when a fracture runs into a joint and irregularity of the joint surfaces blocks movements; loose bodies within the joint may also have this effect.

Secondary osteoarthritis developing within a joint may also reduce movements. This may occur as a result of:

- persisting irregularity of the joint surface leading to accelerated wear
- concurrent traumatic damage to articular cartilage and subchondral bone
- avascular necrosis
- malalignment of the fracture leading to abnormal joint stresses, again accelerating wear.

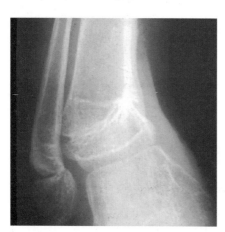

Fig. 1 **Malunited ankle fracture with separation of the malleoli and secondary osteoarthritis.**

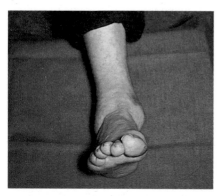

Fig. 2 **Partial epiphyseal growth arrest with tilting of the plane of the ankle.**

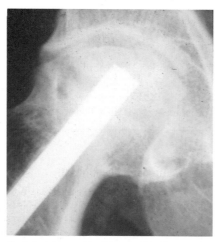

Fig. 3 **An intracapsular fracture of the femoral neck, treated by nailing, has developed a segmental avascular necrosis which has resulted in deformity of the weight-bearing portion of the femoral head.**

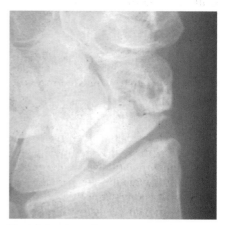

Fig. 4 **Deformity and increased density of the proximal part of the scaphoid due to avascular necrosis.** Unusually the scaphoid has also failed to unite (non-union).

Periarticular factors

The factors lying close to a joint which may result in loss of movement include:

- persistent angulation of a fracture, e.g. an uncorrected Colles' fracture deformity may lead to a loss of palmar flexion at the wrist (sometimes with a corresponding gain in dorsiflexion)
- persistent displacement of a fracture which may produce a mechanical block to movement
- adhesion of muscles and tendons to developing callus, tethering the joint
- fibrosis occurring in joint capsule as a result of direct injury, disuse, passive stretching or Sudeck's atrophy (reflex sympathetic dystrophy)
- myositis ossificans resulting in a mechanical block to movement.

Remote factors

Muscles and tendons which adhere to callus in diaphyseal fractures may also cause loss of movement through tethering; this effect is greatest when a fracture lies close to a joint. It is a common problem in fractures of the distal third of the femur where adhesions between the quadriceps muscle and the fracture lead to restriction of knee flexion (and sometimes extension).

Post ischaemic fibrosis in muscles may also lead to reduction in movements and sometimes deformity (e.g. Volkmann's ischaemic contracture); this may be the result of arterial obstruction, such as may occur in a supracondylar fracture, or from a compartment syndrome.

PREVENTION OF JOINT STIFFNESS

- Where indicated, carry out and maintain as accurate a reduction as possible.
- Immobilise only those joints necessary to the security of the fracture and mobilise the others without delay.
- Any joint which is immobilised should be placed in a position conducive to recovery of function (e.g. in an ankle fracture being treated in a cast, the joint should be placed in the neutral position and not in plantar flexion).
- Elevate the affected limb, especially in the early stages, to reduce the deleterious effects of chronic peripheral oedema.
- Reduce, modify or remove the splintage as soon as the stability of union will permit.
- Unless there is no significant loss of movements, and function is excellent, commence physiotherapy (and where indicated, occupational therapy) as soon as possible and continue with this treatment until there is no further gain.
- If non-union is suspected, avoid procrastination.
- In some situations the importance of an excellent recovery of movements may influence the decision not only to use internal fixation, but to choose a method which will permit early joint mobilisation.
- In some circumstances, continuous passive movements, mediated by machine, may be employed. Note however that passive stretching of the elbow may result in myositis ossificans and must be scrupulously avoided.

Treatment of established stiffness

Methods of dealing with loss of movements which have failed to respond to physiotherapy are limited. In some cases, once the position has become static, manipulation of the joint under a general anaesthetic may occasionally result in some gain. At the knee, where there is serious restriction of knee flexion due to quadriceps tethering, a quadricepsplasty operation may be helpful. Where myositis ossificans has produced a mechanical block, delayed excision of the bone mass may be undertaken with benefit. Where the loss is due to an intra-articular cause, such as gross irregularity or secondary osteoarthritis, joint replacement may have to be considered.

SUDECK'S ATROPHY (REFLEX SYMPATHETIC DYSTROPHY)

This curious condition, which is considered to be due to an abnormal peripheral autonomic response to injury, is seen most often at the wrist after Colles' fractures. It is also common in the foot and ankle (Fig. 5) after fractures of the fifth metatarsal base or the malleoli. It can occur after soft tissue injuries alone; this is often the case about the knee where its effects can be particularly severe.

In the most common instance, after a Colles' fracture, there is complaint of pain in the wrist and fingers which are swollen, tender, pink and warm. Movement in the joints of the fingers is often severely restricted, rendering the hand almost useless. The condition may not come to light until some weeks after the initial injury, when the cast is removed in anticipation of union. At first it may be thought that the fracture has failed to unite, but if radiographs are taken these will show not only union, but the gross peripheral decalcification characteristic of the condition. The findings are similar when the condition occurs at other sites.

The factors leading to this abnormal response to trauma are not often clear. It may follow the use of a cast which is too tight or too slack, where there is a prolonged period of high pressure within a related muscle compartment or where there is failure to elevate the injured limb and peripheral oedema becomes prominent.

While it is usually self-limiting, resolving over a course of 4–12 months, it is essential that mobilisation is pursued with vigour as some joint stiffness is common. Sympathetic blockade, using guanethidine sulphate, may be used to confirm the diagnosis and in the treatment of severe cases.

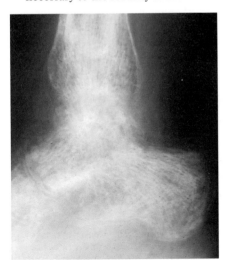

Fig. 5 **Gross Sudeck's atrophy of the ankle.**

Fracture complications (II)

- Malunion may affect the appearance and function of a limb, and is generally avoidable.
- Avascular necrosis of bone is seen most often after intracapsular fractures of the femoral neck and after fractures of the scaphoid and talus.
- The possibility of permanent joint stiffness should be borne in mind at all stages of fracture treatment, and affected and related joints should be mobilised as soon as possible.
- Unexpected pain and joint stiffness in convalescence should raise the possibility of Sudeck's atrophy.

FRACTURE COMPLICATIONS (III) / PRIORITIES OF TREATMENT

MYOSITIS OSSIFICANS

In the most common form of this condition an extensive calcified mass appears in the soft tissues near a joint and this leads to a severe mechanical block to movement. It is most common near the elbow (Fig. 1) and may follow a period of ill-advised passive stretching of a stiff joint. It is also found at the shoulder, the hip and the knee. It is often seen in paraplegics and those suffering from head injuries where good intentioned passive movements of spastic joints may be a contributory factor. While surgical excision of the bony mass is often possible and the obvious treatment, this must be delayed for 6–12 months, otherwise recurrence is inevitable.

OSTEITIS

Infection of bone is extremely rare in closed fractures, although it is occasionally seen (as a result of blood borne organisms) in patients suffering from rheumatoid arthritis. This is most likely in those who are being treated with anti-inflammatory drugs. Osteitis is essentially the feared complication of open fractures (Fig. 2) and of internal fixation in closed fractures. The techniques employed in these procedures are aimed at reducing the risks of this complication.

If infection supervenes in a fracture, it should be dealt with promptly by the administration of appropriate antibiotics (systemically and/or locally by irrigation or the use of antibiotic impregnated acrylic beads), by maintaining good fixation of the fracture and usually by establishing adequate drainage. Once union has occurred, any internal fixation device (which may be acting as a foreign body) can be removed to further improve the prospects of healing.

FAT EMBOLISM

This complication is thought to be due to microparticles of fat escaping into the circulation from the region of the fracture, although a disturbance of lipid metabolism may account for other common features. It is seen most often after fractures of the femoral shaft and pelvis, and in the former inadequate fixation of the fracture is sometimes a factor. It may declare itself some days after the initial trauma by an elevation of temperature and the appearance of petechiae in the skin. The patient may become confused or become unconscious and there may be evidence of renal failure. Radiographs of the chest may reveal mottling of the lung fields.

Preventative measures include ensuring meticulous fluid replacement after trauma and the rigid internal fixation of femoral shaft fractures, especially in cases of multiple trauma. In the established case the routine measures of administering intravenous fluids and oxygen should be pursued; in severe cases where the blood gas levels are disturbed, intubation and the use of a ventilator may be required. If further deterioration occurs, surgical stabilisation of any femoral fracture must be considered.

IMPLANT COMPLICATIONS

Implants may give rise to mechanical difficulties, cause problems from corrosion and provide a nidus which may prevent the healing of a local infection.

If an internal fixation device is unable to withstand the forces to which it is subjected, it may fail; screws may pull out of bone and become ineffective; screws, plates (Fig. 3) and intramedullary nails may fracture, sometimes as a result of fatigue from repeated stressing. If mechanical failure happens before union, deformity may occur and further surgery may become necessary (e.g. to replace the failed device).

Long plates and intramedullary nails reduce the elasticity of that part of the bone they span and cause stress concentrations at their ends; as a result there is an increased tendency for further fracture in these areas.

Although all the materials for implants are carefully chosen, some are less biologically inert than others. Corrosion, especially occurring between plates and

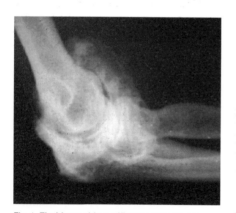

Fig. 1 **Florid myositis ossificans at the elbow.**

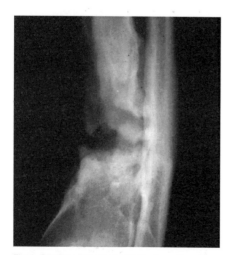

Fig. 2 **Osteitis of the tibia with the formation of a large abscess cavity and a sinus, secondary to an open fracture.**

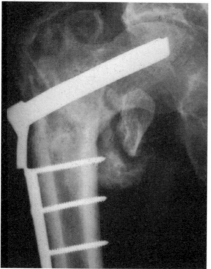

Fig. 3 **Failure of a nail-plate used to hold an extracapsular fracture of the femoral neck.** The fracture has united with lateral angulation (coxa vara).

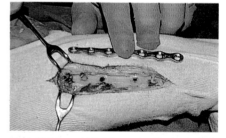

Fig. 4 **Stainless steel plate removed because of local pain.** The fracture has united, but note the tissue staining.

screws where there is fretting, may lead to local staining of the tissues and cause aching pain in the area (Fig. 4). Microscopic metallic debris on rare occasions has been known to cause neoplastic tissue change, and there is sometimes concern about the rare but possible distal effects of substances such as chromium and aluminium (leached from alloys containing them) when they enter the transport system.

Because of these factors, as a general rule internal fixation devices should be removed after they have served their purpose in all patients under the age of 40. In older patients the indication for the routine removal of internal fixation materials is less clear; nevertheless this is advisable when the implants are the source of local symptoms or where they are contributing to the continuance of a local infection. It is also probably best to remove intramedullary nails from the femur to reduce the risks of subsequent femoral neck fractures.

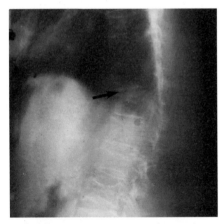

Fig. 5 **Osteoporosis of the spine, with a wedge fracture which has caused an angulatory kyphosis.** There are also several disc herniations into the soft vertebral bodies.

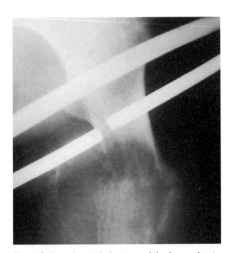

Fig. 6 **Subtrochanteric fracture of the femur due to a metastatic deposit.** The fracture is being treated in a Thomas splint and is uniting.

PATHOLOGICAL FRACTURES

A pathological fracture is one which has occurred in a bone which is abnormal or diseased. In many cases the abnormality has led to loss of bone strength; by far the most common example is osteoporosis, which is an underlying factor in many fractures of the wrist, femoral neck and spine (Fig. 5). Fractures in these regions are particularly common in postmenopausal women. Where the bone has become greatly weakened, as for example in the presence of a destructive metastatic bone deposit (Fig. 6) the force required to produce the fracture may be trivial.

In many other conditions the pathological process may not materially affect the bone strength; it may be a local manifestation of a generalised disease process which is revealed by the radiographs taken of the part.

In the treatment of pathological fractures, attention is first directed to the fracture itself which is usually dealt with by conventional methods. Thereafter any additional treatment is dependent on the nature of the disease process.

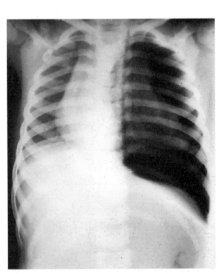

Fig. 7 **Tension pneumothorax, with mediastinal shift, requiring immediate decompression.**

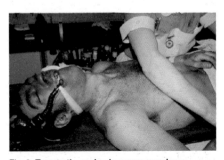

Fig. 8 **Traumatic asphyxia accompanying a fracture of the femoral shaft.** Note the cyanosis and supraclavicular skin haemorrhages. Prompt, initial treatment of the former (by intubation and assisted respiration) resulted in full recovery.

PRIORITIES OF TREATMENT

Other conditions may require attention before the definitive treatment of a fracture is undertaken. The majority of fractures do not suffer if there is a delay of hours or even days in their treatment (although there should be no procrastination in the handling of open fractures or those where there is loss of the distal arterial supply). A number of other conditions, which may be potentially life threatening, may have to be dealt with first. These problems may be *respiratory* (e.g. obstruction or impairment, Figs 7 and 8), *cranial* (e.g. head injury with raised intracranial pressure requiring decompression), *cardiac* (e.g. tamponade or intrathoracic rupture of the aorta), *visceral* (e.g. rupture of the spleen, liver or bowel) or *circulatory* (with haemorrhage leading to oligaemic shock). In the latter case it is important to note that internal haemorrhage in closed fractures can be high, requiring scrupulous observation and prompt measures to ensure adequate replacement. This is especially so in fractures of the pelvis and femora and blood loss when these fractures are open is even higher.

While those conditions which require prior attention are being dealt with, bleeding from open wounds should be controlled (usually the application of local pressure will suffice), open wounds should be covered to reduce the risk of infection and fractures should be temporarily splinted to reduce further soft tissue damage and local haemorrhage. Once those conditions requiring prior management have been dealt with, and the patient's general condition will allow, then direct treatment of the fracture may be commenced.

Fracture complications (III) / Priorities of treatment

- Rapid deterioration in a patient's general condition some days after a fracture of the femur or pelvis should suggest the possibility of fat embolism.
- If a fracture has resulted from a trivial injury, the possibility of it being pathological must be considered.
- Osteoporosis is the most common cause of pathological fracture.
- The most common neoplasm responsible for fracture is the metastatic deposit.
- Life threatening conditions take precedence in the treatment of any fracture.

TREATMENT OF FRACTURES

The primary aims of fracture treatment are in essence quite simple:

- sound bony union with no (or minimal) deformity
- restoration of function so that the patient is able to return to his former occupation, and pursue any physical activity that he desires
- these to be achieved as quickly as possible, and without significant risk of early or late complications.

The sometimes rather bewildering range of methods available for the treatment of any fracture is due to differences in the interpretation of these factors and their particular application in the case under consideration.

ELEMENTS OF FRACTURE TREATMENT

1. Decide whether the fracture requires reduction

Reduction is obviously not needed if the fracture is virtually undisplaced. Accurate reduction is however essential in fractures involving joint surfaces, or where there is severe angulation or rotation. Correction of displacement in diaphyseal fractures is often of less importance, especially in the case of children where the powers of remodelling are good.

2. If reduction is required, decide how this should be carried out

In the majority of fractures and dislocations the deformity may be corrected by closed methods. The techniques employed have evolved over many years and the arts of the bone setter have always enjoyed a certain (although largely undeserved) mystique. Where dislocations are concerned, the methods which have proved consistently effective are quite distinct for each major joint.

In the case of fractures, the initial (and sometimes the only) element required is the application of traction. This disimpacts the fragments and serves to align the proximal and distal parts of the limb. Traction may have to be assisted by manipulation of the fragments; in many cases this is simply the correction of any residual angulation by pressing the distal fragment in the correct direction while a hand is held under the fracture to provide a fulcrum.

Closed reduction of a fracture may fail due to a number of causes, including soft tissues becoming trapped between

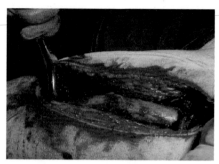

Fig. 1 **Fracture of the femoral shaft being openly reduced, using bone clamps, prior to intramedullary nailing.**

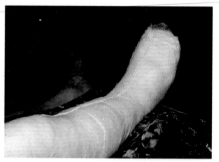

Fig. 2 **Fracture of the mid tibial shaft treated with plaster.** The cast has been split down to the wool padding and the limb will be elevated. Note the inclusion of the joints above and below the fracture.

the bone ends. If this happens, then it may become necessary to expose the fracture surgically and reduce the fracture under vision (Fig. 1). Open reduction may also be required in a number of other cases where great accuracy in the reduction is essential: this applies particularly to fractures involving joints

3. Decide how to hold the fracture

Whether a fracture has required reduction or not, thought must be given on how loss of alignment may be prevented while it is uniting, so that the line of treatment most appropriate to the fracture is adopted.

(a) No support required. In some cases the risks of secondary displacement are minimal and, apart from the relief of pain and swelling, no definitive support for the fracture is needed; many avulsion, terminal phalangeal and hairline fractures come within this category, as do some minor vertebral compression fractures.

(b) Non-rigid supports. Where a fracture is inherently stable (e.g. in many impacted fractures) the only protection that may be required is from the stresses of excessive movement or weight bearing. This may be achieved by the use of slings, local bandaging or strapping: e.g. many fractures in the region of the neck of the humerus may be successfully treated with a broad arm sling and body bandage to limit movements at the shoulder, while in the lower limb crutches may give adequate protection.

(c) Traction. Unopposed muscle spasm may cause redisplacement of a fracture, a problem most frequently encountered in fractures of the femoral

shaft. There it is common to maintain traction until union is well advanced (continuous traction), with the limb supported in a Thomas splint. (This device consists of two side irons attached to a ring; the latter is padded and fits into the groin. Slings of canvas or other material run between the side irons and support the limb.)

(d) Casts. The position of most fractures may be satisfactorily held with a suitable cast. Plaster of Paris bandages are most versatile and widely used; others employing synthetic resins and other materials, while more expensive, have in some circumstances advantages in terms of durability, water resistance and lightness. Prior to the application of the cast the skin and bony prominences must be protected by the use of appropriate materials (e.g. stockingette and wool padding). Usually the joints above and below the level of the fracture are included, although exceptions are often made when the fracture lies close to a joint. The joints supported must be placed in a position which contributes to the stability of the fracture yet does not interfere with recovery of movements. Allowance must be made for post-injury swelling of the limb. Measures include the initial use of a half cast bandaged to the limb, generous padding, splitting of the plaster to allow expansion (Fig. 2) and elevation of the limb. Frequent plaster and circulatory checks are imperative.

(e) External fixators. These are of particular value in supporting open fractures of the tibia (Fig. 3), but they are also used in treating other long bone fractures (including the metacarpals and phalanges) and certain fractures of the pelvis. At least two pins are inserted the local bone contours (Fig. 4). The holes through which the fixing screws are inserted may be designed to provide a degree of compression of the bone surfaces; this may increase the degree of rigidity of the fixation and encourage union. In dealing with fractures close to the bone ends, the support of the plate may be extended into the epiphysis by a large screw in an integral housing (*nail-plates*, *screw-plates*) or by an extension of the plate itself (*blade plates*). *Intramedullary nails* may be used to treat long bone fractures — particularly of the femur, tibia and humerus — and give excellent control of displacement and angulation. Prevention of rotation may be dependent on friction between the bone fragments or between the nail and the walls of the medullary cavity; this may be improved by reaming the medullary cavity and inserting a close-fitting nail. Transverse screws, passed through both bone and nail, give better control of rotation (*interlocking nails*).

(g) Primary joint replacement. In some cases, where the damage to articular surfaces is beyond repair, a primary joint replacement may be carried out. This line of treatment may also be used in carefully selected cases of femoral neck fracture where the risks of non-union or avascular necrosis is considered to be particularly high.

4. Decide how and when to mobilise
To reduce the risks of joint stiffness, unsupported joints should be mobilised from the start, and others at the earliest possible opportunity. Where an external support (such as a plaster cast) has been used, this may not be possible until the fracture has united. (This is usually judged to have occurred when there is no tenderness or movement at the fracture site, and radiographs have confirmed the union.) In other cases it may be possible to proceed to mobilise before union is complete, so long as some support of the fracture is maintained (e.g. by freeing one of the joints enclosed in a cast, by using a removable support or by using a hinged cast-brace). Where rigid internal fixation has been employed, it may be possible to commence mobilisation at a very early stage. It is customary to continue with physiotherapy until either a good functional result has been achieved or a static position has been reached. Significant loss of movement, with its work and leisure implications, may have to be accepted, although in a number of situations surgery may lead to improvement (e.g. quadricepsplasty for loss of

knee movements following fractures of the femoral shaft or removal of a bony obstruction due to myositis ossificans).

TREATMENT OF OPEN FRACTURES

First measures include taking a bacteriology swab from the wound, covering it with sterile dressings to reduce the risks of secondary infection, commencing a short course of appropriate antibiotics and applying temporary splintage.

Definitive treatment is dictated by the degree of tissue damage, skin loss and contamination. All necrotic tissue is excised and the wound thoroughly irrigated. The fracture is reduced and fixed appropriately; an external fixator is often suitable. In most cases it is best to pack the wound open and inspect it on the second or third day, carrying out a further debridement if necessary. The aim is to obtain bone and skin cover as soon as possible, and certainly in under 2 weeks; plastic surgical procedures may be required to achieve this (Fig. 5).

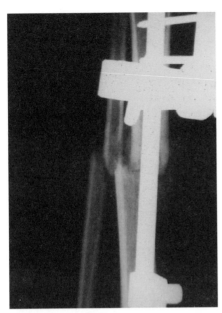

Fig. 3 **Uniting fracture of the tibia treated with an external fixator.** The upper tibial pins and the connectors can be seen in the film.

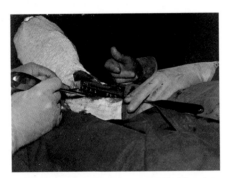

Fig. 4 **Well-reduced tibial fracture held with a plate and 6 screws.** There should be a minimum of two screws on either side of the fracture.

through the skin into sound bone on either side of the fracture; the fracture is reduced and the pins held in rigid alignment with specially designed clamping devices (fixators).

(f) Internal fixation. The majority of internal fixation devices are made of stainless steel, although a number of other materials (e.g. chrome cobalt alloys, carbon fibre and biodegradables) are employed. There is an almost infinite range of devices. *Cortical screws* are designed to grip cortical bone; the bone in which they are engaged is first threaded with a tap, or self threading screws may be used. They are often used to fix plates to bone or to hold together major bone fragments. *Cancellous screws* have coarse threads designed to grip spongy bone; they are used in the metaphyseal or epiphyseal areas. *Plates* come in a great number of shapes, sizes and degrees of rigidity so that any situation may be dealt with; metal plates can also be bent to fit

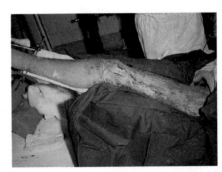

Fig. 5 **De-gloving injury of thigh with a fracture of the femur.** Skeletal traction in a Thomas splint was preferred to primary intramedullary nailing or the use of a fixator because of the extent of the skin damage and the contamination. At this wound inspection, the extensive split skin grafts are seen to have taken.

Treatment of fractures
- The definitive treatment of a fracture may have to be deferred until more serious injuries have been dealt with.
- Where treatment is going to be delayed, the fracture should be supported and any open wounds covered.
- The three pillars of fracture treatment are:
  i) reduction of the fracture (if required)
  ii) support of the fracture, and the prevention of displacement (until the fracture unites)
  iii) mobilisation of the related joints and of the patient as early as possible.

SCOLIOSIS

When viewed from the side the normal spine is seen to consist of a series of inter-linked curves: in the cervical and lumbar regions the convexity of each curve lies anteriorly (lordosis), whilst in the thoracic and sacral regions the convexities lie posteriorly (kyphosis). When viewed from the front or back (i.e. in the coronal plane), the spine should be straight. In the erect position the centre of gravity lies a little in front of the second sacral vertebra, and in the face of any spinal deformity, compensatory mechanisms come into play to maintain the normal orientation of the head. Scoliosis is defined as a curvature of the spine in the lateral or coronal plane. It may be *non-structural* or *structural*.

NON-STRUCTURAL SCOLIOSIS

In this form of scoliosis the vertebrae have a normal appearance and the curvature of the spine may be purely *postural* in origin (this being seen most commonly in adolescent girls); it may be *compensatory*, resulting from shortening of a limb or deformity of the pelvis; or it may be *sciatic*, due to protective muscle spasm (e.g. in a prolapsed intervertebral disc). In postural scoliosis the curve may be seen to disappear when the patient bends forwards; if there is shortening of a leg, the spine straightens when the patient is seated; and in sciatic scoliosis the curve disappears when the underlying condition resolves.

STRUCTURAL SCOLIOSIS

One or more vertebrae are altered in shape, and the deformity cannot be corrected by alteration of the posture. Spinal movements in the area of the deformed vertebrae are affected, leading to a fixed (non-mobile) or *primary* curve. *Secondary*, mobile curves develop above and below any primary curve in order to maintain the alignment of the head and pelvis (Fig. 1). In the primary curves there is usually an additional element of vertebral rotation, and with growth the curvature often gets worse. Where the deformity becomes severe, respiratory and cardiac function can be seriously affected, leading to chronic invalidity and a reduction in life expectancy. There may be anaesthetic problems if surgery is being contemplated.

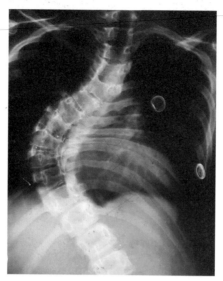

Fig. 1 **Idiopathic scoliosis with a primary thoracic curve of nearly 90 degrees and secondary curves above and below.**

There are three main types:

- **Idiopathic**. (a) infantile: onset from birth to 3 years; (b) juvenile: from 3 years to puberty; (c) adolescent: occurs at or shortly after puberty.
- **Congenital**. Associated with a vertebral anomaly.
- **Neuromuscular**. Associated with specific medical conditions, e.g. cerebral palsy, muscular dystrophy or poliomyelitis.

At the time of initial assessment full length radiographs of the spine are taken so that the severity of the primary curvature(s) can be made, using one or more geometric constructions of which the Cobb method is most widely used (Fig. 2). In infants the rib–vertebral angle is measured. Any bony anomalies are noted. These investigations may allow a firm diagnosis to be made; they may also indicate a prognosis and suggest a plan of further observation and treatment. It should be remembered that a patient with scoliosis requires follow up until skeletal maturity; thereafter progression is unlikely (although this may occur as a result of disc degeneration and vertebral subluxation). In adult life those who have suffered from scoliosis are prone to suffer from mechanical back pain.

IDIOPATHIC SCOLIOSIS

This type is by far the most common type of structural scoliosis. Its cause is thought to be multifactorial, with genetic,

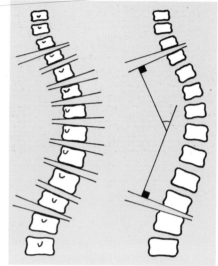

Fig. 2 **Measuring scoliosis (Cobb method).** The vertebrae at the extremes of the curve are identified (by noting where the disc space wedging changes); the angle between perpendiculars erected from them defines the scoliosis.

metabolic and growth disorders all playing a part. There is a 2–3 fold increase in the incidence in first-degree relatives, who should be screened. As a general rule, the higher the level of the primary curve and the earlier the age of onset the worse the prognosis. Screening of all schoolchildren has been instituted in most areas of the UK, and any with suspected anomalies are sent for specialist assessment.

Adolescent type

This is the most common variety of idiopathic scoliosis, and has a female to male ratio of at least 3:1. The likelihood of having a progressive curve is greater in females. Sometimes the deformity may not be obvious as there may be only a minor asymmetry of the torso. Rotational deformity in the thoracic region alters the shape of the rib cage, producing a so-called rib hump which is most obvious when the patient bends forward (Fig. 3). Note that scoliosis at its onset is normally painfree, and that the most common cause of a *painful* scoliosis is an osteoid osteoma of a vertebral pedicle.

Treatment is dependent on the severity at the time of presentation. In mild cases (curves of < 20 degrees) a watching policy (with serial radiographs) can be adopted until growth has finished. With larger curves, or where there is deterioration of a mild one, bracing becomes necessary. There are a variety of types, but the Boston brace is widely

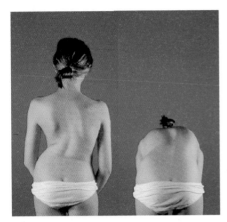

Fig. 3 **Lower thoracic scoliosis convex to the right with some asymmetry of the rib cage on forward flexion.**

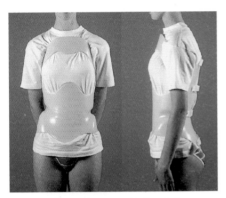

Fig. 4 **The Boston brace, used primarily for lumbar and lower thoracic scolioses.**

used and the most cosmetically acceptable (Fig. 4). Bracing is fulltime (with one hour off per day for hygiene purposes) and must be maintained until growth ceases. In severe curves (> 40 degrees), spinal fusion of the primary curve will be required, usually with some form of internal fixation to maintain the correction until fusion is established.

Infantile

Unlike the adolescent variety, infantile scoliosis is more common in males than females and, although it may be significant at presentation, 70–80% resolve without treatment. Unfortunately the remainder may progress to severe deformity. Favourable factors are left-sided curves occurring in the first year of life in males, with a rib–vertebral angle of less than 20 degrees. Treatment should be started as soon as possible; this is usually in the form of bracing if the child will tolerate it. Surgery should be postponed for as long as possible because of the inevitable stunting of growth which occurs after spinal fusion. There are some who use internal fixation alone; this allows some growth whilst still correcting the deformity. However, when growth ceases, a fusion remains likely.

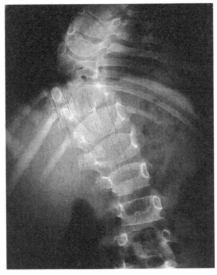

Fig. 5 **Congenital scoliosis.** Note the hemivertebra with its own rib.

Juvenile

The deformity is very similar to the adolescent variety and has a similar sex ratio. Many of the curves are progressive but some can resolve with bracing. Surgical instrumentation without fusion may be useful if the curve progresses despite bracing.

CONGENITAL SCOLIOSIS

This type of scoliosis is always caused by a malformation of the vertebral bodies. This can be in the form of a unilateral growth anomaly such as hemivertebra which causes a lateral wedging deformity of the spine (Fig. 5). It may result from a failure of segmentation where the vertebrae remain as a block instead of splitting into their component parts. As growth proceeds the deformities usually worsen and thus early recognition is helpful. The degree of the deformity (and how obvious it may be) is dependent on the site and magnitude of the spinal angulation. Associated bony anomalies such as rib fusions and elevated scapulae (Sprengel's shoulder) are common. In addition, there is a high incidence of genitourinary and cardiac anomalies

estimated to be around 15–20%. **Diastematomyelia** is a rarer cause of congenital scoliosis. It is characterised by a bony spur (or spurs) which protrudes into the spinal canal and which the spinal cord may actually straddle. Initially there may be no problem, but as the child grows the spinal cord can be tethered by the spur causing a progressive neurological deficit.

As in idiopathic scoliosis, the prime investigation is by plain radiographs of the spine to establish a diagnosis and serve as a guide to prognosis and treatment. This is best started early and follows the same lines as the other types of scoliosis. Although most curves tend to progress with growth, if a curve is mild, regular observation or bracing may be sufficient. Once the curve exceeds 40 degrees or is progressing rapidly, surgical treatment becomes necessary. This is usually in the form of localised surgical fusion to abolish growth in the affected area and may include some form of internal fixation.

NEUROMUSCULAR SCOLIOSIS

Severe spinal deformity may occur in association with neuromuscular disorders: these include poliomyelitis, cerebral atrophy, muscular dystrophies and spinal muscle atrophies. The deformity is due primarily to muscle imbalance or weakness. Each condition may have a characteristic age of onset and produce different patterns of curvature with varying rates of progression. All patients with neuromuscular disorders should be carefully monitored on the assumption that a deformity will occur. Once a curve has developed, evolution may be rapid. Bracing can be used, but the results are less predictable than in other forms of scoliosis; nevertheless this may slow the progress of the deformity in the younger child. Treatment by spinal fusion is frequently required, but because of the relative risks of surgery in this class of patient the procedure used must be carefully tailored to the particular case.

Scoliosis

- Scoliosis is a curvature of the spine in the coronal plane and is usually accompanied by a rotational deformity.
- The most common type is adolescent idiopathic scoliosis.
- Continuous assessment is required until skeletal maturity is reached.
- Bracing is used for minor curves.
- Surgical fusion is necessary where primary curves are severe or progressive.

MECHANICAL BACK PAIN

'Mechanical back pain' is a catch-all diagnosis for patients with low back pain where a specific pathological process has not been identified with any degree of certainty. It is the most common category of back pain and is often the most difficult to treat.

In the majority of cases the pain is short-lived and settles within 4–6 weeks. There are, however, patients who have persistent symptoms which are resistant to all forms of treatment. They require careful assessment to ensure that serious pathology is not missed; this can be time consuming.

The pain is usually confined to the back, but may have some radiation to the buttocks or posterior aspects of the thighs (if, however, it goes below the knee and is in the sciatic distribution, suspect a distal intervertebral disc prolapse).

The pain always has a characteristic pattern and is rarely present all the time. There is usually a history of morning stiffness, which settles or improves after a period of activity. It may then worsen as the day progresses, ranging from a mild ache to pain of a more severe degree; this is usually dependent on how active the patient has been and how much stress the back has been subjected to. A period of rest may be sufficient to alleviate the pain, at least for a short time. There is often some disturbance of the patient's sleep pattern. (If the pain is severe, and apparently present all the time, then you must be alert to the possibility of a malignant infiltration. However, symptoms of this nature may also have a psychogenic basis or be due to malingering. It is clear that great care must be taken in differentiating between these conditions, even although this may be difficult and time consuming.)

ACUTE MECHANICAL BACK PAIN

Frequently, there is no specific precipitant apart from what seems like a minor event, e.g. bending forward or twisting suddenly. In an appreciable number of cases a faulty technique has been used in a single or repeated lift. The patient is often distressed and dismayed that a minor occurrence can lead to so much disability. Fortunately, most cases resolve with conservative treatment and reassurance.

Alternatively, severe pain may follow the application of more significant flexion

forces to the spine. Such may occur in head-on pattern road traffic accidents, falls from a height or heavy blows across the shoulders (e.g. from falling weights). The onset of symptoms is, of course, acute and, assuming that no fracture has been caused, is usually presumed to be due to injuries to the spinal muscles or ligamentous structures. Symptoms in these circumstances can linger for many weeks or months and are often resistant to standard treatment regimes.

CHRONIC MECHANICAL BACK PAIN

In these cases the onset is slow and there is often a long history of intermittent backache over many years. The problem is usually an acquired one, most often resulting from a mechanically unstable spinal segment, degenerative disease (lumbar spondylosis) or a combination of both. This is the most common type of mechanical back pain and can be resistant to treatment. It may lead to prolonged or permanent employment difficulties and causes more lost work days per annum than any other pathology.

In these cases the source of the pain in the back is somewhat controversial and much research has been done to try and clarify the situation. Although the facet joints, major ligamentous structures and parts of the disc are probably the main culprits, this is by no means certain. Muscular spasm, which is a normal protective mechanism, can itself produce much discomfort, although this tends to resolve in step with the primary pathology.

Clinical features

In the acute stages the patient is distressed and there is much muscular spasm. Careful examination will reveal that the range of movement is restricted. Sometimes patients can flex reasonably well but cannot extend easily without an abnormal 'writhing' manoeuvre; this is suggestive of facet joint pathology. Neurological examination is usually normal, but although the straight leg raising (SLR) may be restricted, it usually only causes back pain (remember that SLR is only positive for root tension if it causes pain in the distribution of the stretched root).

Further investigation

This is often unnecessary and, as radiographs of the lumbar spine pick up significant pathology in less than 5% of cases, it is to some extent arguable if these should be taken routinely. Nonetheless, patients 'expect' an X-ray

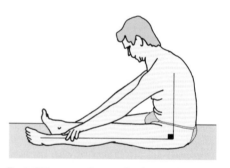

Fig. 1 **Sitting up on the examination couch with the knees extended is equivalent to straight leg raising in the order of 90 degrees.**

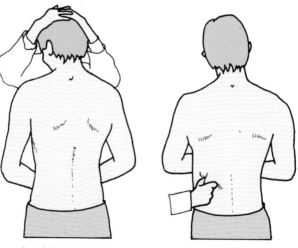

Fig. 2 **Axial compression of the spine by applying pressure to the head, and skin pinching in either flank should not produce pain from any of the deep seated structures.**

and this can be difficult to resist. On the other hand, a negative radiograph may help to reassure the patient and make an indirect contribution to recovery.

Treatment

This is mainly conservative, consisting of reassurance, analgesics and muscle relaxants, at least during the acute phase. Where pain is severe, bedrest can be useful, but should be curtailed as soon as possible (prolonged recumbency encourages muscle wasting which in itself may help to perpetuate the problem, as the spine thereby progressively loses its muscular support and protection). Physiotherapy can often produce dramatic early relief of pain and improved mobility. Lumbar corset supports should be reserved for the spine with degenerative changes and are not suitable for obese patients.

Pain clinics have become fashionable; in these, patients with chronic back problems are assessed by a multidisciplinary team which usually includes an orthopaedic surgeon, an anaesthetist, a physiotherapist and a clinical psychologist. In this way all avenues can be investigated and individual treatment regimes planned. Epidural steroid injections, or local anaesthesia to specific sites, can often identify the location of the pathology and allow better targeting of

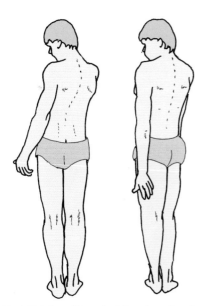

Fig. 3 **Rotation of the spine takes place almost entirely in the *thoracic spine*.** If this causes complaint of pain, note the position of the shoulders when it occurs. Repeat the examination after asking the patient to hold their arms and hands tightly at the sides, and see if and when they complain of pain again (rotation here is simulated as it now occurs in the joints of the lower limb rather than the spine, where it is blocked).

treatment. Steroid injections can also be therapeutic in so far as they may give the patient a 4–6 week period of complete relief.

PSYCHOGENIC BACKACHE

Psychological factors do not in themselves cause backache, but tend to lead to exaggerated symptoms, prolongation of disability and abnormal responses to examination.

History

In many cases this may reveal particular stresses at work or in the patient's personal life. If possible, the social history should be clarified. Undoubtedly, patients can become 'trapped' in their disability as family, friends and work colleagues make adjustments to their lives to accommodate the problem. The extreme case is the one of so-called 'illness behaviour' where a patient has become totally dependent on other members of the family who have, in turn, adapted their own lives and activities. This is usually an irretrievable situation.

The history may also be laced with responses which are inappropriate and full of exaggeration: for example, a patient may complain of excruciating pain, while at the same time being seen to sit or move comfortably around the examination room. In most cases of back pain due to an organic problem, the pain follows a pattern which can be clearly outlined. Where no clear pattern exists, the complaint is less likely to be organic in origin. Complaints of widespread back pain, or of weakness or altered sensation in the whole of a limb, should be considered suspect.

Examination

During the examination, inconsistent reactions may often be easily detected.

This is particularly true during the stretch tests, where a patient may appear to have limited straight leg raising, yet be able to sit upright on the couch with their legs fully extended (see 'flip' test, p. 27 and Fig. 1). A sensory deficit which involves the whole leg is usually abnormal; a so-called pain diagram (where the patient fills in a chart to illustrate the areas affected) may be useful. If the pattern is found to cover the whole leg, back and front, this is highly suggestive of non-organic pain. Axial compression of the spine by pressure on the head (Fig. 2), skin pinching in the flanks (where any stimulus is quite superficial) and simulated rotation (Fig. 3) should not increase pain in the lumbar spine, and may add additional weight to any impression that there is a non-organic component to the patient's complaints.

Investigations

These should if possible be kept to a minimum to avoid reinforcing any tendency to illness behaviour. Nevertheless, it should always be remembered that pathology may be present, and it is important to ensure that this is not missed. There are many patients who overreact in minor ways in their desire to convince whoever is examining them that they have a genuine problem: this is where much difficulty in assessment lies.

Treatment

Treatment of psychogenic backache is difficult and often unsuccessful. Patients often have an unrealistic view of their problem and expect a quick and complete answer, which may not be possible. If traditional methods of therapy make no headway, referral for psychological assessment may be helpful, although many patients will not accept that their psyche is contributing to what they believe to be a purely physical problem.

Mechanical back pain

- 'Mechanical back pain' is a catch-all term which is reserved for patients where no major, specific, pathology has been found.
- It is the most common category of back pain and is usually self-limiting within a period of 4–6 weeks.
- A mainstay of treatment is in the education of the patient (and the public) in proper handling and lifting techniques, particularly those related to employment.
- Psychogenic backache requires careful assessment to avoid missing genuine pathology.
- Sensory or motor involvement of the whole limb is rarely organic in origin.

INTERVERTEBRAL DISC PROLAPSE

Disc prolapses can occur at any level in the spine, although they are very rare in the thoracic region. In the lumbar spine they are most common between the ages of 25 and 45; in the cervical spine they tend to occur in the older patient, are usually more insidious in onset, and are frequently associated with local degenerative changes.

ANATOMY

The disc lies between the vertebral bodies and has two main components, the annulus fibrosus and the nucleus pulposus. The annulus fibrosus consists of concentric sheets of collagen fibres running between adjacent vertebrae. They are strong, help bind the vertebrae together, and limit vertebral movements. Within this dense ring lies the nucleus pulposus which has a gelatinous appearance and consists of 80% water, collagen and proteoglycan. The disc is avascular in the adult, and the cells within it are nourished by diffusion through the central part of the vertebral end plate.

PATHOLOGY

Degenerative changes occur as part of the ageing process or as a result of repeated minor trauma and distort the annulus. Within the nucleus, a gradual reduction in the water and proteoglycan content leads to the loss of structural integrity. Tears develop in the annulus which may allow the nucleus pulposus to herniate; this can be in any direction and of varying degree. In the so-called *contained prolapse* (Fig. 1), escape of the nucleus is restrained by intact fibres at the periphery of the annulus or by the posterior longitudinal ligament. In the *sequestered disc prolapse*, extrusion of the nucleus is usually more extensive, with it being cut off from its central source; it may extend into the spinal canal for several centimetres. The extrusion of the disc (nucleus) may be *central* (Fig. 2). In the lumbar region it may cause bilateral lower limb symptoms and signs; more seriously, it may interfere with bladder or bowel function. If the prolapse is *lateral*, it may press on one of the issuing spinal nerves and affect the corresponding dermatome and myotome.

In the longer term, disc herniation will result in a loss of disc height, seriously impairing its function in relation to vertebral movements. Greater stress is put on the facet joints, which tend to develop secondary osteoarthritic changes.

Degenerative changes start in the discs in the third decade, first with dessication of the nucleus, then with changes in the annulus; later these are followed by arthritic changes in the facet joints. While this natural process may remain entirely painfree, it may be disrupted in a number of ways:

- In the younger patient (15–45 yrs), an acute disc prolapse may occur.
- In the middle-aged (35–70 yrs), symptoms of local spinal instability from degenerative disc disease may present.
- In the elderly patient (over 70), more advanced degenerative changes may lead to nerve root impingement.

LUMBAR DISC PROLAPSE

This is by far the most common acute disc problem. Most patients relate the onset of their complaint to a specific incident, but on closer questioning they often have been aware of milder symptoms over the preceding weeks. While the presentation is variable, most patients complain primarily of back pain radiating down the leg to the foot, i.e. *sciatica*. Pain in the *sciatic distribution* below the knee must be distinguished from pain restricted to the buttock and posterior thigh which commonly occurs in cases of mechanical back pain. The pain is intermittent, but is made worse with activity; it is usually helped by recumbency. Sneezing, coughing and straining during defecation all worsen the symptoms. Paraesthesia is a common accompanying symptom and its distribution may give some idea of which nerve root is affected. Where the pain/paraesthesia is bilateral and involves the perineal area, a central disc prolapse should be suspected.

Motor weakness is a significant symptom in that it has to be quite profound before it is noticed by the patient. It may take the form of a drop foot. The site of any motor, sensory and reflex disturbance (myotomes and dermatomes) may allow the lesion to be localised. Be aware that a very stiff and often scoliotic spine in the young patient under 25 may indicate a significant disc prolapse or, less commonly, an osteoid osteoma of a pedicle.

Clinical features

The commonest levels to be affected are between L4/5 or L5/S1. Muscular spasm can be profound, leading to a scoliosis and restricted flexion. It is important to ensure that the history and any sensory or motor changes are in agreement. Pain produced by the straight leg raising or femoral nerve stretch tests (see page 27) should correspond with the distribution of a specific nerve root. If straight leg raising on the unaffected side produces contralateral pain, this is highly

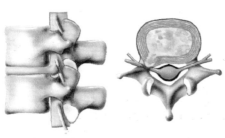

Fig. 1 Ruptured annulus leading to a lateral nucleus protrusion and nerve root pressure.

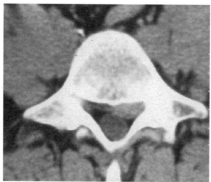

Fig. 2 **CT scan showing a mainly central disc prolapse, with some caudal compression.**

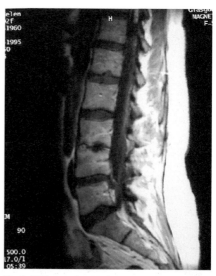

Fig. 3 **MRI scan showing inflammatory changes in the L3/4 disc (discitis) and an L4/5 prolapse.**

suggestive of disc prolapse. Any involvement of the bladder or anal control should be dealt with as an emergency, as without prompt treatment permanent paralysis may occur.

Investigation

Although in an acute lumbar disc prolapse plain radiographs of the lumbar spine are invariably negative, they may be advised (particularly in the older patient) for reassurance and to exclude other pathology. If surgery is contemplated, CT or MRI scanning are the investigations of choice.

Treatment

Prevention is the best remedy, and much effort has been put into the teaching of lifting and handling methods to minimise the likelihood of overstressing the lumbar spine. This is particularly true in hospitals where disc problems are common, particularly amongst nurses and porters. In established cases, the only reliable remedies are rest or surgery. Most acute episodes settle in 4–6 weeks and manipulative therapy – in whatever form – has not been shown to significantly alter the course. *Surgery* is indicated for the following:

- Acute central disc prolapse with bladder involvement – a surgical emergency.
- Progressive neurological weakness despite adequate bed rest.
- Unremitting pain with abnormal neurological signs despite bed rest for 2–3 weeks.
- Marked muscle weakness, e.g. foot drop in a young patient.
- Recurrent episodes of sciatica with only partial relief from conservative treatment.

Surgery involves removing the protruding disc material through a laminotomy or partial laminectomy. Uncommonly, this may be combined with a fusion of the affected segment. Less invasive methods include percutaneous nucleotomy, where a contained disc may be decompressed by laser or instrumentation passed into the disc under X-ray control. In chemonucleolysis, chymopapain (a meat tenderiser) is injected into the disc space to dissolve it; this procedure carries the risk of anaphylaxis and is being used less frequently.

CERVICAL DISC PROLAPSE

The cervical spine is unique in that it has additional uncovertebral joints (joints of Luschka). These are situated at the posterolateral edges of the vertebral bodies and are the main sites of hypertrophic and degenerative change, leading to nerve root impingement. Degenerative changes can produce symptoms similar to those seen in disc prolapse, but their presentation is more chronic. Disc prolapses are less common, and tend to present with severe acute symptoms; they are most frequent at the C5/6 and C6/7 levels. Although rare compared with lumbar disc prolapse, the pathology is similar, and disc herniation and annular degeneration may lead to local instability.

Clinical features

Symptoms can be variable, but usually neck pain is prominent. Pain referred across the shoulders is extremely common and often leads to some confusion as to the site of the primary pathology. Nerve root compression causes pain which radiates down the arm in a dermatomal pattern: when severe there is associated motor weakness (Fig. 4). Remember cervical disc disease can mimic cardiac disease with chest and arm pain. In severe cases of disc prolapse the patient may present with a cervical myelopathy (where the cord itself is compressed). Then the neurological signs may be variable, but usually affect both the upper and lower limbs. Any spasticity, clonus, hyperreflexia or a positive Babinski response should alert the examiner to this possibility.

Investigations

Plain radiographs with oblique views can clearly show degenerative disease but CAT and MRI scans define disc prolapse and root compression with greater accuracy.

Treatment

Conservative treatment is usually tried first using analgesia, rest with a stiff cervical collar and physiotherapy. Cervical traction may be helpful in relieving radicular pain. As the pain settles, progressive mobilisation and strengthening exercises can be implemented. Surgical intervention is reserved for the resistant case or those with worsening neurological signs. An anterior approach is performed, allowing disc excision and, if thought necessary, fusion of the affected segments to maintain stability and avoid recurrent symptoms.

THORACIC DISC DISEASE

This is rare, accounting for less than 0.5% of all cases. It tends to occur in the 5th decade at the T10–T12 level, with a chronic presentation. Symptoms are usually referred to the lower limbs or the abdomen. Occasionally there may be profound weakness and cord compression. Investigation is usually by CAT or MRI scan. Unless the symptoms are mild, surgical decompression is usually advised.

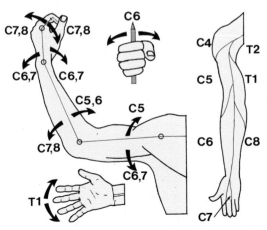

Fig. 4 **Myotomes and dermatomes in the upper limb: C5, 6 control elbow flexion and the biceps jerk, while C7, 8 control extension and the triceps jerk.** Flexion and extension of the wrist and fingers involve two roots only; pronation and supination, and intrinsic finger movement only one. C5 controls shoulder abduction and C6, 7 adduction.

Intervertebral disc prolapse

- A clear history and careful examination can usually define the affected level in a case of disc disease.
- Most cases will settle with conservative treatment.
- MRI and CT scanning are the investigations of choice.
- Progressive neurological change is an indication for urgent surgical intervention, especially where bladder or bowel function are impaired.

SPINAL STENOSIS, LATERAL ROOT STENOSIS, SPONDYLOLISTHESIS

SPINAL STENOSIS

Narrowing of the spinal canal can cause pain and neurological symptoms, often with few clinical signs.

Aetiology and pathology

Congenital forms of the condition are rare. It occurs most commonly in young patients suffering from achondroplasia. *Acquired* types are seen in association with spinal osteoarthritis or fracture, or complicating spondylolisthesis, Paget's disease or previous spinal surgery (especially fusions).

When the spinal canal is narrowed, activity (especially walking) may lead to pain and impaired nerve conduction within the spinal canal. This may be due to venous engorgement and a failure of the arterial supply to cope with increased local demand or to the mechanical effects of spinal rotation in walking.

Symptoms

The main complaints are of pain, paraesthesia and, at times, weakness in the lower limbs; these become evident after a variable walking distance. Typically, on stopping to rest at the onset of pain, the symptoms persist unless the patient flexes his spine by leaning forwards or sitting down; unlike mechanical back pain, it is unusual to have symptoms while sitting or lying. There may be very dramatic leg weakness and even foot drop, which resolve rapidly with rest.

It is important to differentiate the symptoms of spinal stenosis from those of peripheral vascular disease, where exercise-induced pain settles rapidly with rest and is localised to the affected muscle groups in the legs; it is usually cramp-like and not associated with any neurological symptoms. It is possible, however, for the two conditions to coexist, which can lead to difficulty in attributing symptoms.

Diagnosis

Little may be found on clinical examination, although there may be depression of the reflexes. Root tension signs are absent. It is important to examine the peripheral pulses to exclude vascular disease as its treatment may take priority over stenotic symptoms. In confirming the diagnosis, radiculography has been supplanted by the CT scan, with or without radio-opaque dye enhancement, or by the MRI scan. The latter is more

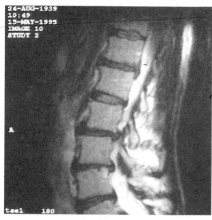

Fig. 1 **MRI scan showing spinal stenosis at two levels (L2/3 & L3/4) secondary to retrolisthesis** (posterior displacement of a vertebra relative to the one below, usually due to facet joint arthritis).

sensitive and, because it does not use X-rays, can be used to visualise the entire spinal column if necessary (Fig. 1).

Treatment

Where the symptoms are marked in a fit patient, surgical decompression, even in the elderly, can significantly increase walking distance and improve quality of life. If surgery is unsuitable, some advice about the aetiology of the problem and the methods of relieving the symptoms (e.g. by stooping or sitting) often suffices.

LATERAL ROOT STENOSIS

The root canal is the narrow channel through which the nerve roots leave the spinal canal. A disc protrusion, degenerative changes in the facet joints or segmental instability can compromise the canal and put pressure on a nerve root. The pain from root entrapment has a segmental distribution similar to that found in prolapsed intervertebral discs with nerve root involvement, but the character is different. It is often more severe and unremitting both by day and night. Unlike the sciatica of disc disease, it tends not to be relieved by lying down (and indeed the patient may pace the floor all night) and is not aggravated by coughing or sneezing (the patient may, however, have a history of previous disc protrusion, although with atypical symptoms). The clinical signs may be sparse and root tension signs (e.g. restricted straight leg raising) are only present in 30% of cases. Lumbar spine radiographs usually show some degenerative changes, but the diagnosis may only be confirmed by CT or MRI scan.

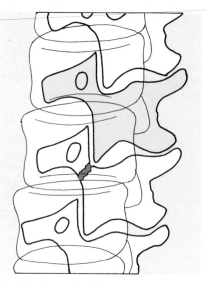

Fig. 2 **The Scotty dog.** The nose is formed by a transverse process, the ear by a superior articular process, the front legs by an inferior articular process and the neck by the pars interarticularis.

Treatment

Severe symptoms require technically exacting surgical decompression. Although pain relief is usually gratifying, some patients may have persisting symptoms secondary to irreversible root damage.

SPONDYLOLYSIS AND SPONDYLOLISTHESIS

Spondylolysis is a congenital or acquired deficiency of the pars interarticularis of the neural arch of a vertebra. It is most common in the lumbar region (involving L4 and L5 especially) and is estimated to be present and asymptomatic in 5–6% of the normal population. *Spondylolisthesis* is present when a vertebral body slips forward on the one below. This may be quantified by noting the percentage loss of bony apposition: in Type 1 spondylolisthesis the slip lies in the 0–25% range; in Type 2, 26–50%; in Type 3, 51–75%; and in Type 4, more than 75%. The main types of the condition are isthmic, degenerative and dysplastic.

ISTHMIC SPONDYLOLISTHESIS

Here the problem is due to fracture (or less commonly elongation) of the pars interarticularis in an otherwise normal spine as a result of trauma or repeated stress. It is common in fast bowlers and other active individuals. In the early stages, spondylolysis precedes any forward slip and standard X-rays may not reveal a defect. Oblique views, however,

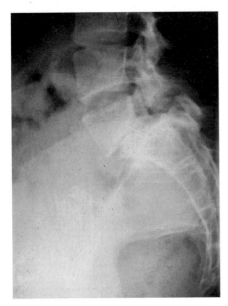

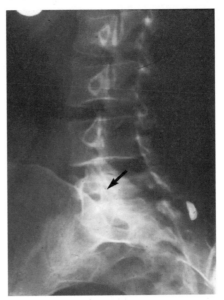

Fig. 3 **Long standing type 1 spondylolisthesis of L5 on S1.** The lateral projection shows a defect in the pars interarticularis, and in the oblique the Scotty dog has been decapitated.

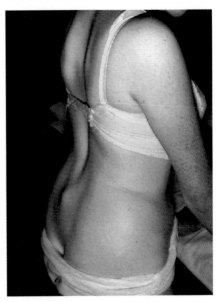

Fig. 4 **Acute spondylolisthesis of L5 on S1.** The spinous process of L5 has been rendered prominent by the forward slip of the body of L5 (which has taken the rest of the spine above with it).

will show elongation of the neck or the presence of a collar on the so-called Scotty dog revealed by this projection (Fig. 2). An isotopic bone scan may reveal a 'hot spot' and be used to confirm the diagnosis and, if repeated, assess if healing is taking place.

Treatment

Acute spondylolysis may be treated by screw fixation or, less predictably, by immobilisation in a plaster jacket. In established cases (Fig. 3) of more than a year, surgical fusion can produce good results. Where displacement has occurred, this often stabilises. Fusion in the male patient should be reserved for those who have not responded to conservative treatment. As further slippage may occur in pregnancy, there are greater indications for fusion in women.

DEGENERATIVE SPONDYLOLISTHESIS

Degenerative changes in the facet joints and the discs, especially in women, may lead to a degree of spondylolisthesis without loss of the integrity of the neural arches. The spinal and root canals may become narrowed, necessitating further investigation by CT or MRI scan. Symptomatic treatment is all that is generally required, but where there are neurological symptoms, decompression with or without a local fusion may be indicated.

DYSPLASTIC SPONDYLOLISTHESIS

A number of congenital defects at the lumbosacral junction may encourage slippage at this level. These include

dysplasia of the neural arch with associated spina bifida, posterior wedging of the fifth lumbar vertebra and poorly formed facet joints. All these factors tend to encourage forward slip. The displacement, while progressive, is slow, although an acute acceleration (Fig. 4) may occur during the phase of rapid growth that occurs at puberty (the so-called 'lumbar crisis'). Usually (but not invariably) this produces much muscular spasm and local pain, associated with an abnormal waddling gait and an increase in lumbar lordosis. Assessment of the severity and progress of the slippage may be made by serial lateral radiographs.

TREATMENT

This is dependent on the presentation and the severity of the slippage. *In the young patient with minimal deformity*, a watching policy can be adopted, taking serial radiographs so that any progression can be identified early. *Where pain is prominent*, an intertransverse fusion generally gives good results. *In cases of lumbar crisis* where there is an acute slip, it is often difficult to reduce severe displacements and a period of preliminary traction is sometimes necessary to improve the position prior to fusion. Internal fixation may be required to maintain position. *In older female patients who have significant symptoms and who may be contemplating pregnancy* it may be advisable to stabilise a displacement early, as increased slippage is a well recognised complication of pregnancy. It should be remembered that there is a 30% incidence of defects in first degree relatives and they should be reviewed.

Spinal stenosis, lateral root stenosis, spondylolisthesis

- Spinal stenosis is usually secondary to degenerative changes in the spine.
- It can produce severe symptoms with few associated physical signs.
- Surgery can produce excellent results.
- Consider lateral root stenosis where severe symptoms are unrelieved by forward flexion or rest, but BEWARE of the possibility of malignant infiltration of nerve roots.
- Spondylolisthesis and spondylolysis are common in the general population and the incidence increases with age; both may be asymptomatic.
- Oblique views of the lumbar spine, in addition to the standard projections, should be taken when either is suspected.
- If there are neurological symptoms, MRI and CT scans are the investigations of choice.
- Most patients can be treated symptomatically, but surgical decompression with fusion is sometimes necessary.

NECK PAIN AND TORTICOLLIS

POSTURAL NECK PAIN

This is the most common of all neck problems and has a typical history and symptomatology. A good history and careful examination should allow a diagnosis to be made without further investigation or imaging. Patients are usually under 40 and may have sedentary jobs (e.g. as typists or computer operators) or ones which require them to drive. Their leisure pursuits are usually of an inactive nature (e.g. reading, or watching television for prolonged periods). There is complaint of pain in the neck and across the shoulders which in many cases can be relieved quickly by change of posture or activity. It does not tend to be troublesome at night. Although there may be a history of a precipitating injury, the condition usually becomes persistent as a result of environmental influences at work or in the home. A striking confirmatory feature (the significance of which often evades the patients) is that in many cases they are asymptomatic over a weekend or during holiday periods. Clinically, there is usually a full range of motion in the neck. The head and neck may be protracted (Fig. 1). If radiographs are taken, these are usually found to be quite normal.

Treatment

The majority of patients will settle with analgesics and physiotherapy. It is important to educate the patients in postural control at work and in the home. This can simply mean raising or lowering their desk or chair to allow a direct view of a computer screen and to avoid prolonged postural indiscretions. In addition, breaking up the day into sedentary periods coupled with more active periods can be helpful in avoiding recurrences.

CERVICAL SPONDYLOSIS

Degenerative change is common to us all as we age, but not all of us become symptomatic. Many patients develop symptoms gradually, whilst in others they may be precipitated by a traumatic incident such as a fall or road traffic accident. The patient is usually over 40, and whilst the pain is primarily in the neck, it may radiate widely to the occiput, scapular region and across the shoulders into the arms. Complaints of paraesthesia and weakness are frequent, but objective neurological signs are less common. Neck movements are usually significantly restricted, even in the absence of spasm, and this helps differentiate it from other causes. Where objective neurological signs are present, these are likely to be related to arthritic encroachment on the neural foramina, sometimes in combination with disc collapse.

In some cases large forward projecting osteophytes may press on the pharynx and lead to difficulty in swallowing. This problem is also common in Forestier's disease, a condition in which there is excessive osteophyte formation and abnormal ligamentous calcification (especially of the anterior longitudinal ligament, Fig. 2).

Investigations

Plain radiographs show changes which may be at multiple levels, the most common being C5/6 (Fig. 3) and C6/7. There may be disc space narrowing and lipping of vertebral bodies. In patients with neurological signs, oblique views allow an assessment of the neural foramina (Fig. 4). CAT and MRI scanning may be helpful in excluding cervical disc prolapse.

Treatment

Conservative treatment is along the same lines as postural neck pain, although symptoms are likely to be more resistant to treatment. A soft or firm cervical collar may be utilised during acute episodes, but should not be worn routinely. Surgical treatment (local decompression and/or intervertebral fusion) is rarely necessary.

RHEUMATOID ARTHRITIS IN THE CERVICAL SPINE

While this is common, many patients are relatively asymptomatic even with severe disease. This is an important fact in the case of any patient who is undergoing surgery, as there is a potential risk if cervical instability is present. This can occur at any level, but is most common at the

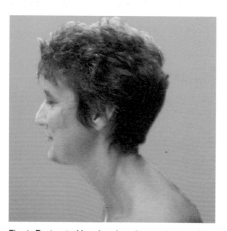

Fig. 1 **Protracted head and neck associated with postural neck pain.**

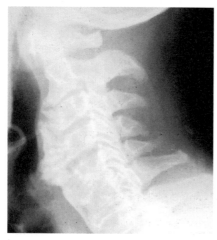

Fig. 2 **Forestier's disease, with osteophyte formation, ligament calcification and dysphagia.**

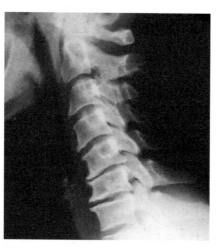

Fig. 3 **Cervical spondylosis, with narrowing of the C5/6 disc and both anterior and posterior lipping.**

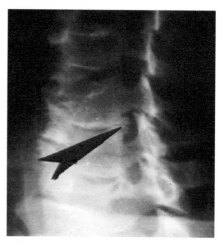

Fig. 4 **Uncovertebral joint lipping (joint of Luschka) leading to narrowing of a neural foramen and root signs.**

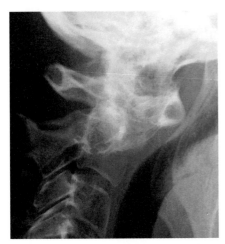
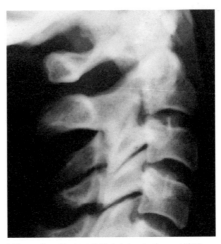
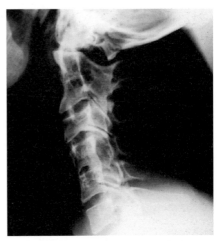

Fig. 5 **Flexion view of the cervical spine showing instability at the atlantoaxial joint due to rheumatoid arthritis.** Note the gap between the odontoid process and the anterior arch of the atlas. A normal cervical spine is shown on the right for comparison.

Fig. 6 **Klippel–Feil syndrome with vertebral fusions at two separate levels.**

atlantoaxial joint. Lateral radiographs in flexion and extension should be taken preoperatively (Fig. 5) whether the patient has symptoms or not, as the neck is particularly vulnerable during intubation and anaesthesia. In a few patients arthritic encroachment on the spinal canal produces upper motor neurone signs in the upper and lower limbs. These can be difficult to detect in a patient with severe disease; a careful examination and urgent investigation with CAT or MRI scanning are necessary, followed by surgical decompression and fusion at the appropriate level.

CONGENITAL MUSCULAR TORTICOLLIS

This is a common problem occurring within the first 2 months of life. It is secondary to a contracture of the sternomastoid muscle, which pulls the head to the affected side and turns the chin to the opposite. The cause is obscure, but may be related to birth trauma or ischaemia from abnormal intrauterine posture (this however does not explain why it is more frequent on the right side, or its 20% association with acetabular dysplasia). In the newborn a small lump may sometimes be palpable in the muscle ('sternomastoid tumour'), but this may resolve before the deformity becomes obvious. If untreated, torticollis may produce some asymmetry and distortion of the face.

Treatment

If a sternomastoid tumour has been felt, it should be assumed that a deformity will occur and daily stretching exercises should be undertaken to minimise any contracture. Occasionally the muscle and deep fascia need to be released, but this should be postponed until the child is 2 or 3.

ACQUIRED TORTICOLLIS

This is less common, but is usually secondary to an atlantoaxial rotatory subluxation where the facet joints are malaligned. It occurs in the older child and can be secondary to trauma or ligamentous laxity following an upper respiratory infection. The head is tilted as previously described and resists attempts at correction. Careful imaging with plain radiographs and CAT scanning may be necessary to demonstrate the problem.

Treatment

Analgesics and collar immobilisation may be all that is required. In the more resistant cases, traction may be needed to obtain a reduction. Surgical correction is rarely necessary.

KLIPPEL–FEIL SYNDROME

Classically the syndrome has three factors: a low posterior hairline, shortening of the neck and restriction of neck motion. The restricted motion is secondary to a congenital fusion in the cervical spine; this can vary in extent from a short segment (Fig. 6) to the whole neck, from occiput to the cervicothoracic junction. If there is a mobile segment, this may develop compensatory hypermobility, with increased susceptibility to neurological compromise, especially in

the upper levels. Clinically, the neck is often very short, with webbing of skin between the neck and the shoulders.

Treatment

In the presence of instability, treatment should be preventive. A supportive collar may be helpful, along with the avoidance of potentially traumatic pursuits. Fusion of the segment is not indicated (unless there is severe neurological involvement), as this may worsen the stresses on the neck. Other anomalies may require appropriate treatment.

SPRENGEL'S SHOULDER (CONGENITAL ELEVATION OF THE SHOULDER)

This is frequently associated with the Klippel–Feil syndrome or other congenital anomalies such as scoliosis, syringomyelia and local bony malformations. The scapula fails to develop properly and is usually small and abnormally elevated. It may be medially rotated and connected to the cervical spine by fibrous bands, cartilage or bone (omovertebral bone). The deformity is clinically obvious, and the surrounding muscles may be hypoplastic. The condition may be hereditary.

Surgical intervention can produce an improvement in appearance and function.

Neck pain and torticollis

- Poor posture is the most common cause of neck pain in the younger patient.
- Cervical spondylosis is more common in the older patient and may be difficult to resolve.
- Preoperative flexion and extension X-rays of the neck are essential (to assess cervical stability) in patients suffering from rheumatoid arthritis.

BRACHIAL PLEXUS INJURIES

Brachial plexus injuries can occur at any age. They may occur during childbirth, when the prognosis is often excellent. In older age groups they may result from penetrating wounds in the neck or traction injuries (e.g. from forces applied to the arm, shoulder or neck, often from falls and road traffic accidents); there the prognosis is often poor, and the permanent disability often profound.

ANATOMY

A sound knowledge of anatomy is necessary to allow assessment of the severity of any injury. Dorsal and ventral nerve roots leave the spinal cord and come together in the spinal canals to form spinal nerves (Fig. 1). There is an intrathecal ganglion on each posterior nerve root. Spinal nerves divide into anterior and posterior rami, and the brachial plexus is formed by the anterior rami of C5–T1 (the so-called roots of the plexus, not to be confused with the roots of the spinal nerves). There are variable contributions from C4 and T2. The trunks of the plexus are formed in the posterior triangle of the neck, with the main sympathetic outflow (postganglionic fibres) to the upper limb being carried in the lower trunk. Each trunk splits into an anterior and posterior division behind the clavicle. The upper and middle anterior divisions form the lateral cord, the anterior division of the lower trunk forms the medial cord, and the three posterior divisions form the posterior cord. These then pass into the axilla and form the individual nerves of the upper limb.

In assessing a brachial plexus injury it is important to examine the rhomboid and serratus anterior muscles as they are supplied by the dorsal scapular (C5) and long thoracic nerves (C5, 6, 7). These nerves arise from the roots of the plexus close to the spine. If they are not functioning it indicates that the damage to the plexus is proximally situated, and is probably due to avulsion of spinal nerve roots from the cord. This is the so-called preganglionic lesion which is not amenable to any form of repair procedure and carries a hopeless prognosis. If the rhomboids and serratus anterior are spared, then the lesion may be assumed to be postganglionic where the potential for recovery or repair is better.

Birth injuries occur during difficult labours and are usually the result of traction often from the overzealous use of forceps.

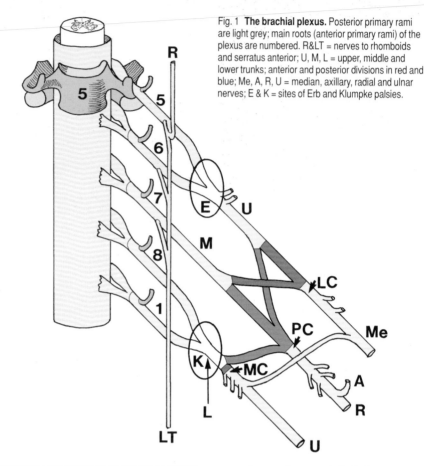

Fig. 1 **The brachial plexus.** Posterior primary rami are light grey; main roots (anterior primary rami) of the plexus are numbered. R&LT = nerves to rhomboids and serratus anterior; U, M, L = upper, middle and lower trunks; anterior and posterior divisions in red and blue; Me, A, R, U = median, axillary, radial and ulnar nerves; E & K = sites of Erb and Klumpke palsies.

ERB'S PALSY (UPPER PLEXUS INJURY)

This is the most common plexus injury, involving the 5th and 6th cervical nerve roots, and very occasionally the 7th. The traction that causes it occurs during childbirth, when the (delivered) head is manipulated whilst a shoulder is still caught. This leads to a relative depression of the shoulder, with lateral flexion of the neck away from the affected side. The palsy may not be obvious initially, although the parents may notice that the limb is not being moved as much as the other unaffected limb. The abductors of the shoulder are paralysed (deltoid and supraspinatus) as are the external rotators (infraspinatus and teres minor) and the elbow flexors (biceps, brachialis and brachioradialis). This produces the typical deformity of an internally rotated adducted upper limb and an extended elbow (waiter's tip deformity).

Treatment

Most injuries will resolve spontaneously. All that is usually necessary is a 3–6 month period of observation during which time the parents are instructed to perform daily stretching exercises (to avoid permanent deformity occurring secondary to the muscle imbalance). In a few instances, resolution does not occur and investigation with possible surgical exploration may become necessary.

KLUMPKE'S PALSY (LOWER PLEXUS INJURY)

This relatively uncommon injury usually occurs when a trailing arm is caught during a breech delivery; the C8 and T1 roots are damaged by inappropriate traction. This produces paralysis of the flexors of the wrist and fingers, and all of the intrinsic muscles of the hand. There may be a sensory deficit along the ulnar side of the forearm and hand, although it may not be possible to confirm this until the child is older. In addition, there may be a Horner's syndrome (anhydrosis, ptosis and pupillary constriction on the affected side) due to sympathetic nerve damage.

Treatment

Unfortunately this carries a poor prognosis with little likelihood of improvement. Tendon transfers may improve the imbalance of the forearm muscles, but the intrinsic muscle function cannot be restored.

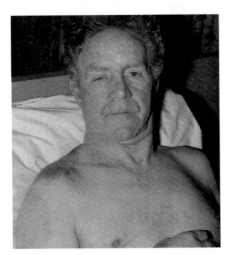

Fig. 2 **Lower plexus lesion resulting from a blow on the shoulder.** Note tell-tale bruising and the ptosis (Horner's).

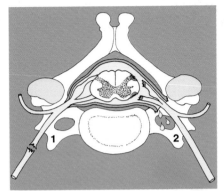

Fig. 3 **Patterns of injury. (1)** Postganglionic divisions or ruptures may respond to suture or grafting. **(2)** Preganglionic lesions are untreatable. Rupture of the dural sleeves may be detected by myelography. **(3)** Lesions in continuity (not shown) generally make a partial or full spontaneous recovery.

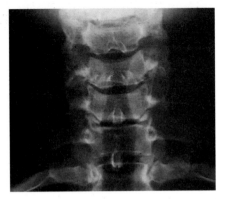

Fig. 4 **Bilateral cervical ribs.**

ADULT BRACHIAL PLEXUS INJURIES

These are most commonly caused by injuries such as falls from a height or from a motorcycle when the shoulder is either forcibly depressed (damaging the upper roots) or forcibly elevated (damaging the lower roots). Injury may also result from stab or gunshot wounds; there the extent and pattern of injury is variable.

Clinical features

There are often associated injuries, including head injuries, which may make initial assessment difficult. It is important to look for supraclavicular bruising, which can be extensive and may occasionally be associated with a vascular disruption. The specific areas of weakness and the sensory deficit (myotomes and dermatomes) indicate which nerve roots are involved, although the sensory pattern may take some hours to become clearly defined. To differentiate a preganglionic from a postganglionic injury it is necessary to test the rhomboids (which retract the shoulders) and serratus anterior (which stabilises the scapula and stops it 'winging'). If both are paralysed it is likely that it is a preganglionic injury, normally associated with a very poor prognosis. In addition, these more significant plexus involvements may be associated with severe and unremitting pain. A Horner's syndrome may be evident if the T1 root is involved (Fig. 2).

Investigations

In the acute case, a cervical spine X-ray is essential as there can be fractures of the transverse processes at the affected levels, a poor prognostic sign. At a later stage, neurophysiological tests, myelography (to show any avulsed dural spinal nerve sleeves) or MRI scanning can help to define which roots are involved and the anatomical site.

Treatment

The most important aspect of treatment is clear counselling of the patient so that it is understood that regardless of treatment, restoration of normal limb function is very unlikely. Without this, false expectations may be raised, leading to later difficulties. In addition, the prognosis cannot be defined until 18–24 months have passed.

In lesions caused by a direct injury such as a stab wound, suture may be possible. In the case of cord avulsions (Fig. 3), direct suture is not possible. More distal nerve injuries can sometimes be repaired and any gaps bridged by nerve grafting; the clinical results are however very variable. Repair of the upper roots may produce some restoration of shoulder and elbow motion, but the lower roots in the adult never improve and consequently are often used as the source of nerve grafts. Exploration is usually delayed for at least 6 weeks to allow any local swelling to settle and to complete the investigations. Some surgeons advocate earlier surgery on the basis of improved results, but controversy remains.

THORACIC OUTLET SYNDROME

This results from compression of the lower trunk of the plexus, with or without vascular compromise. It is usually caused by a cervical rib (Fig. 4)(or one of its fibrous attachments) or the drooping shoulders which are so common in the general population. Other less common causes include an abnormal scalenus anterior or medius, local trauma, or anomalies of the first rib or clavicle. A rare but important cause is an apical tumour of the lung which invades the T1 root, leading to typical wasting of all the small muscles of the hand. The clinical findings may be subtle, or there may be marked weakness or sensory symptoms. Unremitting pain should alert the examiner to the possibility of malignant infiltration.

Investigations

These should include routine chest and cervical spine X-rays, neurophysiological tests, and arteriography if vascular involvement is suspected. It should be noted that cervical ribs are common in the general population and are only occasionally symptomatic.

Treatment

In the uncomplicated case physiotherapy can solve the postural problems and commonly alleviate symptoms. In a few cases surgery to decompress the plexus by excision of a cervical rib or freeing of a tight scalene band may be indicated.

Brachial plexus injuries

- Brachial plexus injuries are uncommon, but may lead to permanent disability.
- Birth injuries can be difficult to assess, and careful observation is necessary.
- It is important to differentiate preganglionic from postganglionic lesions, as the former carry a much poorer prognosis.
- The thoracic outlet syndrome can be caused by a variety of conditions, but the most common is a cervical rib.

SPINAL INJURIES: CERVICAL SPINE (I)

As a rule, the prime concern in any spinal injury is not the damage to the vertebrae or their ligaments but the involvement of the related neurological structures (the spinal cord, the cauda equina, the nerve roots and the spinal nerves). In those cases where the cord has been transected, so that the neurological damage is complete and irreversible, the manner in which the spinal injury is dealt with is not critical; but in other cases the concern is that with improper handling, neurological damage may be caused or, if already present, made worse.

With this in mind it is important to make an early assessment of presence or otherwise of mechanical or neurological instability. To do this it is necessary to have a knowledge of the structural elements of the spine and how they may have been affected. For the sake of simplicity, the spine may be considered as having three supporting columns, one or more of which may become compromised. The *anterior column* is formed by the anterior longitudinal ligament and

the anterior halves of the vertebral bodies and the related annular ligament; the *middle column* from the posterior longitudinal ligament and the remainder of the vertebral bodies and the annular ligaments; and the *posterior column* from the neural arches, pedicles, spinous processes and their related ligaments (the so-called posterior ligament complex) (Fig. 1). Note that the axis of movement between any two vertebrae is generally situated at the centre of the corresponding intervertebral disc.

CLASSIFICATION

Most spinal injuries can be classified into one of four categories, in which the three columns may be variously involved.

1. Compression fractures

Simple compression fractures, the most common of spinal fractures, involve the anterior column (anterior wedge fractures) and are generally stable. The anterior part of the vertebra (or less commonly the lateral aspect in so-called lateral wedge fractures) is crushed; the posterior part (or the other side in lateral wedge fractures) maintains its normal height (Fig. 2). These fractures are impacted and involve cancellous bone, so that they heal rapidly, usually within 6 weeks.

If however the causal violence is more severe, the middle column may also become affected, so that the fracture

in effect becomes a burst fracture (see below). This may be suspected if the degree of wedging exceeds 15 degrees or if there is a decrease in the height of the posterior part of the vertebra compared with the ones above and below.

2. Burst fractures

These fractures involve both the anterior and middle columns of the spine. They may occur as the result of axial loading of the spine, e.g. from a heavy object falling on the head or from a fall from a height landing on the heels. Burst fractures may result from flexion injuries, which, if less severe, would have resulted in involvement of the anterior column alone. In this pattern of fracture the vertebral body is split vertically; fragments of bone may be extruded backwards into the spinal canal, putting its contents at risk (Fig. 3).

3. Seat belt or tension fractures

In the event of a head-on pattern road traffic accident, the vehicle decelerates and the body flexes forwards (due to its inertia). The lap strap of a seat belt (especially if there is no diagonal strap) may move the axis of flexion of the spine forwards. This leads to posterior tension forces which may cause the posterior and the middle columns to fail. The resulting lesions may involve either bone, ligaments (Fig. 4), or a combination of both.

4. Fracture dislocations

In these potentially most serious injuries, all three columns fail, so that at one level at least there is loss of all the constraints which link the vertebrae together: this may then result in dislocation or subluxation. Various patterns are seen (Fig. 5).

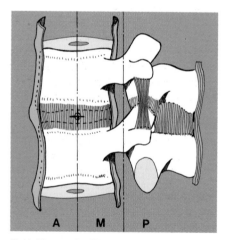

Fig. 1 **The anterior (A), middle (M) and posterior (P) spinal columns.**

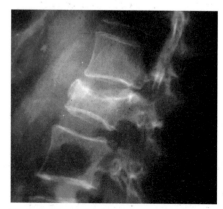

Fig. 2 **Stable anterior wedge fracture of a lumbar vertebra, with some bulging of the disc into the centre of the vertebral body.**

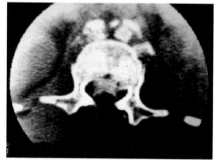

Fig. 3 **CAT scan showing extrusion of bony fragments into the spinal canal.**

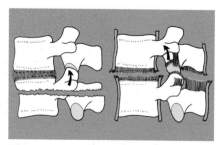

Fig. 4 **Some patterns of tension fracture.**

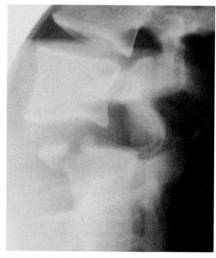

Fig. 5 **Unstable fracture dislocation of L5 on S1.**

CERVICAL SPINE INJURIES

Suspect a cervical spine injury if, following a traumatic incident (e.g. after a road traffic accident), there is:

- complaint of neck, shoulder or occipital pain
- torticollis or restricted neck movements
- if the patient has had a head injury.

In the acute case, protect the neck from any movement which might jeopardise the integrity of the neural structures (or further damage them) by applying a cervical collar — regular or improvised — or in the stretcher case by placing sandbags at either side of the head. Do not attempt to check the range of movement in the neck at this stage, and personally supervise the taking of radiographs.

The standard X-ray projections comprise a lateral and two APs (one of the upper two cervical vertebrae, taken through the open mouth, and the other of the lower cervical vertebrae). If these fail to show any abnormality, and if symptoms are marked, further investigation is indicated: this might include additional laterals taken in flexion and extension, oblique projections and CT scans. If no abnormality is detected, then the patient may be treated expectantly in a collar, with review after a short interval. On the other hand, one of the following may be found.

A stable anterior wedge fracture

This pattern of injury is relatively uncommon in the cervical spine and results from pure flexion of the spine. Before being confidently diagnosed, damage to the posterior ligament complex must be excluded by careful study of both the plain radiographs (for avulsion fractures of the spinous processes), and of the flexion and extension laterals for evidence of anterior subluxation of the

spine on flexion. If uncomplicated, a 6 week period of rest in a cervical collar is indicated.

Flexion–rotation injuries of the cervical spine in the most severe cases involve all three columns. There may be associated fractures so that they can be considered truly as fracture dislocations, but in many cases, although there may be gross instability, the damage is confined to the soft tissue structures.

Unilateral facet joint dislocation

Here one facet joint dislocates while the corresponding articular surfaces on the other side preserve their normal alignment, e.g. the facet joints on the right at C5–6 may dislocate, while those on the left at the same level appear undisturbed. Due to the shape of the articular facets, they become locked in the dislocated position. The extent of the damage to the posterior ligament complex is rather variable, and a number of cases are stable after reduction. This does not always hold, and instability must always be presumed if there is an associated fracture.

Clinically, the head is tilted and rotated away from the side of the dislocated facet and there is intense protective muscle spasm. The diagnosis can usually be confirmed by oblique X-ray projections of the cervical spine which throw the facet joints into profile. If there is any neurological abnormality then further investigation (preferably by MRI scan) should be undertaken. In most cases any neurological involvement is confined to the spinal nerve related to the dislocated facet, but sometimes the cord is compromised by an intervertebral disc prolapse. If so, this should be dealt with by an anterior decompression prior to reduction of the dislocation.

Treatment

Prior to reduction of the dislocation the head should be supported with a collar or sandbags. Manipulative reduction is

generally a straightforward procedure, but of course requires great care and a clear understanding of the technique. It is performed with X-ray control under general anaesthesia; during the latter, precautions must be taken during induction to avoid excessive movement of the neck (especially extension during intubation). Others prefer to apply skull traction under local anaesthesia and after sedation supervise the slow unlocking of the facets under X-ray control.

After reduction the neck may be supported in a collar for some weeks unless there is evidence of instability, when a formal local fusion will be required.

Bilateral facet joint dislocation

This is a serious injury with disruption of all three columns. There may be a fracture of a spinous process, but more often no fracture is present. The spine may be slightly or moderately subluxed at one level or there may be a frank dislocation with the facet joints on both sides becoming locked (Fig. 6). Neurological involvement may be absent or profound (at the higher levels, death occurs from paralysis of the diaphragm and the other respiratory muscles; lower down, there may be quadriplegia).

If there is paralysis which is not permanent and complete, then it is imperative that any further loss is avoided. A common method of definitive treatment is firstly to apply skull traction and then, under X-ray control, to unlock the facets by adjusting the direction and amount of the traction. The spine may then be gently extended and the weights reduced to complete the reduction. In the recently injured patient this process may be completed within a half hour period. Where treatment is delayed, the process may take several days; rarely, open reduction may be necessary. Later, as a cold procedure, a local fusion may be required to stabilise the spine. Any neurological problem will create its own demands.

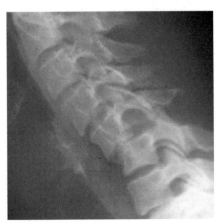

Fig. 6 **Bilateral facet joint subluxation (C5 on C6).**

Spinal injuries: cervical spine (I)

- In any spinal injury the possibility of neurological involvement is the main concern.
- Always make an assessment of spinal stability.
- The most common fracture of the spine is a stable anterior wedge fracture.
- Burst fractures may endanger the cord through the extrusion of bony fragments into the spinal canal.
- The cord is at most serious risk in unstable fracture dislocations.
- In any suspected neck injury apply a collar or other support until the diagnosis has been clarified.
- Unilateral facet joint dislocations may be stable, but bilateral facet joint subluxations never are.

SPINAL INJURIES: CERVICAL SPINE (II)

BURST FRACTURES OF THE CERVICAL SPINE

Fractures of this pattern result from axial loading of the spine. This may come about in a number of ways: objects falling on the head, the head striking the roof of a car in road traffic accident and the head striking the bottom of a swimming pool in diving accidents.

When the forces are moderate, a vertical split may occur in a single vertebral body, and the injury is uncomplicated. In more severe cases, the fracture may be comminuted, with backward extrusion of bony fragments causing compression of the cord (Fig. 1). The exact nature of the bony injury should be clarified by CT scans; any neurological involvement requires a full neurological examination.

Neurological assessment

Backwardly extruded vertebral body fragments press first on the anterior part of the cord, affecting the motor supply to the upper limbs before that to the lower limbs. Next to be involved are the spinothalamic tracts carrying pain and temperature and, lastly, the posterior columns carrying proprioception and light touch. A full neurological examination should be carried out on admission, taking these facts into account. The examination should include testing of: (i) all the main muscle groups in the upper and lower limbs; (ii) the skin and tendon reflexes and (iii) the sensory response to pin prick, light touch and proprioception. (The latter is most important as these pathways are the last to be involved.) If paralysis is present, and it is found to be bilateral, symmetrical, complete and corresponding to the level of the spinal injury, testing should be repeated at 6, 12 and 24 hours after the injury. If no recovery from a complete paralysis is found on the last examination, the prognosis is almost certainly hopeless.

If there is an incomplete cord lesion and the neurological state is deteriorating, any bone fragments which have been demonstrated to be pressing on the cord should be removed by an anterior decompression. Some also advise decompression procedures even if the neurological picture is static. If on exploration the spine is found to be very unstable, internal fixation using locking spinal plates may be undertaken. Otherwise burst fractures of the cervical spine (involving as they do the cancellous bone of the vertebral bodies) may be treated with 6 weeks' cervical traction.

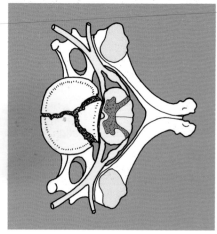

Fig. 1 **Burst fracture with involvement of the cord.**

EXTENSION INJURIES OF THE CERVICAL SPINE

Unlike flexion, which stops when the chin contacts the chest, limitation of excessive extension movement is completely dependent on the ligamentous structures of the neck; when these fail, the resultant injuries may be severe. They commonly result from backward directed blows on the forehead, e.g. when someone falls going down stairs and strikes the front of the head against the ground. Occasionally in front impact car accidents they result if the head hits the roof, fascia or bonnet and the trunk flexes beneath the fixed head. More commonly, they occur in rear impact car accidents when the head stays in position, due to its inertia, as the trunk moves forwards beneath it (see also later). In the first two instances bruising of the forehead is a characteristic finding.

In severe cases extension of the spine leads to rupture of the anterior longitudinal ligament (or sometimes avulsion of the anterior osteophytes to which it is attached). The effects of extension tend to be greater if the stresses are concentrated at one level, often the case where there is a mobile segment remaining in a spine which has otherwise become stiff from osteoarthritis (Fig. 2), rheumatoid arthritis, ankylosing spondylitis or congenital neck ankyloses. The cord may be stretched and spinal vessels injured, leading to spreading thrombosis (within the cord). In the older patient, osteophytes projecting backwards from the vertebral bodies may cause further neurological damage. The intervertebral discs may be affected and there may be nerve root involvement.

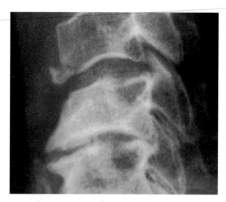

Fig. 2 **Extension injury in an arthritic cervical spine, with an avulsion fracture of an osteophyte.**

Diagnosis

A typical history of injury and complaint of pain and stiffness in the neck should alert you to the possibility of this pattern of injury. In more severe cases there may be weakness of the upper limbs or more serious neurological involvement which sometimes deteriorates (occasionally with a fatal outcome) as thrombosis spreads within the cord. There may be forehead bruising, anterior osteophyte avulsion or evidence of anterior longitudinal ligament rupture on MRI scanning.

The local injury is generally stable and may be treated with a cervical collar; there may be some permanent neurological disturbance which resists treatment.

WHIPLASH INJURIES

This emotive term was first used to describe injuries of the neck which had resulted from the cervical spine being violently extended and then flexed, such as may occur to a car occupant whose vehicle is struck from behind and which then collides with another ahead. Over the years it has been repeatedly devalued so that some now use it to refer to virtually any soft tissue injury of the neck. The point has been made that there is a considerable difference between flexion and extension injuries of the cervical spine and many would prefer the term 'whiplash' to remain restricted to soft tissue extension injuries.

Extension injuries of the neck from rear impact car accidents are common and have a characteristic symptomatology. The onset of symptoms may be delayed for some hours but there is invariably complaint of pain in the neck, often with radiation of pain into the shoulders, arms, head and, curiously, the mid-thoracic and low back region. There may be paraesthesia in the arms.

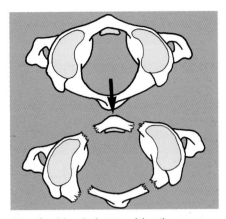

Fig. 3 **Quadripartite fracture of the atlas.**

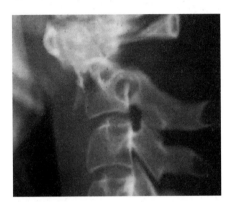

Fig. 4 **Odontoid process fractured and flexed forwards.**

Infrequently there may be motor and sensory signs in the upper limbs which follow a segmental pattern. Rarely there may be vertigo, tinnitus, ocular problems and facial pain (Barré-Lieou syndrome) which may be due to sympathetic nerve involvement at the C3-4 level.

After other pathology has been excluded by X-ray examination of the cervical spine, these injuries are usually treated initially with a cervical collar and analgesics. If there is no improvement after 6 weeks other measures, such as cervical traction, may be tried. In about a third of cases symptoms are intrusive, prolonged and often permanent. Adverse prognostic factors include pre-existing cervical spondylosis, prolonged cervical muscle spasm with reversal of the normal cervical curvature in the radiographs and abnormal neurological findings. Only rarely, and after further investigation, is surgery advised (e.g. by anterior discectomy and local fusion in the case of the Barré-Lieou syndrome).

OTHER CERVICAL SPINE INJURIES
Fractures of the atlas

The most common injury which affects the atlas is a quadripartite bursting fracture (Fig. 3); this often results when a heavy object falls on the head, causing pressure on the atlas through force transmitted through the occipital condyles.

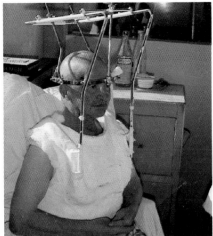

Fig. 5 **Halo-pelvic traction.**

These fractures cannot be reduced and the neck must be supported until union occurs. In most cases this involves a 6 week period of in-patient treatment with skull traction.

Fractures of the odontoid process

The odontoid process may be fractured as the result of sudden flexion or extension of the neck and become displaced accordingly: flexion (Fig. 4) and extension pattern fractures. If not immediately fatal, the cord is at risk and these injuries must be treated with great respect.

The fracture usually shows in the plain lateral and the through-the-mouth views of C1 and C2. Congenital abnormalities such as hypoplasia or persistent non-fusion of its ossification centre may cause some difficulty in diagnosis, but CAT scans may be helpful if there is any doubt.

The usual treatment is to apply skull calipers and reduce the fracture by adjustment of the direction and the amount of traction (taking care to avoid distraction). The neck must be supported for a minimum of 8 weeks. This may be achieved by continuing traction,

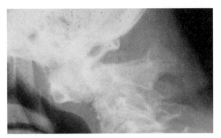

Fig. 6 **Rupture of a transverse ligament in rheumatoid arthritis.**

by the use of a Minerva plaster or by halopelvic traction (Fig. 5). Stability is then checked with flexion and extension radiographs. If instability or non-union (which is least common in fractures through the odontoid base) persists, then a C1–C2 spinal fusion may be required.

Rupture of the transverse ligament

The transverse ligament holds the odontoid process in check and separates it from the cord. It may be torn as a result of sudden flexion, or become attenuated as a result of the local effects of rheumatoid arthritis. C1 tends to slip forwards on C2 and a gap appears between the anterior arch of the atlas and the odontoid process, visible in the lateral radiographs (Fig. 6). If there is doubt, well supervised flexion and extension views and CT scans may be obtained.

Acute traumatic cases may be treated by a period of skull traction followed by halopelvic traction for 8 weeks. If at the end of this period any persisting instability is demonstrated by flexion and extension views of the spine, then fusion (C1–C2) is indicated. Cases due to rheumatoid arthritis are best dealt with by fusion, and it is sometimes necessary, because of local bone fragility, to extend the fusion to the occiput. In children, especially where the problem has arisen from an infective process in the neck, a 6 week period of traction alone may suffice in restoring stability.

Spinal injuries: cervical spine (II)

- In burst fractures of the cervical spine the earliest neurological sign is muscle weakness in the upper limbs.
- The last structures to be involved (the posterior columns) lead to disturbance of proprioception and light touch.
- Bruising of the forehead may be the only external sign of a serious extension injury of the cervical spine.
- If you are going to use the term 'whiplash injury', reserve it for extension injuries of the cervical spine.
- Fractures of the atlas usually result from blows on the vertex, and are often quadripartite.
- Flexion and extension radiographs may be necessary to identify ruptures of the transverse ligament and fractures of the odontoid process; the taking of these films must always be most carefully supervised.

LUMBAR AND THORACIC SPINE FRACTURES / PARAPLEGIA

Fractures of the thoracic or lumbar spine most commonly result from flexion injuries, with or without an element of rotation. They may result from a fall from a height on to the feet (which causes the spine to jack-knife), from a blow across the shoulders from a falling object or from severe flexion stresses sustained in road traffic accidents. The thoracolumbar junction (where the mobile lumbar spine meets the relatively fixed thoracic spine) is especially vulnerable. Where the strength of the spine is greatly reduced (e.g. by osteoporosis) a fracture may result from lifting something heavy. With even greater weakness of the spine (e.g. where there are metastatic deposits) the forces required to produce fracture may be trivial. There are many different patterns of injury (see p. 60) but the most common are anterior or lateral wedge fractures. In all cases the primary aim is to achieve the optimum neurological outcome; at the acute stage it is vital to ensure that the handling of the patient does not produce or aggravate any neurological damage.

DIAGNOSIS

The aims are to recognise the presence, site and nature of the fracture and whether the injury is stable or not. Where there is any neurological involvement it is vital to distinguish between complete, irrecoverable lesions and any others.

Fracture of the spine should be suspected if there is complaint of localised back pain after a traumatic incident. This is especially the case if there is local tenderness, deformity or boggy swelling on palpation of the interspinous spaces; and certainly if there are abnormal neurological symptoms and signs. Movement of the patient must be minimised and always rigorously supervised (e.g. by using scoop stretchers and avoiding flexing the spine).

Plain radiographs generally allow an adequate assessment of the injury, but a CT scan may provide valuable additional information, especially on any spinal canal encroachment (e.g. in the case of burst fractures).

STABLE WEDGE FRACTURES

The anterior column only is involved and the cancellous bone of the vertebral body is compressed at the front (anterior wedge fracture) or to one side (lateral wedge fracture). The cord is not at risk, but in lateral wedge fractures there may be nerve root compression; these injuries often do less well in terms of functional recovery and freedom from pain.

As these fractures involve cancellous bone they are usually soundly united within 6 weeks. Extension exercises should be performed to build up the supporting paraspinal muscles and a period of bed rest, certainly during the acute phase, is advised.

The forward tilting of the spine (which inevitably persists) is compensated for by extension of the spine below the level of the fracture; this may lead to mechanical low back pain for which a corset support is often helpful.

UNSTABLE WEDGE FRACTURES

Instability in a wedge fracture may be suspected if:

- the degree of wedging exceeds 15 degrees or the height of the anterior part of the vertebra is reduced by more than a third
- there is a reduction of height in the posterior part of the vertebral body, perhaps with backwards bulging or extrusion of bone into the vertebral canal (Fig. 1)
- if there is evidence of damage to the posterior column: this may be suspected on clinical grounds by palpation, while the radiographs may show fracture or separation of the spinous processes or avulsion fractures of the interspinous ligament attachments.

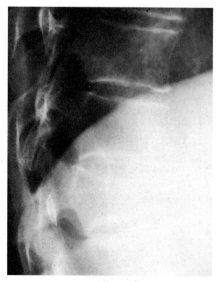

Fig. 1 **Unstable anterior wedge fracture with backward bulging.**

OTHER UNSTABLE FRACTURES

In a number of other spinal fractures there is loss of alignment in the spinal column: i.e. there is movement of one vertebra relative to its neighbour. This is indicative of the involvement of all three columns.

Common patterns (Fig. 2) include:

(i)   fractures involving the facet joints or pedicles
(ii) shearing fractures of the vertebral bodies
(iii) fractures through the neural arches
(iv) rotational fractures, where one or both facet joints are fractured or dislocated.

Treatment
With incomplete or no neurological involvement

The aim is to reduce any displacement and prevent its recurrence until stability is achieved. The latter generally occurs when any fracture present unites or if there is a spontaneous anterior fusion. If a reduction can be obtained by closed methods, treatment by conservative methods may be continued. In many cases careful nursing in a Stryker frame can preserve the necessary degree of spinal immobility during the period of healing. In the later stages a plaster jacket support may allow the patient to be mobilised.

Where the damage is mainly ligamentous, instability may persist and in those cases a local spinal fusion is often advised. Fusion is also usually carried out when persisting deformity necessitates open reduction, with or without internal fixation. Methods of internal fixation include various forms of plating, internal fixators and pedicle screw devices.

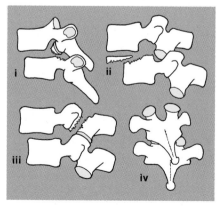

Fig. 2 **Unstable injuries of the spine.**

With complete neurological involvement

If the spine is grossly unstable, internal fixation may be advised to facilitate nursing and permit earlier mobilisation; it also helps minimise the final degree of spinal deformity and prevent pain from local nerve root involvement. If the instability is not severe, then the indications for internal fixation are less clearly defined.

NEUROLOGICAL LESIONS

Spinal concussion is generally a patchy, temporary loss of conduction within the cord and recovery is rapid; if there is a complete spinal lesion persisting for more than 12 hours after the injury then the cause is not spinal concussion.

The spinal cord ends at the level of the first lumbar vertebra (Fig. 3); if there is a complete neurological lesion below this, then it is the cauda equina that is involved. (Note that injuries to the cauda and to isolated nerve roots have at least in theory some potential for recovery.) Injuries at the thoracolumbar junction may cause involvement of either the cord, the nerve roots forming the cauda or both. Above the thoracolumbar junction, complete spinal lesions are due to transection of the cord.

Diagnosis

A thorough neurological examination is essential on discovery of a defect and it should be confirmed that this corresponds in terms of level and character with any bony injury. Sensation to pin prick, light touch and proprioception should be scrupulously tested in the entire affected area. Muscle activity and power should be assessed, along with the tendon, plantar, anal and glans-bulbar reflexes. Any response below the affected level shows that the lesion is incomplete and reinforces the need for vigilance in treatment. The examination should be repeated at regular intervals; if there is no response after 24 hours, the lesion is almost certainly complete and, if the cord is involved, it will be permanent.

TREATMENT OF PARAPLEGIA

The aim of treatment is to achieve maximal physical independence and mental readjustment to the disability. There is no doubt that these aims are best served in a specialised paraplegic unit to which the patient's admission should be arranged at the earliest opportunity. Besides attention to the fracture and to measures which will reduce the risks of complications, the patient will receive physical and mental stimulation from intensive and frequently competitive physiotherapy and occupational therapy. Pending transfer, however, attention must be paid to the skin and bladder.

Care of the skin

This is an important and complex matter; intractable bed sores which may ultimately prove fatal must be avoided at all costs. Basically, attention must be paid to how long the skin is subjected to pressure, how the loads applied to the skin may be spread and how the skin's cleanliness and freedom from infection can be encouraged.

In practice, particularly in the initial stages, the patient must be turned every 2 hours (e.g. by rotation in a Stryker frame) between the prone and supine positions. If the patient is being nursed in a bed he should be supported on pillows and cycled through supine, lateral, prone and lateral positions. There must be no delay in the setting up of this regime. The bony prominences (e.g. the malleoli, heels, knees, trochanters, sacrum) must be protected (e.g. by pillows and other forms of padding). Skin hygiene must be maintained by frequent washing with soap and water, thorough drying (with the judicious use of alcohol rubs and talc) and care must be taken in avoiding contact with starched or otherwise abrasive bed linen.

Care of the bladder

Complete spinal lesions isolate the bladder control centres (in the S2 & S3 levels in the cord) so that the ability to appreciate when the bladder is full and to initiate emptying are lost. If the problem is due to a cord transection above the sacral centres, in ideal circumstances and after about 4 weeks a so-called automatic bladder becomes established (Fig. 3). With this, there is a coordinated contraction of the bladder wall and relaxation of the sphincter (which can often be initiated by pressure over the bladder or other stimuli). This is mediated through the now independent but still preserved autonomic nerves and sacral centres. If the sacral centres or the cauda are damaged, an autonomous bladder with incomplete and irregular emptying results. The priorities in initial management are to reduce the risks of urinary tract infection and prevent overstretching of the bladder wall. Most commonly an indwelling catheter is inserted, with the usual aseptic precautions, until spontaneous emptying routines become established.

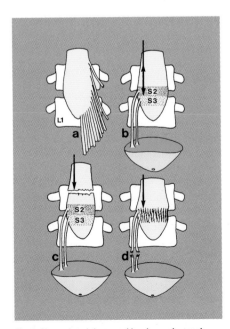

Fig. 3 **Normal and damaged lumbar spine and bladder control. (a)** The cord and cauda; **(b)** spinal centres and autonomic nerves for the bladder and sphincter; **(c)** automatic bladder; **(d)** autonomous bladder.

Lumbar and thoracic spine fractures / paraplegia

- Suspect instability in an anterior compression fracture if the wedging is severe, if the height of the posterior aspect of the vertebral body is reduced, or if there is an additional fracture.
- Unstable injuries must be stabilised, either by surgical or conservative methods.
- If paraplegia is complete, internal fixation may still be required to facilitate nursing, to reduce the risks of root pain, to allow earlier mobilisation, and to minimise the final deformity.
- Spinal concussion is seldom complete and is usually of short duration.
- Paraplegia cannot be judged to be complete without full neurological examinations (including testing proprioception) repeated over a 24 hour period.
- The most common problems in the management of paraplegia are related to the care of the skin and the bladder.

SHOULDER IMPINGEMENT SYNDROMES

There is no denying the complexity of the shoulder, which comprises a number of joints whose movements interlap in a normally smooth and well-coordinated manner. The main component is the glenohumeral joint, which has an excellent range of movement; this is achieved through a glenoid socket which is small in relation to the humeral head. The inherent instability of this arrangement is compensated for by the extent and strength of the musculotendinous shoulder cuff surrounding the joint. (This comprises the supraspinatus, infraspinatus, subscapularis and teres minor. Note that the supraspinatus passes through a canal whose roof is formed by the acromion, coracoacromial ligament and the coracoid.)

When the shoulder is abducted, movement comes to a stop when the greater tuberosity comes in contact with the upper margin of the glenoid; this can be delayed by external rotation of the shoulder which carries the tuberosity posteriorly. While deltoid plays the major part in abduction, the *initiation* of abduction requires the additional contraction of supraspinatus. Abduction beyond 90 degrees is dependent on movement between the scapula and the thoracic cage; this tilts the plane of the glenohumeral joint, giving another 80 degrees approximately. Towards full abduction there is often an increase in lumbar lordosis. The scapula is tethered by the clavicle through the acromioclavicular and sternoclavicular joints. Note that the translation from glenohumeral to scapulothoracic movements is not abrupt but gradual (often commencing at 60 degrees or less), and that this may be disturbed in the presence of shoulder pathology.

IMPINGEMENT SYNDROMES

Painful impingement may occur during glenohumeral joint movement if part of the rotator cuff is compressed between the humeral head and the acromion, the acromioclavicular joint and the coracoacromial ligament. The lesions vary from minor inflammatory changes in the cuff to partial or complete tears. The impingement can be acute or chronic, and involve one or more of three common sites:

Subacromial. This is by far the most most common site of impingement. It is

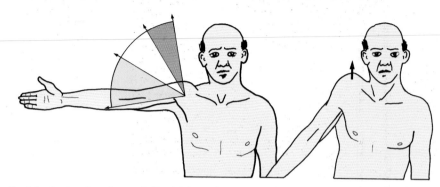

Fig. 1 **Impingement syndromes. Left:** painful arcs of movement seen in subacromial impingement (blue) and acromioclavicular joint arthritis (red). **Right:** 'hitch' at start of abduction.

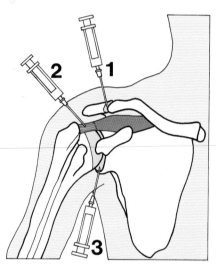

Fig. 2 **Sequence of diagnostic injections of local anaesthetic (at 5–10 minute intervals) into the AC joint (1), the shoulder cuff (2) and the glenohumeral joint (3).**

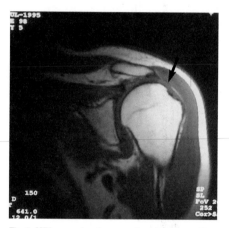

Fig. 3 **MRI scan showing massive shoulder cuff rupture.**

usually caused by an acromial osteophyte arising from AC joint arthritis, or from a hooked deformity of the acromion. There is typically a painful arc of movement between 70 and 120 degrees of abduction, with minimal or no pain on either side (Fig. 1).

Subacromioclavicular joint. This is also common, usually in association with degenerative change in the joint which is invariably prominent and distorted. Here the painful arc tends to be exacerbated during the last 30 degrees of abduction (Fig. 1). Degenerative change in the AC joint may produce similar symptoms without impingement, then joint pain can be clinically exacerbated by adducting the arm whilst it is extended.

Coracoacromial ligament. This may also be responsible for causing impinge-

ment symptoms. It cannot be separated from the other two and is likely to coexist with them.

Clinical features

In all three types the scapulothoracic rhythm will be disturbed. This is evident when the shoulder is abducted. The patient may 'hitch' up (elevate or shrug the shoulder, often with a grimace), before abduction proceeds (Fig. 1).

The *acute* type tends to result from overuse in the young sportsman involved in throwing or racquet sports. The range of movement is often normal, but with a painful arc in the mid-range. Nonspecific, localised tenderness may be present, and the radiographs are normal. The *chronic* type is found in the older patient and is normally secondary to a degenerative problem of the acromion, AC joint, coracoacromial ligament or the rotator cuff itself. There may be pain at rest, and usually during some part of the range of motion.

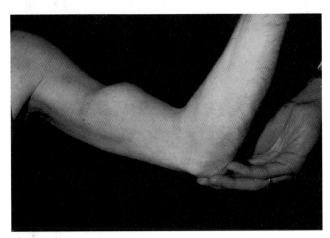

Fig. 4 **Rupture of the long head of biceps.**

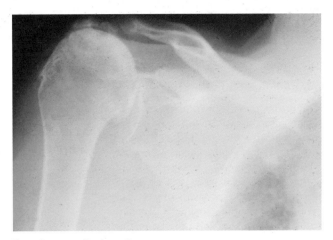

Fig. 5 **Rotator cuff arthropathy.**

Investigation

AP and axial (tangential) lateral radiographs will usually give sufficient information on the state of the glenohumeral and AC joints.

Treatment

In the young athlete, rest, if it can be enforced, is usually curative. In addition, modification of the particular sporting activity may be needed to reduce the provocation. In the chronic type, physiotherapy and analgesics can be helpful. Steroid injections may be required but should be limited to a maximum of three. Sequential lignocaine injections can be given into the AC joint, the subacromial space and, if necessary, the shoulder joint (Fig. 2). If one relieves the pain, steroid may be injected at the same site. For persistent symptoms surgical intervention may be required. The most common procedure is a decompression of the subacromial space; this can include an excision arthroplasty of the AC joint with removal of osteophytes, excision of the deep surface of the anterior part of the acromion, and excision of the coracoacromial ligament. Recovery can be prolonged and requires intensive physiotherapy.

ROTATOR CUFF RUPTURES

These usually result from chronic impingement and attrition. The onset may be insidious, but a traumatic incident may complete a tear causing a sudden increase in disability with reduced active movement. Occasionally a rupture occurs in a young athlete after a significant incident, e.g. a skier sustaining a forced adduction injury in a fall. Clinically, the diagnosis is based on finding a reduction of active motion with weakness of external rotation of the shoulder. *Passive motion is usually full, but patients cannot initiate abduction without trick movements.*

Investigation

Plain radiographs may show a decrease in the space between the head of the humerus and the acromion. Double contrast radiography, ultrasound and MRI scans may help confirm the diagnosis (Fig. 3).

Treatment

In essence, most acute tears require surgical repair to ensure an improvement in function. If there is an associated impingement problem (which is often the case in the older patient) this may also have to be dealt with. Graduated, supervised mobilisation exercises are necessary in all cases to ensure the integrity of the repair is maintained.

RUPTURE OF THE LONG HEAD OF BICEPS TENDON

Rupture at the proximal end is most common. The tendon (which arises from the supraglenoid tubercle), is completely invested in synovium while it traverses the glenohumeral joint on its way to the bicipital groove; it is therefore subject to inflammatory and degenerative changes and ultimately rupture. Clinically, the patient is usually aware of something 'snapping' in the arm combined with the appearance of a defect in the upper arm and a swelling proximal to the elbow (the retracted muscle belly, Fig. 4).

Treatment

This is symptomatic, as reattachment of the tendon proximally is unrewarding. If there is an associated rotator cuff rupture, this may require appropriate surgical repair.

ROTATOR CUFF TEAR ARTHROPATHY

Some patients have a complete rupture of the rotator cuff and the diagnosis is delayed or missed. In this situation there may be a degree of joint instability which results in degeneration of the articular cartilage covering the humeral head, often with local bony collapse. The radiographs show superior subluxation of the humeral head, erosion of the inferior surface of the acromion and adjacent humerus, and marked degeneration of the glenohumeral joint (Fig. 5).

Treatment

This is generally symptomatic, but in some severe cases joint replacement may be considered.

Shoulder impingement syndromes

- Impingement syndromes are common, but require careful assessment to define the site of pain.
- Sequential injections of local anaesthetic may be useful in defining the site of a shoulder impingement, and subsequent steroid injections may help to modify the symptoms.
- Rupture of the long head of biceps requires no treatment, but may be indicative of some rotator cuff degeneration.
- Chronic rotator cuff tears may lead to degenerative change in the glenohumeral joint.

CALCIFYING TENDINITIS AND ARTHRITIS OF THE SHOULDER

CALCIFYING TENDINITIS (CALCIFYING SUPRASPINATUS TENDINITIS)

This is a comparatively common problem which often presents with such severe pain that it is mistaken for a septic arthritis. It has a peak incidence in the 5th decade, with men said to be more commonly affected than women. The onset is often rapid and without warning. When the patient seeks help, he has often had sleepless nights and been unable to work; he may be afraid to move the arm or permit examination. Acute localised tenderness may be present. In view of the sudden onset it is important to exclude infection and metabolic diseases such as gout. It should be remembered that there may be coexisting pathologies, and a careful assessment is necessary. The striking radiographic anomaly is a calcific deposit in the rotator cuff (Fig. 1), usually near the insertion of the supraspinatus tendon. There is often little or no pain during the formative phase of the calcification but it is thought that acute symptoms occur during resolution and may be the result of the calcified material encroaching and irritating the subdeltoid bursa.

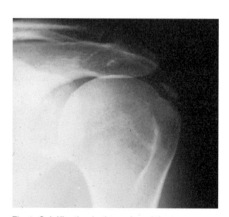

Fig. 1 **Calcification in the region of the supraspinatus tendon.**

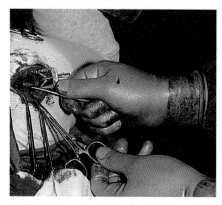

Fig. 2 **Curettage of calcifying tendinitis through a superior approach: note white material in the curette.**

Treatment

Although the natural history is towards resolution, this may take many painful months. Treatment for mild cases is symptomatic with anti-inflammatories and physiotherapy. Where more severe symptoms are present, an attempt should be made to aspirate the affected area (the material may be of milky or, more frequently, a cheesy consistency). A general anaesthetic may be required because of the severity of local tenderness. Whether the tap is productive or not, it should be followed by a long acting steroid injection. In the (rare) intractable case, curettage of the area may be necessary (Fig. 2).

FROZEN SHOULDER (ADHESIVE CAPSULITIS)

The terms 'frozen shoulder' and 'adhesive capsulitis' are often used for any painful condition about the shoulder associated with loss of movement, and it is important for treatment reasons to differentiate it from other conditions affecting the joint. The aetiology is frequently obscure, although there is often a history of preceding trauma or a period of immobility. It can follow any shoulder or neck pathology in a predisposed individual.

Clinical features

It is characterised by a reduction in glenohumeral motion (particularly abduction and internal rotation), accompanied by distressing pain. Typically it affects the 40–60 age range, with women being twice as commonly afflicted as men. Strangely it is more common in the non-dominant shoulder. It normally passes through three distinct phases: firstly, there is a gradual onset of pain,

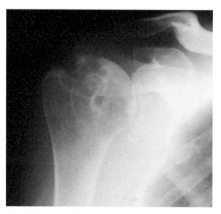

Fig. 3 **Rheumatoid arthritis of the shoulder with multiple cysts in the humeral head.**

which becomes severe and is accompanied by slowly worsening stiffness (freezing stage); secondly, the pain recedes and the stiffness predominates, producing a severe functional deficit (the frozen phase); thirdly, there is a gradual return to normal function (thawing phase) which in some may not be complete. The condition is self-limiting over 1–3 years, with the average duration being 18 months. In general terms, each phase lasts 6–9 months, although this is extremely variable. The pathology in the active phase is one of an intense fibrous reaction within the capsule, leading to thickening and contraction.

Investigations

Radiographs of the shoulder are invariably normal: indeed if they are not, other pathology should be considered. Arthrography can confirm the contracted capsule so typical of this condition.

Treatment

If the diagnosis is certain, it may suffice to reassure the patient and prescribe analgesics and physiotherapy. In many cases impatience and/or despair prevail, and steroid injections then may afford some relief. Manipulation should only be done in the frozen phase and requires great care to avoid humeral fracture. Surgical release is rarely necessary.

ARTHRITIS IN THE SHOULDER

Any pain or stiffness in the shoulder can cause a significant functional deficit in the whole of the upper limb as the stable base for movement is disrupted. Any form of arthropathy can occur, but by far the most common are rheumatoid arthritis and post-traumatic arthritis.

RHEUMATOID ARTHRITIS

Two-thirds of rheumatoid patients will have shoulder involvement to a greater or lesser extent. It is important to make a careful assessment as to which of several joints about the shoulder are involved, as this will obviously influence treatment. The glenohumeral and acromioclavicular joints are most commonly involved and, as in other conditions, sequential local anaesthetic injections can help define the site. Although pain is the predominant symptom, its localisation may not reflect the site of the pathology. Restriction of movement (particularly

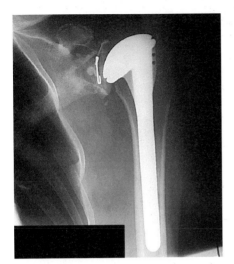

Fig. 4 **Total shoulder joint replacement.**

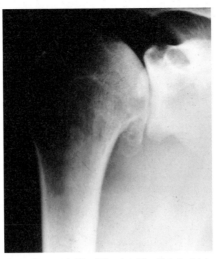

Fig. 5 **Osteoarthritis of the shoulder.** Note the joint space narrowing, marginal sclerosis and new bone formation.

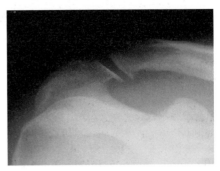

Fig. 6 **Osteoarthritis of the acromioclavicular joint.**

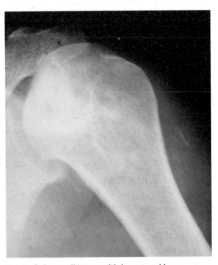

Fig. 7 **Caisson disease with increased bone density in the inferomedial quadrant of the humeral head.**

abduction and rotation) is the major cause of loss of function. The radiographs typically show cysts and erosions (Fig. 3), superior subluxation of the humeral head and, ultimately, destruction of the humeral head.

In juvenile chronic arthritis the shoulder is frequently affected and the assessment and treatment are similar.

Treatment

Medical treatment is always the first to be tried, although intra-articular injections can alleviate symptoms for prolonged periods. Any surgical treatment must be targeted to the source of the pain. Much of the pain may be from subacromial impingement and the acromioclavicular joint, and decompression procedures may be dramatically effective. Where the glenohumeral joint is severely diseased, total shoulder joint replacement will produce pain relief and improved function (Fig. 4).

OSTEOARTHRITIS

Primary osteoarthritis of the glenohumeral joint is rare (Fig. 5); when osteoarthritis occurs in the shoulder it is generally secondary and post-traumatic in origin. The acromioclavicular joint (Fig. 6) is often the source of pain, and selective injections are again helpful in deciding the best form of treatment. Conservative therapy is more likely to be effective, although decompression procedures may sometimes be beneficial.

CRYSTAL ARTHROPATHY

Crystal synovitis is relatively uncommon and pseudogout is more frequent than gout. Patients with gout usually present acutely with a painful, swollen joint which can be mistaken for a septic arthritis; pseudogout can have a more chronic presentation. In gout, hyperuricaemia may be present. To establish a diagnosis, joint aspiration and polarised light microscopy may be necessary. In gout the typical sodium urate crystal will be seen, whilst in pseudogout birefringent calcium pyrophosphate crystals are evident. The radiographs may show erosions, but in pseudogout linear calcific opacities can sometimes be seen deposited within the articular cartilage.

Treatment

Treatment is medical, with anti-inflammatories being used to settle the acute episode. Long-term uricosuric agents such as allopurinol may be required if there are recurrent attacks of gout.

AVASCULAR NECROSIS OF THE HUMERAL HEAD

This is relatively uncommon and results from a disturbance of the blood supply to the humeral head. This is most common after comminuted (multifragmented) fractures, but is also found in association with the inflammatory arthropathies such as systemic lupus erythematosus and rheumatoid arthritis, particularly if the patients have been given steroids to control the underlying disease. The problem is also seen in caisson workers and deep-sea divers (especially where decompression rituals are lax) and sometimes in aviators flying in unpressurised conditions. The femoral heads may be involved in a similar manner. Unfortunately in most cases the process may be well advanced at the time of presentation, as the onset of symptoms may be delayed until after there is significant bony collapse. Avascular necrosis becomes evident on the plain radiographs (Fig. 7) after some delay (but usually before bony collapse). MRI scans may also be helpful in defining the lesions. Treatment in the first instance is conservative, but if destruction of the humeral head occurs, joint replacement may be required.

Calcifying tendinitis and arthritis of the shoulder

- Acute calcific tendinitis can present with such severe symptoms that sepsis may be suspected.
- 'Frozen shoulder' is overdiagnosed and the term often attributed to any painful condition of the shoulder.
- The shoulder is a common site of degenerative or inflammatory arthropathies and crystal synovitis.

INJURIES ABOUT THE SHOULDER GIRDLE

FRACTURES OF THE CLAVICLE

The clavicle may be fractured as a result of a fall on the out-stretched hand, but much more frequently from a fall on the side. It is a common injury, particularly in children and in the middle aged. Fortunately the clavicle has a quite remarkable potential for rapid union, healing of clavicular fractures being unmatched by any other long bone.

It is impossible to immobilise displaced fractures by closed methods, but in spite of repeated movement at the fracture site (which is a consequence of this), non-union is extremely rare. The power of remodelling is also good, even in the adult. For these reasons it is not necessary to strive to obtain a full reduction of any clavicular fracture and there is very seldom call for any form of internal fixation.

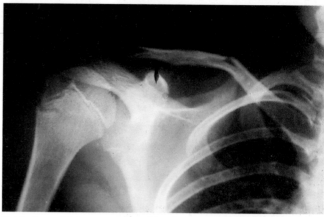

Fig. 1 **Greenstick fracture of the clavicle.**

FRACTURE PATTERNS

Undisplaced fractures

In children, especially in the younger age groups, the fracture may be a greenstick one, with local kinking of the clavicular contours or angulation (Fig. 1). Healing of this type of fracture is rapid (often in 2–3 weeks), and the injury may be treated by a short period of rest in a broad arm sling.

Displaced fractures

With greater violence in older bones the clavicle fractures and displaces. The proximal end, under the influence of the sternomastoid, is often elevated, while the distal fragment becomes depressed with the weight of the limb; the fragments may overlap (Fig. 2). As much of the clavicle is subcutaneous, the bone ends may become quite prominent and bleeding from them often results in local bruising.

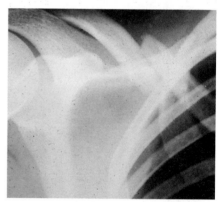

Fig. 2 **Fracture of the clavicle with overlapping bone ends.**

Treatment

An attempt may be made to minimise overlapping by the use of padded clavicular rings or a brace, although the benefits are regarded by some to be outweighed by the risks of developing skin problems in the axilla. In all cases it is customary to support the weight of the limb with a broad arm sling.

The arm should be removed from the sling daily to allow the elbow to be exercised. The broad arm sling may usually be discarded after 2 weeks and any other support by 4 to 5 weeks. Physiotherapy is seldom required, except occasionally in the elderly patient if the shoulder has become stiff.

Note that most fractures in the outer third of the clavicle are akin to acromioclavicular dislocations and may generally be treated by the use of a broad arm sling alone.

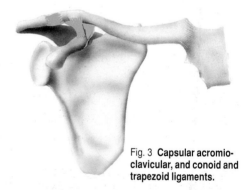

Fig. 3 **Capsular acromio-clavicular, and conoid and trapezoid ligaments.**

ACROMIOCLAVICULAR DISLOCATION

The clavicle guides the scapula in its movements round the chest wall and is attached to it by the capsular ligaments of the acromioclavicular joint and by the conoid and trapezoid ligaments (which run between the coracoid and the clavicle) (Fig. 3).

The acromioclavicular joint may be injured as a result of a fall or blow on the point of the shoulder. In minor injuries the capsular ligaments are stretched or torn and there is some joint subluxation so that the outer end of the clavicle becomes prominent. In more major disruptions the conoid and trapezoid ligaments are ruptured, so that there is greater displacement of the outer end of the clavicle. In very severe cases the muscle attachments of the trapezius and deltoid are involved, and the clavicle becomes wildly unstable.

Diagnosis

In all cases there is tenderness over the outer end of the clavicle, which is often quite obviously prominent. The diagnosis is confirmed by X-ray, but there is an important point to keep in mind: acromioclavicular dislocations usually reduce when the patient lies down, so that radiographs taken with the patient in the supine position may

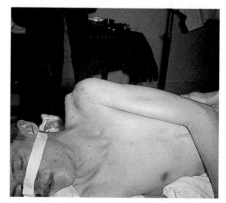

Fig. 4 **Gross acromioclavicular displacement about to undergo surgical repair.**

appear quite normal. The rule is that in cases of suspected acromioclavicular dislocation the radiographs should be taken with the patient standing, preferably holding something heavy (such as a book). It is also often useful to take comparison films of the other side at the same time. In interpreting the radiographs, displacement of the lateral end of the clavicle by its own diameter or more is suggestive of complete ligamentous disruption.

Treatment

The majority of acromioclavicular dislocations may be treated successfully by

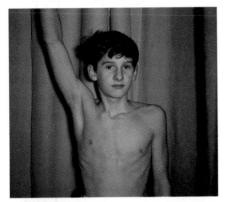

Fig. 5 **Dislocation of the right sternoclavicular joint.**

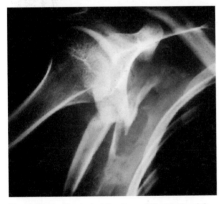

Fig. 6 **Markedly angled fracture of the blade of the scapula.**

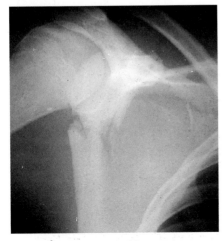

Fig. 7 **Fracture of the neck of the scapula.**

the use of a broad arm sling under the clothes for 4–6 weeks. Where displacement and instability are severe (Fig. 4), operative treatment may be considered. (A common procedure is to run a cancellous lag screw between the clavicle and coracoid to stabilise the clavicle. The acromioclavicular joint may be reinforced with absorbable transarticular sutures; tears in the deltoid and trapezius are then repaired. Note however that any screws placed between the clavicle and the coracoid need to be removed at about 6 weeks before the shoulder is mobilised.)

STERNOCLAVICULAR DISLOCATION

Although dislocations of the sternoclavicular joint are sometimes seen without any history of injury, they generally follow a blow on the shoulder or a fall on the outstretched hand. The contours marking the medial ends of the clavicles become asymmetrical and in some cases the resulting alteration in the appearance of the suprasternal notch may be rendered more obvious by abduction of the shoulder (Fig. 5). In acute cases there is local tenderness; rarely the medial end of the clavicle may come to lie behind the sternum, thereby endangering the great vessels; associated swelling may conceal the deformity. The diagnosis is made on clinical grounds following a careful clinical examination. Plain radiographs of this area are very difficult to interpret, but CT scans may be helpful in confirming both the plane and extent of any displacement.

Treatment

Minor anterior displacements should be accepted and treated symptomatically with a few weeks' rest of the arm in a broad arm sling. Gross displacement should be reduced; this may be carried out under general anaesthesia by placing a sandbag between the shoulder blades and pressing the shoulders backwards. Marked instability following reduction

should be treated by surgical repair using fascia lata slings. Irreducible retrosternal dislocations may require open reduction, which can be a hazardous procedure.

FRACTURES OF THE SCAPULA

Fractures of the scapula are relatively uncommon.

The blade and the spine (including the acromion) may be injured by direct violence; fractures of the neck and of the glenoid itself may result from forces transmitted up the arm.

Treatment

Fractures of the **blade** of the scapula may be markedly displaced or angled (Fig. 6). Where the displacement is particularly marked, some advocate operative reduction and internal fixation to reduce the risks of stiffness and discomfort. In the majority of cases good results are obtained by conservative treatment, first resting the arm in a sling and then mobilising the shoulder once the acute symptoms have settled.

Fractures of the **spine** of the scapula are generally splinted by the supraspinatus and infraspinatus muscles, so that displacement is uncommon. They should also be treated by rest in a sling for a short period.

Fractures of the **neck** of the scapula (Fig. 7) involve a large area of cancellous bone so that their union is rapid. They are also splinted by the muscles surrounding the neck so that minimal additional support is required. Again the position should be accepted and early mobilisation commenced after a short period of rest in a sling.

Fractures of the **glenoid** with involvement of the glenohumeral joint may in the majority of cases be treated conservatively with rest and early mobilisation. If the fragments are badly displaced with disruption of the joint, then surgery should be considered (e.g. open reduction and internal fixation).

Injuries about the shoulder girdle

- Union in fractures of the clavicle is nearly always rapid and non-union is rare.
- Accurate reduction of clavicular fractures is not necessary for a good result.
- In any case of suspected acromioclavicular dislocation, be sure to check that the X-ray films are taken with the patient in the erect position.
- Only the most unstable of acromioclavicular dislocations should be considered for internal fixation.
- Sternoclavicular dislocation is diagnosed in most cases on clinical grounds; CT scans may be required for confirmation.
- The majority of scapular fractures may be treated successfully by a short period of rest in a sling followed by early mobilisation.

DISLOCATIONS OF THE SHOULDER / FRACTURES OF THE PROXIMAL HUMERUS

ANTERIOR DISLOCATION OF THE SHOULDER

This is by far the most common of all shoulder dislocations. Its highest incidence is in the 15–25 age group as a result of sporting activities (such as rugby) and in the elderly from heavy falls on the outstretched hand. In both instances dislocation follows violent external rotation of the arm, with or without abduction of the shoulder.

At the front of the joint the capsule of the glenohumeral joint and the glenoid labrum are torn or avulsed from their attachments to the glenoid margin, so that the head of the humerus is free to dislocate anteriorly; it comes to lie in front of the glenoid (and also often slightly medially and inferior to it)(Fig. 1).

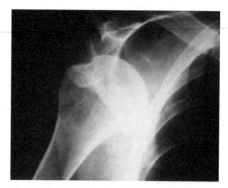

Fig. 1 **Anterior dislocation of the shoulder.**

Diagnosis

In acute cases there is a clear history of injury. The patient complains of severe pain in the shoulder and is unable to move it and use the arm. The lateral contour of the joint is often slightly disturbed, with some 'squaring' of the shoulder and a little hollowing distal to the acromion; in some cases the displacement of the humeral head may be detected by palpation. An X-ray examination, with films in two planes, is mandatory. (Note that fractures of the neck of the humerus are often mistaken for dislocations of the shoulder and that dislocations of the shoulder are often accompanied by fractures, particularly of the greater tuberosity.) The clinical examination must include a search for the signs of the neurovascular complications which are known to complicate anterior dislocation of the shoulder; the findings should be recorded prior to manipulation (see later).

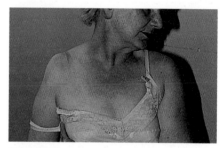

Fig. 2 **Wasting of the right deltoid muscle due to an axillary nerve palsy complicating an anterior dislocation of the shoulder.**

Treatment

A manipulative reduction of the dislocation should be carried out. To obtain the necessary relaxation heavy sedation or general anaesthesia is usually required. There are two common techniques of manipulating the shoulder. In the *Hippocratic method* the shoulder is abducted and the head of the humerus levered back into the glenoid, using the stockinged heel of the surgeon, placed in the patient's axilla, as a fulcrum. In the *Köcher method* the elbow is flexed to a right angle and held at the side while the arm is slowly and fully externally rotated; then the shoulder is rapidly adducted and internally rotated. X-rays are taken to check the reduction and the arm supported in a broad arm sling under the clothes. There is some controversy as to how long the arm should be supported before mobilisation is commenced; a 4 week period is often advised in those under 40 in the belief that this will facilitate healing of the torn soft tissues and minimise the risks of recurrence; a shorter period, to avoid stiffness, is advisable in the older patient.

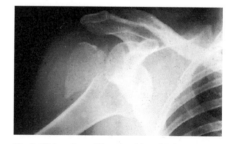

Fig. 3 **Dislocation of the shoulder with fracture of the greater tuberosity.**

Early complications

Damage to the brachial plexus. By far the most common injury is a lesion in continuity of the axillary nerve; this results in sensory loss over the so-called 'Regimental Badge' area of the shoulder and paralysis and wasting of the deltoid muscle (Fig. 2). This complication is generally treated expectantly, the first signs of recovery usually (but by no means invariably) appearing at about 6 weeks. Delay merits further investigation as does more extensive neurological involvement. In every case physiotherapy is necessary to mobilise the shoulder while it remains partially paralysed, and must be prolonged and intensive.

Pressure of the humeral head on the axillary artery. This may lead to an absent radial pulse and progressive paralysis and loss of sensation in all the arm. Prompt reduction generally leads to rapid restoration of the circulation.

Fracture complicating the dislocation. The most common by far is one of the greater tuberosity (Fig. 3) to which the rotator cuff is attached. The treatment is straightforward: reduction of the dislocation usually results in the reduction of the tuberosity; if not, then open reduction and internal fixation of the fracture with a cancellous bone screw may be required. Where a shoulder dislocation is accompanied by a fracture of

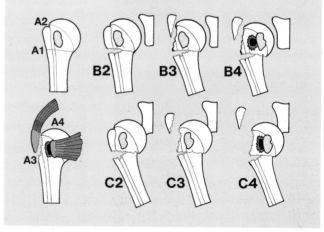

Fig. 4 **Fractures of the proximal humerus.**

A: Possible levels of fracture:
1 surgical neck
2 anatomical neck
3 greater tuberosity
4 lesser tuberosity

B: 2-part fracture
3-part fracture
4-part fracture

C: 2-part fracture-dislocation
3-part fracture-dislocation
4-part fracture-dislocation

the neck or head of the humerus, treatment is often highly specialised, with each case requiring the most careful individual assessment.

Late complications

Recurrent dislocation is potentially the most serious complication of anterior dislocation of the shoulder. This is usually due to attrition of the shoulder cuff at the front of the joint and the failure of the glenoid labrum and anterior capsule to become re-anchored to the anterior glenoid margin; there is little to retain the head of the humerus in its socket and the joint regularly re-dislocates. Eventually the joint may dislocate under the most trivial circumstances (e.g. putting on a jacket) and in a number of cases the patient learns the trick of reducing the dislocation himself. An axial X-ray projection may confirm the diagnosis by revealing a defect in the humeral head (the Hill–Sachs lesion). Apart from the pain and inconvenience, and the risks of secondary osteoarthritis, in some occupations or situations the patient's safety and even life may be put in jeopardy. Surgical treatment is usually advised by the time of the fourth dislocation and the success rate is high.

OTHER DISLOCATIONS OF THE SHOULDER

Posterior dislocation

This is uncommon, but is also often missed as it may not be obvious in a single (AP) view of the joint: it invariably shows up in an axial, translateral or apical oblique projection. Posterior dislocation may accompany obstetrical and Erb's palsies. Reduction by traction in 90 degrees abduction is generally easy; if, however, the joint is unstable afterwards, a 4 week period in a plaster shoulder spica may be necessary. Treatment of recurrent posterior dislocation is specialised. Surgical reconstruction and re-attachment of the damaged soft tissues

(using techniques similar to those employed in anterior dislocation of the shoulder) may be used; occasionally it is necessary to buttress the posterior aspect of the glenoid with a block of bone attached to its posterior margin.

Luxatio erecta

Here the head of the humerus dislocates inferiorly and the arm is held dramatically in full abduction. Neurovascular complications should be looked for and reduction carried out without delay.

Habitual dislocation

Here the patient may be able to voluntarily dislocate and reduce the dislocation without pain. There is frequently a history of a joint laxity syndrome (which should be looked for) or of psychosis. Arthroscopy or arthrography shows a capacious joint with none of the features of recurrent dislocation. There is no Hill–Sachs lesion as in recurrent dislocation. Surgery is unrewarding, and the usual treatment advocated is re-education of the shoulder muscles using biofeedback techniques.

FRACTURES OF THE PROXIMAL HUMERUS

There is a bewildering number of fracture patterns in this area and their classification (Fig. 4) can be confusing; but note the following points:

- The proximal humerus fractures most often through its surgical neck (Fig. 5). This is filled with cancellous bone and union is usually rapid, especially if the fragments are impacted.
- Fractures through the anatomical neck, for mechanical reasons, are much less common, but may imperil the blood supply to the humeral head. This however is not as great a problem as it is in the hip.
- The greater tuberosity may be avulsed by the pull of the supraspinatus.
- The lesser tuberosity may be avulsed by subscapularis.

- Any of these injuries may occur in isolation or combination; in the simplest, there is a single fracture with two elements (2-part fracture); in the most complex, all the elements are involved (4-part fracture)
- Any of these fractures may be accompanied by a dislocation of the head of the humerus (2-, 3- and 4-part fracture-dislocations).

Treatment guidelines

In children. Greenstick fractures of the surgical neck are common, and a short period of rest with the arm in a sling inside the clothes is the usual method of treatment.

In adults. The most common injury is an impacted or moderately displaced fracture of the surgical neck (Fig. 5). The arm may be placed in a broad-arm sling under the clothes, reinforced with a body bandage. Mobilisation should be encouraged as early as possible to avoid permanent stiffness of the shoulder. In practical terms the body bandage may usually be discarded after 2 weeks when the elbow should be exercised fully (by temporary removal of the arm from the sling). At the same time gentle rocking movements of the shoulder may be commenced. At about 4 weeks the sling may be put outside the clothes and discarded at about 6 weeks. Physiotherapy should be started as soon as symptoms allow.

If there is severe displacement of the fracture manipulative reduction may be attempted, and if this fails open reduction and internal fixation may be considered. The technical difficulty increases with the complexity of the fracture and the amount of comminution, and results are less reliable in the older patient.

In the case of a fracture-dislocation, the humeral head must be reduced, which in many cases can only be achieved by open methods. Where the fracture is proximally situated, or the head fragmented, a primary hemiarthroplasty should be considered.

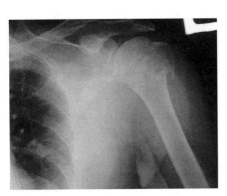

Fig. 5 **Undisplaced, impacted 3-part fracture of the proximal humerus in an adult.**

Dislocations of the shoulder / fractures of the proximal humerus

- Anterior dislocation is the most common of shoulder joint dislocations.
- Axillary nerve palsy and fracture of the greater tuberosity are the two most common immediate complications of anterior dislocation of the shoulder.
- Apart from joint stiffness in the elderly, recurrent dislocation of the shoulder is the most common late complication of anterior dislocation of the shoulder.
- Distinguish between recurrent dislocation and habitual dislocation of the shoulder.
- The majority of fractures of the proximal humerus may be successfully treated by conservative methods, but early mobilisation is essential if stiffness of the shoulder is to be avoided.

FRACTURES OF THE SHAFT AND DISTAL END OF THE HUMERUS

FRACTURE OF THE SHAFT

The shaft of the humerus may fracture as the result of a fall or blow on the side of the arm or from a fall on the outstretched hand. There is usually no problem with the diagnosis as in the majority of cases there is obvious local deformity and loss of function in the arm. The diagnosis is confirmed with appropriate radiographs.

Initial complications

In the mid-shaft region of the humerus the radial nerve lies close to the bone in the region of the musculospiral groove. Although some fibres of the brachialis muscle offer it appreciable protection, it is nevertheless sometimes damaged, resulting in a drop wrist deformity accompanied by a small area of sensory impairment on the dorsolateral surface of the hand.

The lesion is generally one of continuity (a neuropraxia) and may be treated expectantly with a drop-wrist (and preferably lively) splint. Some early signs of recovery may be seen about the sixth or seventh week, after which progress to complete recovery is rapid. Should this expected recovery not occur, further investigation (e.g. by electromyography or exploration) will be required.

In some cases major damage to the nerve may be suspected from the beginning (e.g. where there is gross fracture displacement with much local comminution) which would be an indication for

exploration, internal fixation of the fracture and, if appropriate, primary nerve suture.

Where the humeral fracture is accompanied by other injuries (especially to the chest) which confine the patient to bed, internal fixation is often the best management: conservative measures are most successful when employed in the ambulant patient who can adopt the vertical posture, where gravity acting on the weight of the arm acts as a form of traction.

Conservative treatment

Humeral fractures may be supported by means of plaster casts and broad arm slings. With the patient seated, and after the application of suitable padding round the arm, either a well moulded U-plaster or a hanging cast may be applied (Fig. 1). The arm is then supported in a sling which should be worn under the clothes. After the first few weeks it is often possible to replace the cast with a polythene functional brace. Union may be sufficiently far advanced by 9 weeks to discard splintage, continuing with only a sling for a further 2 weeks. Physiotherapy for mobilisation of both the shoulder and the elbow is often required.

Operative treatment

Open reduction and internal fixation may be combined with inspection of the radial nerve if there is an associated radial nerve palsy. Methods of fixation include: (i) plating of the posterior surface of the humerus and, depending on the configuration, with a lag screw across the fracture; (ii) intra-medullary nailing, with the nail being passed proximally from an entry point just above the olecranon fossa and (iii) intra-medullary nailing, with the nail being passed distally from an opening made in the region of the greater tuberosity (Fig. 2).

In the case of open fractures (Fig. 3), especially where contamination is marked, an external fixator may be employed.

FRACTURE OF THE DISTAL END

In a *supracondylar fracture*, the fracture line lies just proximal to the strong bone masses of the trochlea and capitulum (capitellum), and passes across the floors of the olecranon and coronoid fossae (Fig. 4). The fracture may range from a mere hair line to one where there is complete loss of bone contact. When the injury is more than minimal, the direction of the forces involved most frequently result in an extension pattern of fracture where the distal fragment is tilted backwards (anterior angulation). At the same time, it may be displaced both posteriorly and laterally and it may be externally rotated. Rarely, the distal fragment is displaced anteriorly (anterior supracondylar fracture or flexion type supracondylar fracture).

Supracondylar fractures of the humerus are seen most often in children and generally result from a fall on the outstretched hand. They are of particular importance because of their frequency and the complications with which they may be associated. These complications fall into two categories: vascular complications and those related to persisting deformity.

Vascular complications. In displaced supracondylar fractures the brachial artery may suffer kinking, compression, intimal damage or even division from contact with the spiky end of the proximal fragment (Fig. 5). At the same time, haemorrhage from the bone ends may cause tense swelling within the tissues at the front of the elbow; this, especially if the elbow is excessively flexed, will additionally affect the distal circulation. In the most severe cases the blood supply to the forearm muscles may be completely

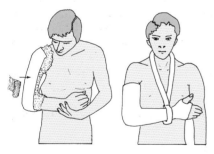

Fig. 1 **U-slab support (left) and hanging cast (right).**

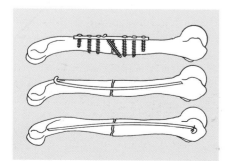

Fig. 2 **Screwing and plating, and intra-medullary nailing of mid-shaft humeral fractures.**

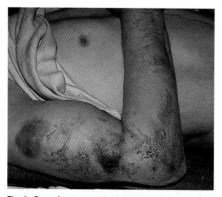

Fig. 3 **Open fracture of the humeral shaft.**

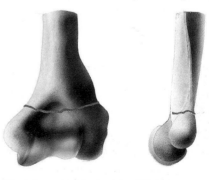

Fig. 4 **Supracondylar fracture of the humerus.**

cut off so that they become necrotic and rendered functionally useless. Over the ensuing months they are replaced with fibrous tissue which slowly contracts, pulling the hand and fingers into a position of gross deformity (Volkmann's ischaemic contracture). Such a catastrophe can and must be avoided by prompt and appropriate treatment.

Complications of malunion. Persisting posterior displacement and backward tilting of the distal fragment lead to loss of elbow flexion (due to the coronoid process impinging on the mass of new bone which forms at the front of the elbow). In the child the processes of remodelling are such that this restriction usually (but not invariably) resolves over the course of a year, although it is obviously desirable to avoid this problem altogether by obtaining a good reduction at the start.

The carrying angle of the elbow may be affected as a result of some inaccuracy in reduction (and cubitus varus or valgus is difficult to assess both clinically and by X-ray when the elbow is in a flexed position); it may also be disturbed by abnormal epiphyseal growth. Cubitus varus is often particularly unsightly (gunstock deformity). In the long term, cubitus valgus in particular may be followed by impairment of conduction in the ulnar nerve as it passes behind the medial epicondyle (tardy ulnar nerve palsy).

Diagnosis
While a careful clinical examination may help to distinguish a supracondylar fracture from other injuries in the area (e.g. dislocation of the elbow, fractures of the capitulum etc), in practice the diagnosis is always established as a result of careful study of the X-rays of the elbow; these should always be taken when there is any suspicion of significant injury in this region. Radiographs can be difficult to interpret due to the changes in the epiphyseal appearances with growth (see p. 76), and if there is any doubt, take radiographs of the other side for comparison.

It is imperative that the vascular status of the limb should be assessed and recorded. Feel for the radial pulse; if this cannot be found, look for other signs suggestive of loss of the distal arterial supply (pallor and coldness of the limb, pain and paraesthesia in the forearm, progressive muscular weakness and paralysis of the forearm muscles). Note also the presence of excessive bruising and swelling round the elbow.

If there is evidence of arterial obstruction the situation should be handled promptly and without procrastination. Fortunately, in the great majority of cases, reduction of the fracture leads to restoration of the circulation. If however this is unsuccessful, the opinion of an experienced vascular surgeon should be sought without delay so that exploration and appropriate treatment may be carried out.

Treatment
Manipulative reduction should be undertaken without delay as a primary measure in all cases where there is a vascular impairment and in other supracondylar fractures where there is significant loss of alignment, i.e. where there is loss of 50% or more of bony contact, or where there is medial or lateral tilting of 10 degrees or more, or where the epiphyseal complex is tilted backwards (as opposed to its normal 45 degree anterior tilt). The technique is straightforward: under general anaesthesia traction is applied with the elbow in about 20 degrees of flexion to disimpact the fracture; the elbow is then flexed, while maintaining traction, just short of where the radial pulse starts to fade. This position should be maintained with a sling, preferably supplemented with a dorsal plaster slab. A complete plaster cast should never be applied. Check radiographs should be obtained and ideally the arm should be elevated and the child admitted for circulatory observation for 24 hours.

Where the radial pulse has been found absent prior to manipulation, in the majority of cases reduction of the fracture leads to its restoration. In an appreciable number of other cases, although the radial pulse remains absent, the peripheral tissues remain well perfused and there are no other signs of arterial obstruction. Under those circumstances the arm should be elevated, with the elbow flexed to no more than 90 degrees, and the circulation most carefully observed at frequent intervals. In the majority of cases no deterioration occurs and the radial pulse re-appears 2–3 days later. If however ischaemic signs appear, or if they are present initially and unrelieved by manipulation, then exploration will be required.

Management of reduction failure
Manipulation beyond the third attempt is not advised because of the risks of increasing the swelling round the elbow to a dangerous level. If an image intensifier is available the problem may often be found to be one of extreme instability: i.e. while the fracture may be readily reduced it almost immediately slips out of alignment. If this is the case, then it may be stabilised by means of two percutaneous Kirschner wires, passed from the lateral side across the fracture line or crossed. Open reduction is advocated by some and may be helpful in reducing the risks of cubitus varus.

In other cases, if the alignment of the fracture can be corrected, gross displacements can often be reluctantly accepted, relying on remodelling over the course of the next year or so for restoration of function.

After care
Assess union at about 3–4 weeks for a child of 4, and at 4–5 weeks for a child of eight. If union is considered adequate, local supports should be discarded and the arm mobilised from a sling. Passive movements of the joint are contraindicated. If there is any cubitus varus or valgus deformity this should be measured, and the child seen at yearly intervals for re-assessment.

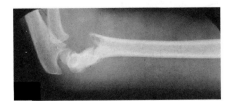

Fig. 5 **Supracondylar fracture with spiky proximal fragment endangering the brachial artery.**

Fractures of the shaft and distal end of the humerus

- In any fracture of the humeral shaft, be on the lookout for an associated radial nerve palsy.
- The majority of humeral shaft fractures may be treated conservatively by the use of external supportive measures such as casts, slings and functional braces.
- Internal fixation of humeral shaft fractures should be considered in cases of multiple injuries or where there is a radial nerve injury which is likely to be more than a lesion in continuity.
- In any supracondylar fracture of the humerus remain alert to the risks of serious circulatory complications.
- Tardy ulnar nerve palsy may occur as a late complication of supracondylar fracture.

OTHER DISTAL HUMERAL FRACTURES / DISLOCATION OF THE ELBOW

The interpretation of radiographs of the elbow in adults is not usually difficult, but in children problems sometimes arise due to lack of familiarity with growth changes. In the newly born child the distal end of the humerus is formed entirely of radio-translucent cartilage. As a child grows, ossification centres appear. As they increase in number and size they progressively reveal more of the shape of this part of the humerus (Fig. 1). The absence, displacement or mutual separation of these ossification centres may indicate the presence and severity of a fracture.

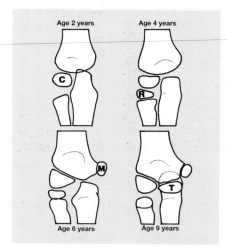

Fig. 1 **Radiographic appearance of the capitulum (C), radial head (R), medial epicondyle (M) and trochlea (T) at ages 2, 4, 6 and 9.**

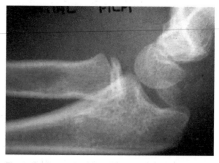

Fig. 2 **Radiograph of the elbow of an 8-year-old child showing medial epicondyle trapped in the joint.**

FRACTURE OF THE MEDIAL EPICONDYLE

This injury commonly results from forcible abduction of the elbow and is of particular importance in children. The ulnar collateral ligament of the elbow is stretched and may avulse the medial epicondyle to which it is attached. As the inside of the elbow opens out, the medial epicondyle may be sucked into the joint where it can be trapped as the pressure is released. If undetected, the function of the elbow will be seriously and permanently impaired. This injury is most common in children of 6 and over, by which time the centre of ossification has appeared. The rule is that if the radiographs of the elbow of a child of 6 or over fail to show the medial epicondyle in the AP view and the epiphysis is visible in the lateral, where it cannot normally be seen (see Fig. 2), then it is trapped in the joint.

Diagnosis and treatment

Suspect this injury if there is bruising and/or tenderness on the medial side of the elbow and confirm it by careful interpretation of the radiographs. Check that there is no associated damage to the ulnar nerve (usually a neuropraxia or lesion in continuity). The trapped epicondyle may often be freed by manipulation or electrical stimulation of the forearm muscles which are attached to it, but sometimes open reduction and internal fixation with a Kirschner wire may be necessary.

FRACTURES OF THE LATERAL EPICONDYLE IN CHILDREN

These injuries are uncommon (the ossification centre appears between the ages of 11 and 14). Only very rarely does the lateral epicondyle become trapped in the joint, when methods similar to those for the medial epicondyle may be used. In adults, epicondylar fractures generally result from direct violence and require symptomatic treatment only.

LATERAL CONDYLAR INJURIES IN CHILDREN

The fracture usually includes the whole of the capitulum, nearly half the trochlea and often a fragment of the metaphysis. The distal fragment may be undisplaced, shifted laterally or rotated by the pull of the extensor muscles (Fig. 3).

Treatment

If there is no displacement, treat conservatively by a period of immobilisation in plaster. If displaced, an accurate reduction is essential, which in most cases entails an open reduction and fixation with Kirschner wires.

UNICONDYLAR FRACTURES IN ADULTS

The main distal articular mass of the humerus remains in continuity with the shaft. When the lateral side of the humerus is involved (either may be affected), the patterns of fracture are similar to those seen in lateral condylar injuries in children.

Treatment

While undisplaced fractures may be treated conservatively, with a period in plaster followed by early mobilisation, displaced fractures require accurate reduction of the articular surface by open operation and internal fixation.

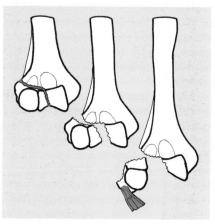

Fig. 3 **Fractures of the lateral condyle with common displacements.**

FRACTURE OF THE ARTICULAR SURFACE OF THE CAPITULUM

Force transmitted up the radial shaft (for example from a fall on the outstretched hand) may result in crushing of the cartilaginous surface of the capitulum and/or some compression of the underlying bone; this may in the long term lead to osteoarthritis. Apart from initial rest, no active treatment is required or likely to be effective.

In some instances a portion of the articular surface of the capitulum may be shorn off (Fig. 4). If this is detected and the fragment is of a substantial size it should be fixed; if it is small, it should be excised.

BICONDYLAR, T- OR Y- FRACTURES

Here the fracture line splits the trochlea vertically and then forks medially and laterally with the creation of three main fragments: the humeral shaft, the medial condyle and the lateral condyle (Fig. 5). Treatment may be difficult due to the problem of reducing and holding the comparatively small fragments in alignment so that the joint may be mobilised

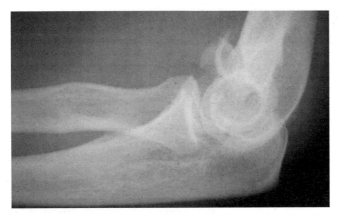

Fig. 4 **Fracture of the articular surface of the capitulum (capitellum).**

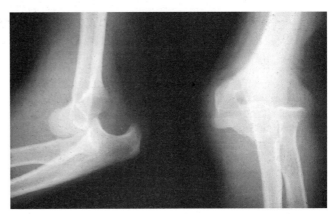

Fig. 6 **Posterolateral dislocation of the elbow.**

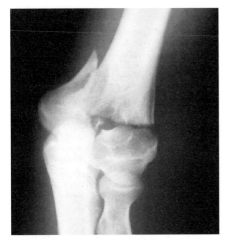

Fig. 5 **Y-fracture of the distal humerus.**

Table 1 **General measures in the management of elbow injuries**

- In the early stages of any elbow injury, a broad arm sling may be used to give support and help relieve pain.
- While a sling is being employed, movements of the fingers, wrist and shoulder must be encouraged.
- A sling should be discarded as soon as it has served its purpose, and movements of the unsupported joints should be continued.
- The complex nature of the articulating surfaces of the elbow joint and its tiny mechanical clearances ensure that any malalignment of its components or any intra-articular adhesions will result in a disproportionate loss of movement. It follows that a good reduction and early mobilisation are essential.
- In children, a good reduction is also of importance so that any disturbance of growth in the epiphyseal complex may be minimised; neglect may result in the long term in an unsightly appearance of the joint (from a cubitus valgus or cubitus varus deformity) and possibly in a tardy ulnar nerve palsy.
- Myositis ossificans is a feared complication of elbow injuries, leading to gross restriction of movement in the joint. As a general rule, to reduce the risks of its occurrence, any surgical procedure should be carried out without delay (comminution of the radial head complicating elbow dislocation is an exception) and passive stretching exercise of the joint must be scrupulously avoided.

without delay; without early mobilisation the elbow will become permanently stiff. In most cases the two condylar fragments are first reduced and held with interfragmentary screws; this in essence converts the injury into a supracondylar fracture which may then be held with a medially applied contoured plate (with an additional lateral plate if there is much comminution)

POSTEROLATERAL DISLOCATION OF THE ELBOW

Most commonly the radius and ulna dislocate both posteriorly and laterally (Fig. 6), often as result of a fall on the outstretched hand. Although usually uncomplicated, on occasion there may be involvement of the brachial artery or the ulnar or median nerves (usually a neuropraxia). There may be associated fractures of the medial epicondyle, the lateral condyle, the radial head or the coronoid.

Treatment

If uncomplicated, the dislocation should be reduced under general anaesthesia by applying strong traction. The joint may be rested in a sling until settling symptoms will permit mobilisation (usually within 2–3 weeks and almost immediately in a stable injury); later, physiotherapy may sometimes be required, especially in the older patient. Vascular complications are usually resolved by reduction of the dislocation; otherwise they may be dealt with along the lines taken in the management of complicated supracondylar fractures. Nerve lesions may generally be treated expectantly.

Where there is an accompanying fracture, the dislocation should be reduced and the fracture then dealt with by methods appropriate to its pattern. In the case of an elbow dislocation complicated by a highly fragmented fracture of the radial head (as opposed to an isolated radial head fracture), many advise delaying surgery for 4–8 weeks to reduce the risks of myositis ossificans, although others recommend immediate excision. Prosthetic replacement of the radial head may be considered if instability is a problem. If the coronoid process is involved, and the bony fragment large, then the reduction may be unstable; operative fixation of the fragment may then be desirable.

Other distal humeral fractures / dislocation of the elbow

- A knowledge of the changing appearance of the epiphyses throughout growth is necessary for the correct interpretation of radiographs of the elbow in children. If there is any doubt, it is justifiable to obtain films of the other side for comparison.
- Fractures of the medial epicondyle trapped within the elbow joint have serious consequences if not promptly diagnosed and treated.
- Displaced fractures of the lateral condyle of the elbow in children must be accurately reduced if stiffness, growth disturbance and non-union are to be avoided.
- In displaced Y-fractures of the distal humerus in adults, unless fragmentation is gross, an attempt should be made at open reduction and internal fixation so that mobilisation may be started as soon as possible.
- Nerve lesions accompanying dislocations of the elbow may generally be treated expectantly.
- The elbow should never be mobilised by forcible passive movements: the risks of myositis ossificans are too high.

RHEUMATOID ARTHRITIS AND OTHER DISORDERS AT THE ELBOW

The elbow plays a vital role in upper limb function: without its excellent range of motion, the arm is significantly disabled. Stiffness is common after injury, and unless a painless range of flexion of 90 degrees or more can be achieved, the ability to work, feed and groom oneself may be seriously impaired. As even a minor anomaly may create difficulties, timely and effective treatment is most important, however difficult this may be to achieve in practice.

RHEUMATOID ARTHRITIS

The elbow is frequently affected by rheumatoid arthritis, and the degree of disability is dependent on the extent of the disease. Symptoms may be mild or severe depending on the degree of joint destruction and instability. Clinically, there may be marked synovitis, with painful restriction of motion and a gradually worsening fixed flexion deformity. In addition, if the radiohumeral joint is affected, pronation and supination may be severely limited. It is important to remember that pain on rotation of the forearm may also have its origin in the distal radioulnar joint, and that it can be clinically difficult to be certain which is responsible: both may be significantly diseased. In the most severe cases, where the integrity of the joint is destroyed, the ulnar nerve may be affected, causing problems (sensory and often motor as well) in the area of its distribution.

Radiologically, the joint space is almost invariably narrowed, with peripheral erosions, cystic changes and progressively severe porosis (Fig. 1). In the end stage, joint integrity may be lost, leading to a flail elbow with its inevitable functional consequences.

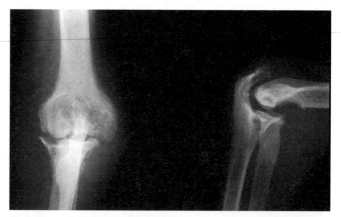

Fig. 1 **Rheumatoid arthritis of the elbow with osteoporosis, cyst formation and joint disorganisation.**

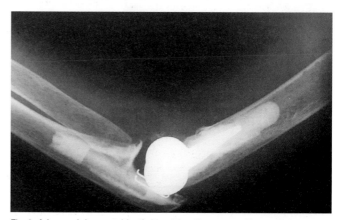

Fig. 2 **Advanced rheumatoid arthritis of the elbow treated by total joint replacement.**

Treatment

In mild cases, medical treatment will suffice, but this may have to be supplemented by intra-articular steroid injections from time to time when control is lost. Surgical intervention is required once symptoms become severe. Synovectomy and radial head excision are effective in combination. Total joint replacement (Fig. 2) is reserved for the mechanically deranged joint.

OSTEOARTHRITIS OF THE ELBOW

It is not uncommon for a patient to be found to have a markedly degenerate elbow with a restricted range of motion and for the diagnosis to come as a surprise: in contrast to rheumatoid arthritis, pain is not usually a prominent feature. Stiffness associated with joint disorganisation is the most common presenting symptom. Osteoarthritis of the elbow is almost always secondary to previous trauma or to osteochondritis dissecans. Both of these are common in manual workers, especially those who do much hammering or who use vibrating tools (e.g. caulkers). As a consequence of either of these conditions loose bodies may form in the joint, and 'locking' may be a presenting symptom. The joint may 'lock' in any position, and the patient usually learns to manipulate the elbow to release it. Radiographs usually reveal the extent and nature of the disease; there is usually loss of joint space, marginal sclerosis and marked osteophyte formation. Where loose bodies are present, defects in the capitulum or the head of the radius may indicate a previous osteochondritis dissecans (Fig. 3).

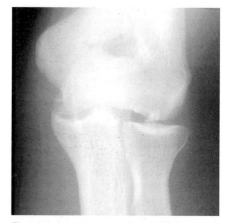

Fig. 3 **Loose body in the elbow secondary to osteochondritis of the capitulum.**

Treatment

In the first instance, analgesics may be sufficient to control the symptoms. Physiotherapy can be employed, but it rarely improves the range of motion. Surgical intervention is largely confined to removal of loose bodies when they become symptomatic. Joint replacement is rarely indicated, because the physical demands of a patient suffering from osteoarthritis of the elbow are generally much greater than those of the patient with rheumatoid arthritis, and are likely to exceed the capabilities of any current prosthesis.

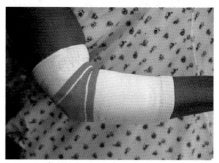

Fig. 4 **Orthosis for tennis elbow.**

TENNIS ELBOW (LATERAL EPICONDYLITIS)

This is the most common of all elbow complaints and is one of the most difficult to cure. Its aetiology still remains a little uncertain, but the most common view is that it may result from single or multiple small tears of the tendinous origin of common extensor muscles of the forearm at their site of origin at the lateral epicondyle. The part related to extensor carpi radialis brevis may be particularly affected. Another view is that the condition is a periostitis secondary to recurrent stresses. The pain is usually well localised to the lateral side of the elbow and is aggravated by gripping objects, forcibly extending the wrist or supinating the forearm. The onset may be gradual or sudden. Although anyone may be affected it is particularly common in manual workers (e.g. joiners and plumbers) and those taking part in sports.

Normally on examination the range of movements in the elbow is full and there is no instability. There is usually well-localised tenderness in the area of the lateral epicondyle corresponding to the site of the pain and the supposed pathology. In addition, resisted extension of the wrist may reproduce the pain at the elbow. Radiographs are usually quite normal. In the absence of treatment the condition tends to be self-limiting over 12–18 months, but avoidance of strenuous activities is necessary to avoid exacerbations.

Treatment

As a first measure the patient is given advice about the likely nature of the condition and its natural history. In sportsmen there may be a flawed technique necessitating correction, and this in combination with a period of rest may be all that is required. If there is no significant improvement, local anaesthetic/steroid injections into the point of maximal tenderness usually modify the symptoms but do not necessarily guarantee resolution. The symptoms are usually significantly changed 10 minutes after the local anaesthetic injection; if not, the injection site may have been inappropriate or the diagnosis may have to be reviewed. In patients where simple measures do not produce benefit an elbow clasp may be helpful (Fig. 4), with or without other measures. (The theory of the clasp is that it redirects the pull of the extensors thus resting the affected proximal part.) In resistant cases, surgical release of part or all of the common extensor origin may become necessary, although even this procedure is not always successful in relieving the symptoms.

GOLFER'S ELBOW (MEDIAL EPICONDYLITIS)

This is similar in character to tennis elbow but involves the flexor muscle origin in the region of the medial epicondyle. It is much less common and usually responds to a period of rest; only occasionally are steroid injections required.

OLECRANON BURSITIS

The olecranon bursa lies over the point of the elbow, between the skin and the tendinous insertion of triceps. It may swell in response to local pressure or friction (e.g. in carpet layers and welders) and sometimes becomes inflamed, especially if the overlying skin is broken. Clinically, the bursa is usually fluctuant, but sometimes the swelling is so tense that a solid lesion is suspected (Fig. 5).

Aspiration can be attempted for both therapeutic and diagnostic purposes. Unfortunately these bursal swellings tend to recur and, if troublesome, excision should be considered. Remember that rheumatoid nodules are common on the extensor surfaces of the proximal part of the forearm and elbow and should not be mistaken for olecranon bursae.

POST-TRAUMATIC ELBOW STIFFNESS

The complex mechanism of the elbow may be disturbed by even a minor injury, with extension of the joint being the first to suffer. Isolated loss of a little extension of the elbow (fixed flexion deformity) of 10 degrees or so seldom results in significant disability and may even pass unnoticed by the patient. Loss of flexion is more important, and if this is reduced to 90 degrees or less the loss of function is always severe. Forearm rotation is often retained, but if it too is restricted, there will be even greater loss of function.

The cause of the restriction of motion can be multifactorial: there may be incongruity of the joint surfaces after a fracture, or there may be soft tissue contractures or heterotopic ossification (myositis ossificans). In the latter, a block of new bone can form a bridge between the humerus and forearm, preventing any flexion (Fig. 6). Ultimately degenerative changes become superimposed, and these will be obvious on radiological examination.

Treatment

Physiotherapy may be helpful in preventing stiffness in the period immediately following an elbow injury. A stiff elbow presenting at a late stage, however, is unlikely to improve with physiotherapy. Passive stretching in particular should be avoided as this may result in heterotopic ossification. Surgical intervention, with arthrolysis (division of contracted soft tissues) and intensive physiotherapy, can produce improvement. Where heterotopic ossification is present, benefit may follow excision of any abnormal bone mass; this however must be delayed for 6 months or a year, otherwise recurrence is inevitable.

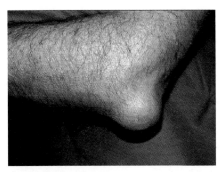

Fig. 5 **Tense olecranon bursitis.**

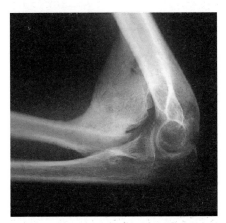

Fig. 6 **Myositis ossificans of the elbow with large bone block.**

Rheumatoid arthritis and other disorders at the elbow

- Tennis elbow is the most common cause of pain about the elbow.
- Two-thirds of patients with rheumatoid arthritis have elbow joint involvement.
- Osteoarthritis of the elbow generally occurs as a sequel to fracture or osteochondritis dissecans.
- Heterotopic ossification may form after an injury and cause restricted motion.

PROXIMAL FRACTURES OF THE RADIUS AND ULNA

FRACTURE OF THE RADIAL HEAD

Although the radial head is often fractured by direct violence (e.g. a blow on the side of the elbow), injury may also follow falls on the outstretched hand. When the hand contacts the ground, the force of impact is transmitted up the radial shaft; the radial head then fractures when it strikes the capitulum (Fig. 1). In the latter case, if the violence is severe, the inferior radioulnar joint subluxes, the interosseous membrane tears, and there is a highly comminuted fracture of the radial head (the so-called Essex–Lopresti fracture dislocation).

A large number of fracture patterns are seen, but the main decision to be made is whether the fracture is highly comminuted and displaced or not; this is established by careful examination of the radiographs.

Treatment

If the fracture is highly comminuted (Fig. 2), the fragments should be excised without delay, preferably within the first 48 hours after injury, to lessen the risks of myositis ossificans. After operation the elbow is rested in a sling for 2–3 weeks before being mobilised. If there is much additional soft tissue damage (e.g. if the elbow has been dislocated as well or if there has been an injury of the Essex–Lopresti type) or if there is a delay in making the diagnosis, then excision is best left until after the fracture has united.

If the radial head is removed there is always a tendency for the radius to drift in a proximal direction in order to close the gap between the radial neck and the capitulum. This may result in subluxation of the inferior radioulnar joint; the distal end of the ulna may become rather prominent and the wrist may become weak and painful. To avoid this risk some surgeons favour the insertion of a prosthetic radial head replacement.

If the fracture is hair-line in pattern or only slightly displaced (Fig. 3) the arm may be rested in a sling and mobilised once the acute symptoms have settled — usually within 3 weeks. Ultimately, an excellent result is usually achieved, although it may take many months before the joint is capable of full extension.

If the fracture is not comminuted, but is nevertheless badly displaced, some advocate immediate operative reduction; others prefer to treat the injury expectantly, only performing late excision if there is persisting severe restriction of movement after an adequately long period of mobilisation.

FRACTURE OF THE RADIAL NECK

The radial neck may be fractured by the same mechanisms which can cause the head to fracture. In some cases the fracture is hair-line or only slightly displaced; in others there is considerable angulation; and in children the epiphysis of the head may be completely separated and badly displaced (Fig. 4). The fracture is diagnosed and assessed by radiographs. Note that the plane of the radial head is at right angles to a line passing through the centre of the radial neck.

Treatment

Hair-line and minimally angled fractures may be treated by resting the arm in a sling for 2–3 weeks before commencing mobilisation. If the fracture is more severely angled, it may be manipulated by applying pressure over the area of the radial head on the lateral aspect of the elbow while pronating and supinating the arm. In grossly displaced epiphyseal injuries (Fig. 5) the fracture must be reduced. This can sometimes be achieved without open operation by inserting a Kirschner wire into the radial head and levering it back into position under intensifier control. After reduction the fragments may lock together; otherwise they may be stabilised using percutaneous Kirschner wires.

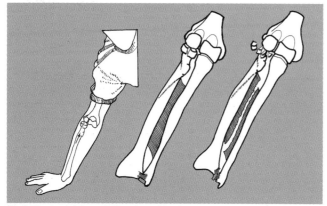

Fig. 1 Fracture of the radial head resulting from a fall on the outstretched hand.

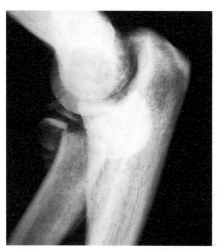

Fig. 2 Displaced, comminuted fracture of the radial head.

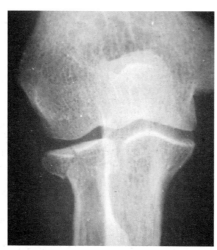

Fig. 3 Minimally displaced marginal fracture of the radial head.

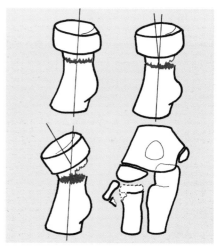

Fig. 4 Fractures of the radial neck.

FRACTURES OF THE OLECRANON

The olecranon may be fractured as a result of a fall on the point of the elbow or from a sudden contraction of the triceps muscle. There is local tenderness which is often accompanied by bruising and skin abrasion. The diagnosis is confirmed by X-ray. It is important to be able to distinguish between a normal epiphyseal line and a fracture and, if a fracture is present, the size of the proximal fragment and whether it has become displaced as a result of triceps muscle pull. If the fracture is hair line and undisplaced, it may be treated conservatively in a plaster cast until united. If the fragment is displaced and small, it may be excised and the triceps expansion repaired. If the fragment is substantial and displaced (Fig. 6), then it should be reduced and internally fixed. The methods available include tension band wiring, screwing and plating.

ANTERIOR FRACTURE–DISLOCATION OF THE ELBOW

This uncommon injury most frequently occurs as a result of a fall in which the upper forearm is pushed forwards, fracturing the proximal part of the ulna or the olecranon (Fig. 7). Less commonly it may be seen in company with a fracture of the humeral shaft and one or both of the forearm bones in so-called 'baby car' or side-swipe fracture. (This occurs when a driver rests his elbow on his car's window ledge and is struck by a passing vehicle.) Reduction may be achieved by applying traction and extending the joint; thereafter it is generally advisable to secure the joint from late subluxation by internal fixation of the fracture. In the management of side-swipe injuries it is vital to reduce the elbow dislocation immediately and to stabilise the proximal

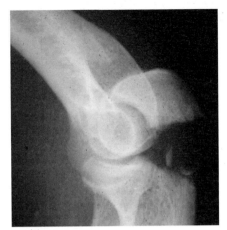

Fig. 6 **Displaced fracture of the olecranon with a large proximal fragment.**

ulnar fracture either by a plaster cast, with the elbow in extension, for 2–3 weeks prior to internal fixation or, preferably, by immediate internal fixation. The other fractures may be treated with less urgency by conservative or surgical means. It is not always possible (or desirable) to attempt the immediate internal fixation of all the elements of this very severe injury.

PULLED ELBOW

This injury is seen in children, usually between the ages of 2 and 6. The child is fretful, complains of pain in the elbow and refuses to use or move the joint. There is lateral tenderness and supination is restricted. The onset is sudden and there is usually a clear history of a traumatic incident involving traction on the arm — commonly when a parent suddenly pulls on a child's hand to restrain it from running on to a road. The history of injury allows it to be distinguished from, for example, infections or other pathology in the region. It is

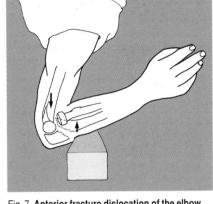

Fig. 7 **Anterior fracture dislocation of the elbow.**

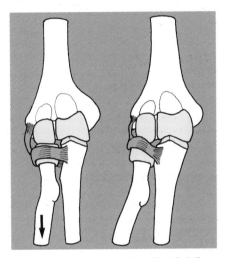

Fig. 8 **Subluxation of the radial head in pulled elbow.**

considered that the lesion is one of the radial head stretching and slipping out from under cover of the annular ligament (Fig. 8). As it is essentially a soft tissue injury, the radiographs seldom show any abnormality. This subluxation reduces spontaneously if the arm is rested in a sling for 48 hours, but some prefer to carry out an immediate reduction by rapidly pronating and supinating the forearm.

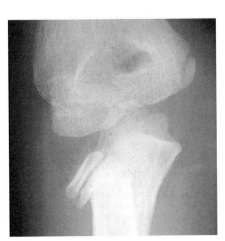

Fig. 5 **Gross displacement of the epiphysis of the radial head.**

Proximal fractures of the radius and ulna

- The majority of fractures of the radial head may be treated conservatively.
- In most cases of radial head fracture there is good recovery of pronation and supination, but elbow extension may be long delayed.
- If an excision of a fractured radial head is being planned, this should be done either within 48 hours of the injury, or delayed until after the fracture has united.
- Small displaced fractures of the olecranon may be dealt with by excision, but large fragments should be reduced and internally fixed so that triceps function is restored and there is no joint instability.
- The radius and ulna can only dislocate anteriorly if there is a fracture of the proximal part of the ulna.
- If there is an anterior dislocation of the elbow, it is usually necessary to internally fix the accompanying ulnar fracture to obtain stability.
- The diagnosis of pulled elbow is made on clinical grounds alone.

FRACTURES OF THE FOREARM BONES

The radius and ulna are linked closely to one another at both ends (by the superior and inferior radioulnar joints) and throughout their length by the interosseous membrane. It follows that both must share the effects of any indirect violence applied to the limb (e.g. from a fall on the outstretched hand). In practice, what this means is that either both will fracture ('fracture of both bones of the forearm'), or one will fracture and the articular end of the other will dislocate (Monteggia fracture–dislocation or Galeazzi fracture–dislocation).

In the case of direct violence, it is perfectly possible for the forces to be concentrated on a single forearm bone, leading to its fracture, without the other being affected (a common instance of this is when the ulna is struck by a club or other weapon as the victim tries to ward off a blow to the head).

PATTERNS OF DEFORMITY

In children, the fracture is often (but not always) greenstick in pattern. The deformity then is purely one of angulation. Although this may be quite severe (Fig. 1) the bone ends remain in close contact and reduction of the fracture is easy, being merely a question of correcting the angulation.

In adults (but also sometimes in children), the bone ends may separate and take up positions determined not only by the direction of the forces leading to the fracture, but by the effects of the pull of the muscles inserted into the fragments: the fractures of the radius and ulna may displace, angulate and rotate independently of one another (Fig. 2).

Loss of bony contact, angulation and displacement are easy enough to see and interpret on the radiographs. Although rotation can be difficult to detect, its presence should always be sought. In all fractures of the radius, pronator quadratus tends to pronate the distal fragment and biceps humeri to supinate the proximal fragment. Axial rotation of the bone fragments is greatest in fractures of the proximal third of the radius, when the pull of the biceps is unopposed and pronator quadratus is assisted by pronator teres. The deforming forces are less marked in fractures in the middle or distal thirds, when pronator teres neutralises the pull of biceps and the only deforming force is that of pronator quadratus (Fig. 3). Radiographic clues to the presence of

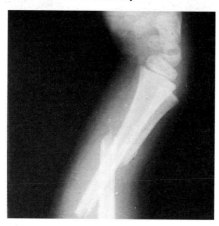

Fig. 1 **Greenstick fracture of both bones of the forearm with marked deformity.**

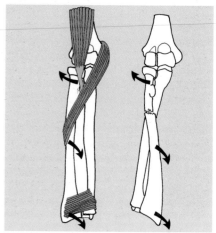

Fig. 2 **Displaced fractures of the radius and ulna.**

rotational deformity may include the relative widths of the bone ends (of the radius) at the fracture site, the relative position of fracture interdigitations and the position of the radial tubercle relative to the radial styloid process.

TREATMENT OF FOREARM FRACTURES

Greenstick fractures

When the fracture is of greenstick pattern, the fracture is manipulated under general anaesthesia and any angulation corrected. Due to the elasticity of the periosteum on the concave side of the fracture there is always a tendency to recurrence of the deformity; this should be borne in mind and is the reason why the position of the fracture should be checked with fresh radiographs at weekly intervals until union is far advanced. To reduce the risks of late recurrence of the deformity, some surgeons advocate momentary overcorrection of the deformity during the manipulation to break the intact periosteum on the concavity of the deformity.

After reduction the arm is put up in a long arm padded plaster in pronation in cases of anterior angulation (posterior tilting) and in supination where there has been posterior angulation.

Displaced fractures in children

The powers of remodelling in children are excellent in the case of off-ending,

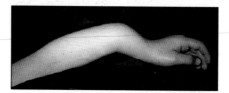

Fig. 3 **Relative effects of biceps, pronator teres and pronator quadratus in the production of axial rotation in radial fractures.**

good in the case of angulation, but fairly poor as far as axial rotation is concerned. The ability to remodel any deformity persisting after a fracture deteriorates with age, particularly beyond the age of 9 or 10. Remodelling tends to be best in the plane of the greatest range of movement and near the epiphyses. This all influences what may or may not be considered to be an acceptable position of a fracture. In practice, displaced children's forearm fractures are treated by traction and attempted manipulative reduction under general anaesthesia. The reduction obtained may then be assessed as follows: (i) persistent displacement, including in the extreme case complete loss of bony contact, may be accepted if this cannot be improved upon; (ii) slight angulation of 10 degrees or less, while undesirable, will correct with remodelling in the younger child, and should be accepted; (iii) where there is gross angulation (20 degrees or more) then the fractures should be remanipulated.

After care. A long arm plaster slab with the forearm in the appropriate position (completed as soon as the swelling subsides) is the usual form of initial support. Check radiographs should be taken at weekly intervals for 3–4 weeks until stability is achieved. The cast should be changed if it shows any sign of becoming slack. Late slipping of the fracture is not uncommon. Minor degrees of angulation may be accepted, but if there is gross late angulation, the fracture should be re-manipulated, even if this means fracturing any early callus that has appeared; this is especially indicated in the older child.

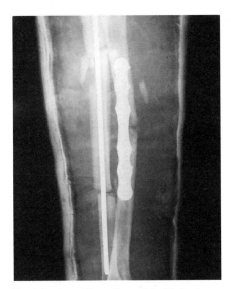

Fig. 4 **Fracture of the radius and double fracture of the ulna treated by plating and intramedullary nailing.**

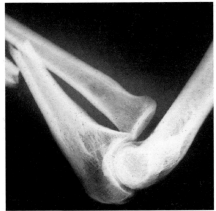

Fig. 5 **Anterior Monteggia fracture.**

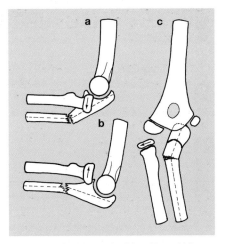

Fig. 6 **Posterior (a), anterior (b) and lateral (c) Monteggia fracture–dislocations.**

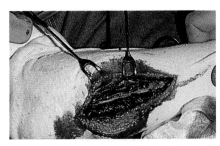

Fig. 7 **Plating of the ulna to stabilise a Monteggia fracture.**

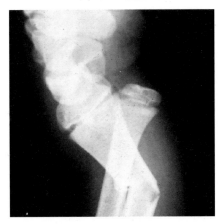

Fig. 8 **Galeazzi fracture–dislocation.**

Fractures in adults

In the adult, all but the power of local remodelling is lost, and to reduce and hold a forearm fracture by closed methods can be extremely difficult. While it is reasonable to treat undisplaced fractures by long arm plaster casts (particularly in the case of isolated fractures of the radius or ulnar shafts), great care is needed in the follow-up to detect any slipping that may occur and to deal with it promptly. As a rule the majority of forearm fractures in the adult are best treated by open reduction and internal fixation (Fig. 4). Separate incisions are employed for each fracture to reduce the risks of cross union, a feared complication of forearm fractures.

THE MONTEGGIA FRACTURE–DISLOCATION

This is a fracture of the ulna associated with a dislocation of the radial head and may arise from forced pronation of the forearm or from direct violence. The radial head may dislocate anteriorly (Fig. 5), posteriorly or laterally (in children), in each case with a corresponding angled fracture of the ulna (Fig. 6). The key to the successful management of this fracture is an accurate reduction and fixation of the ulnar fracture; reduction of the dislocated radial head usually follows spontaneously. In children, any greenstick angulation of the ulna should be corrected by manipulation and, in the case of an anterior Monteggia, the arm put up with the elbow in 90 degrees of flexion and in full supination. Posterior Monteggia fractures are often stable in full extension, but the arm should not be held in this position for more than 3 weeks before repositioning in 90 degrees flexion. Frequent check films should be taken and exploration considered if there is any sign of radial head subluxation. In the adult, open reduction and internal fixation of the ulnar fracture is the usual practice, with the radial head only rarely requiring open reduction. In practice it is usual to fix the ulna with a plate or other device (Fig. 7).

THE GALEAZZI FRACTURE–DISLOCATION

In this combination of injuries a fracture of the radial shaft is associated with a dislocation of the inferior radioulnar joint (Fig. 8). In children this may be treated by manipulative reduction, with the arm being put up in plaster in full supination. Open reduction is seldom required. In adults, however, it is difficult to reduce and hold this injury by closed methods and poor fixation may be associated with non-union. It is therefore usually best to treat Galeazzi fracture–dislocations in adults by open reduction and plating of the radius.

Fractures of the forearm bones

- Do not accept a fracture of the radius or ulna as being an isolated injury until you have excluded a fracture or dislocation at either end of the other bone.
- Bone remodelling in children's fractures can be remarkable, but decreases significantly at the age of 9–10, until by adolescence it is not much better than in the adult.
- As a rule displaced fractures of the forearm bones are best treated in children by manipulation, and in adults by open reduction and internal fixation.
- Where open reduction of forearm fractures is required, separate incisions must be used for the radius and the ulna to reduce the risks of cross union (which would result in the loss of all pronation and supination).
- Reduction and fixation of the ulnar fracture is the key to the treatment of Monteggia fracture–dislocations.
- Galeazzi fracture–dislocations are best treated in the adult by plating of the radius.

COLLES' FRACTURE

A Colles' fracture is one of the distal radius; it occurs within 2.5 cms of the wrist and has characteristic deformities. Although it is the most common of all fractures, it was not until 1814 that it was first adequately described by Abraham Colles (hence its name).

Aetiology

It almost always results from a fall on the outstretched hand It often occurs when someone trips and involuntarily reaches out in an attempt to prevent their head contacting the ground; the force of impact is taken by the hand and transferred to the radius. The stresses in the radius exceed those it can tolerate and it fractures. The force of the fall and the manner of impact determine the nature and severity of the displacement of the fracture. This is a fracture which occurs in adults. Although similar violence in children may also result in fracture, the presence of the radial epiphysis and the elasticity of their bones generally produce a different pattern of injury. In the young adult Colles' fractures are not particularly common but should be treated with respect as they are usually of high energy pattern. The fracture is most prevalent in middle-aged and elderly women, often as a result of very minor trauma; there is no doubt that the presence of a degree of osteoporosis is a common aetiological factor.

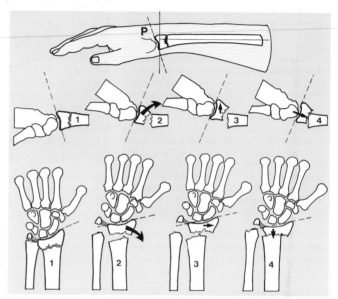

Fig. 1 **The plane of the wrist joint (P) and sequence of deformities in Colles' fracture.** Undisplaced (1); dorsal and radial tilting (2) and displacement (3); impaction (4).

Deformities in Colles' fracture

When the violence involved is minimal, the fracture may in fact remain undisplaced. Such fractures are easily treated (by rest in a plaster cast until union has taken place, usually at about 6 weeks) and unless some complication ensues the results are almost invariably excellent.

With greater violence the distal radial fragment may be displaced and tilted, both in a dorsal and radial direction. The fracture is almost always impacted. The dorsal tilting of the distal fragment affects the plane of the wrist joint. Normally this is not at right angles to the radius, but is tilted anteriorly by about 6 degrees (Fig. 1). This anterior tilting is reduced in the majority of Colles' fractures and, indeed, the plane of the wrist may be inclined posteriorly. If uncorrected, the overall effect is to permanently decrease the range of palmarflexion by at least the amount of angular alteration in the plane of the wrist joint; it may also result in some weakness of the wrist and a greater tendency to the development of carpal tunnel syndrome. Where dorsal displacement and tilting are quite marked, there is conspicuous deformity of the limb. The increase in the convex curvature of the anterior surface of the wrist when viewed with the fingers gives rise to the term 'dinner fork deformity' (Fig. 2).

The radial displacement and tilting of the distal fragment lead to disruption of the inferior radioulnar joint. The distal end of the radius is connected to the ulnar styloid process by the triangular fibrocartilage. In some cases this tears away from the bone and in others it avulses the ulnar styloid itself. This is an important cause of disability following Colles' fracture as the mechanics of the inferior radioulnar joint are disturbed. Pronation and supination may be reduced and become painful at the extremes and the joint may remain tender. As a result of impaction of the fracture and subsequent resorption of bone, the distal radial fragment is moved proximally in relation to the relatively intact ulna; the effect is that on the dorsal surface of the wrist the distal end of the ulna becomes relatively prominent. The ensuing deformity may be conspicuous and the distal end of the ulna may impinge on the carpus.

Diagnosis

Complaint of pain in the wrist after a fall on the outstretched hand in any adult merits a careful clinical and X-ray examination. Tenderness over the distal radius is invariable, and in many cases the characteristic deformity leaves little doubt. Do be careful to eliminate the presence of a scaphoid fracture: in an isolated scaphoid fracture there is no deformity and tenderness is situated over that bone and not over the radius. Remember, however, that on rare occasions the scaphoid may be fractured in conjunction with the

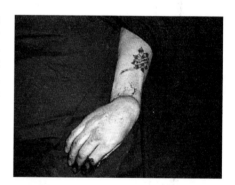

Fig. 2 **Dinner fork deformity of the wrist typical of a badly displaced Colles' fracture.**

distal radius, so always look for both fractures. If there is tenderness over the scaphoid, then specialised X-ray views of the scaphoid will be required.

Treatment

In the majority of cases good results follow conservative treatment by fixation in a plaster cast until the fracture has united. Preliminary reduction will be required if in the lateral projection of the wrist the plane of the wrist has become dorsally inclined (Fig. 3) and/or disruption of the inferior radio-ulnar joint is rendered obvious in the AP radiographs (Fig. 4).

Reduction is carried out under intravenous regional or general anaesthesia. Traction is applied to the limb, and the distal radial fragment realigned with the radial shaft by applying pressure with the heels of the hands. A plaster back shell (to allow for swelling) is then applied (although some advocate a complete plaster cast at this stage). The limb is elevated in a sling. In some cases where there is marked instability as a result of gross comminution of the distal fragment, the reduction may be maintained with an external fixator or percutaneous Kirschner wires.

After care
The reduction is checked with radiographs and the circulation and the fixation reviewed the following day. As a rule subsidence of the swelling will allow completion of the cast within 4 days, when the sling may also be discarded. Some advocate check X-rays at one week, with remanipulation if there is significant loss of position. The shoulder and fingers must be exercised. The cast may be removed when the fracture has united (usually at about 6 weeks) and if there is any significant weakness or stiffness, referral for physiotherapy may be advised. This should be continued until full recovery or until progress has come to a halt.

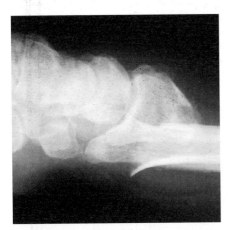

Fig. 3 **Radiograph showing the plane of the wrist tilted dorsally.**

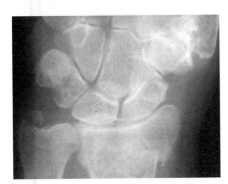

Fig. 4 **Radiograph showing radial displacement and tilting of the distal radial fragment, with avulsion of the ulnar styloid process and disruption of the inferior radioulnar joint.**

COMPLICATIONS OF COLLES' FRACTURE

Stiffness of the wrist and weakness of grip
These are almost always present when the plaster cast is first discarded, but if severe, or if still present to a significant degree 2 weeks later, then physiotherapy should be prescribed.

Malunion
In most Colles' fractures there is absorption of bone at the fracture site in the radius leading to some shortening of that bone; when this is severe, the distal end of the ulna becomes prominent. Persistent 'dinner fork' deformity is usually the result of imperfect reduction of the fracture or a failure to maintain the position after manipulation. Malunion is generally regretfully accepted and, with the exception of the young, corrective osteotomy is seldom recommended.

Sudeck's atrophy / post-traumatic reflex sympathetic dystrophy
This may be first noticed at about 6 weeks when the patient comes out of plaster. The swelling of the fingers, joint stiffness and widespread tenderness may be mistaken for lack of union of the fracture. The diagnosis may be confirmed by X-ray examination (Fig. 5). Intensive physiotherapy is usually indicated and other measures may be advised (see p. 43)

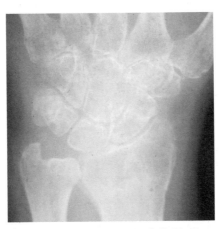

Fig. 5 **Sudeck's atrophy following Colles' fracture.**

Shoulder stiffness
This is a common complication which in most cases can be prevented by the performance of appropriate mobilising exercises starting on the day of injury. The patient should be carefully instructed in these and their importance stressed.

Carpal tunnel syndrome
After a Colles' fracture the median nerve may become compressed in the region of the carpal tunnel; this may be due to a variety of causes including post-traumatic swelling, persisting deformity and local new bone formation. It may cause tingling in the thumb and index and (rarely) weakness of the small muscles of the thumb. If these symptoms appear early, the cast should be checked for tightness. If symptoms persist after union of the fracture, further investigation and carpal tunnel decompression are advised as soon as possible.

Delayed rupture of extensor pollicis longus
Some months after the fracture the patient may lose the ability to extend the distal joint of the thumb due to rupture of the tendon of EPL. (This may be the result of the tendon rubbing against the fracture or from interference with its blood supply.) The usual treatment is operative, by tendon transfer using the tendon of extensor indicis proprius.

Fracture of the scaphoid
If initially a scaphoid fracture is found complicating a Colles' fracture, as a rule the Colles' fracture should be manipulated in the usual fashion and both fractures supported by a scaphoid plaster. A longer period of immobilisation may be required until both fractures have united. If (unusually) the scaphoid fracture in these circumstances is unstable, internal fixation of the scaphoid fracture is desirable; the concurrent Colles' fracture may then be treated by conservative methods.

Colles' fracture
- The Colles' fracture is the most common of all fractures.
- The fracture requires reduction only if significantly displaced.
- Union is usually sufficiently far advanced to allow splintage to be discarded after 5–6 weeks.
- An excellent or very good recovery is the usual outcome.
- Although the chances of problems arising in an individual fracture are low, complications are frequently seen as this fracture is so common and vigilance in its treatment is always required.

SMITH'S AND OTHER FRACTURES OF THE DISTAL RADIUS/WRIST SPRAINS

Apart from Colles' fracture, there are a number of other fractures which commonly occur at the distal end of the radius. Broadly speaking these fall into two categories: other fractures of the distal end of the radius in adults, where the mechanisms of injury may not be the same as those in Colles' fracture; and fractures in children, where the same mechanisms of injury produce different results (due to the malleability of the bones and the presence of the epiphyses).

ADULT FRACTURES OF THE DISTAL END OF THE RADIUS

SMITH'S FRACTURE

This fracture of the distal radius is often referred to as a reversed Colles' fracture as the distal radial fragment is displaced and tilted anteriorly (rather than posteriorly as in a Colles' fracture). A clear history of injury is seldom obtained, but it may result from a fall on the back of the hand (Fig. 1).

Treatment

If the fracture is more than minimally displaced, reduction will be required; this may be difficult to carry out and even harder to maintain. As usual, traction is applied under intravenous regional or general anaesthetic until the distal fragment is disimpacted, and pressure applied with the heels of the hands to reduce the displacement. The wrist is then dorsiflexed and turned into full supination, a position which must be maintained with a long arm plaster, holding the elbow in 90 degrees flexion. The reduction not infrequently slips, and a most careful follow-up is required, with radiographs being taken at weekly intervals; if any slip occurs, re-manipulation may be required. In view of these potential difficulties many surgeons prefer to carry out an open reduction and internal fixation, using a small buttress plate applied to the anterior surface of the radius.

BARTON'S FRACTURE

This is an intra-articular variation of Smith's fracture where the anterior part of the distal radius only is involved. The small fragment becomes displaced anteriorly, with a gap opening up in the articular surface of the radius. The carpus

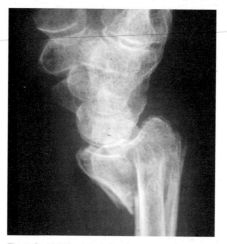
Fig. 1 Smith's fracture following a fall on the back of the hand.

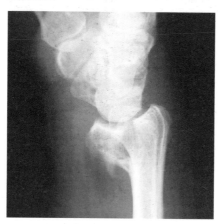
Fig. 2 Barton's fracture resulting in a gap in the distal articular surface of the radius which affects the radiocarpal joint.

tends to follow the anterior fragment and its articulation with the radius is seriously affected (Fig. 2). If uncorrected, radiocarpal osteoarthritis is inevitable, and these injuries are generally treated by open reduction and the application of an anterior buttress plate.

FRACTURE OF THE RADIAL STYLOID PROCESS

This may result from a fall on the outstretched hand or from a kickback when using an engine starting handle. Most are undisplaced (Fig. 3) and do well by simple immobilisation in a Colles' type plaster cast for 6 weeks. Displaced fractures are usually high energy injuries and may be associated with fractures of the scaphoid, with or without carpal instability. The styloid process fracture may be treated by internal screw fixation. Note that there is a high incidence of Sudeck's atrophy (reflex sympathetic dystrophy) following injuries of this pattern.

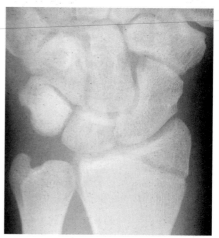
Fig. 3 Undisplaced fracture of the radial styloid process.

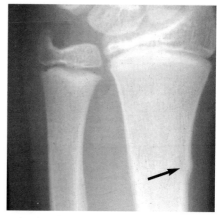
Fig. 4 Greenstick fracture of the distal end of the radius.

CHILDREN'S FRACTURES OF THE DISTAL END OF THE RADIUS

GREENSTICK FRACTURE

The distal end of the radius may fracture without disturbing the epiphysis. The position of the fracture line is rather variable and in the more minor cases may be difficult to detect; local kinking of the cortex of the radius may be the only sign (Fig. 4). In other cases there is deformity, with the distal fragment tilted dorsally as in a Colles' fracture or anteriorly as in a Smith's fracture (Fig. 5). If there is very marked local angulation, manipulation will be required; otherwise a short period (e.g. of about 3 weeks) of immobilisation in a plaster cast is the only treatment that is usually required.

OVERLAPPING RADIAL FRACTURE

In this injury (which also occurs in adults) the radius is cleanly broken (i.e. it

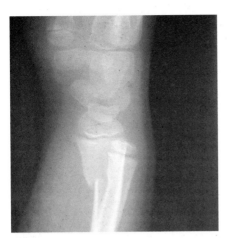

Fig. 5 **Greenstick fracture with the distal fragment tilted anteriorly (Smith-like deformity).**

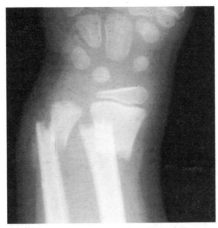

Fig. 6 **Fracture of the distal ends of both radius and ulna in a child.**

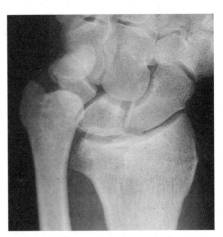

Fig. 8 **Traumatic (radial) epiphyseal arrest, with relative overgrowth of the ulna.**

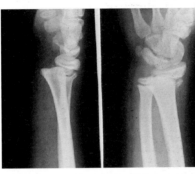

Fig. 7 **Slipped radial epiphysis with juxta-epiphyseal fracture of the distal end of the radial diaphysis.**

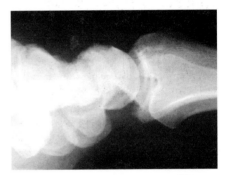

Fig. 9 **Avulsion fracture of carpus from a forcible flexion sprain of the wrist.**

is not a greenstick fracture) and the distal fragment is completely displaced, overlapping the proximal fragment. In addition, the ulna is involved: it often fractures close to the wrist (Fig. 6) or its distal end may dislocate (Galeazzi fracture–dislocation). These fractures can be difficult to reduce as strong traction alone may not be enough to overcome the overlap. There are a number of manipulative techniques which may be tried; if these are unsuccessful, then open reduction will be needed.

FRACTURE DISPLACEMENT OF THE LOWER RADIAL EPIPHYSIS (SLIPPED RADIAL EPIPHYSIS)

In this injury, which is seen in adolescents, the distal radial epiphysis is displaced posteriorly. As it moves out of alignment it usually causes a small fracture of the dorsal surface of the distal radial shaft, and this small bony fragment preserves its relationship with the epiphysis (juxta-epiphyseal fracture) (Fig. 7). Injuries of this pattern are treated like Colles' fractures by manipulative reduction and support in a plaster cast. Delay in reduction should be avoided as after 2 or 3 days rapidly occurring local tissue changes may render manipulative reduction impossible. In some cases growth of the radial epiphysis may be disturbed (traumatic epiphyseal arrest); if the ulna is unaffected, it overgrows (Fig. 8), leading in some cases to pain, weakness and limitation of movement in the wrist.

MINOR AND MAJOR SPRAINS OF THE WRIST

The wrist may be sprained when subjected to stresses which, although quite severe, are not great enough to produce a major fracture. In many cases the mechanisms of injury are similar to those causing fracture (e.g. falls on the front or the back of the hand). They may also occur if the wrist is forcibly dorsiflexed or twisted — for example in the process of manipulating heavy loads. As a result of the forces applied, there may be stretching and some tearing of capsular ligaments. In some cases tension on the carpal ligaments produces minor avulsion fractures of the carpus or radius (seen as tiny bone fragments in the radiographs) (Fig. 9). Clinically there is complaint of pain in the wrist following injury; there may be swelling and there is often widespread tenderness. A careful examination is necessary to exclude other injuries, in particular, fractures of the scaphoid, and an X-ray examination is mandatory in all but the most minor cases. Treatment of these injuries is symptomatic. As pain on movement is a common feature, support in a plaster cast for 2 or 3 weeks is usually advised.

Smith's and other fractures of the distal radius/wrist sprains

- Greenstick fractures of the radius are sometimes difficult to detect in the radiographs and are not infrequently overlooked.
- Overlapping fractures of the distal end of the radius sometimes require open reduction.
- Sudeck's atrophy (reflex sympathetic dystrophy) may follow any injury about the wrist (even when the soft tissues alone are involved), but is comparatively common after radial styloid fractures.
- If possible, the integrity of the articular surface of the distal end of the radius must be maintained; if this is seriously disturbed (e.g. in a Barton's fracture) open reduction and internal fixation are usually indicated.
- Injuries involving the distal radial epiphysis may sometimes be followed by growth disturbance at the wrist.
- Any delay in manipulation of a slipped radial epiphysis may prevent reduction.
- It is important to exclude a fracture of the scaphoid when a sprain of the wrist is suspected.
- Simple wrist sprains, even when complicated by minor avulsion fractures, generally require only symptomatic treatment.

FRACTURES AND DISLOCATIONS OF THE CARPAL BONES

FRACTURES OF THE SCAPHOID

The scaphoid may fracture as a result of a fall on the outstretched hand, from a kickback when using an engine starting-handle or, rarely, from repeated minor stress.

Diagnosis

A fracture may be suspected if there is complaint of pain in the wrist and tenderness is found both in the anatomical snuff box and over the anterior and posterior surfaces of the scaphoid. The diagnosis is confirmed by X-rays. The fracture is often hair-line and frequently difficult to detect. Good quality, well centred films are essential, with a minimum of three projections (AP, lateral and oblique(s)). To ensure that these are taken it is necessary to fill in the request form correctly — i.e. to ask specifically for X-rays of the scaphoid (rather than the wrist). In some cases the fracture may only become visible after 1 or 2 weeks when decalcification at the fracture site renders it more obvious.

Clinical features

The scaphoid is an important component of two major joints (Fig. 1): the radiocarpal joint (which involves the radius and the proximal row of the carpus which consists of the scaphoid, lunate and triquetral); and the joint between the proximal row of the carpus and the distal row (made up of the trapezium, trapezoid, capitate and hamate). As a result of its unique position and the stresses of activity that it normally resists, certain fractures of the scaphoid may be accompanied by carpal instability and/or separation of its fragments (unstable injuries). This, along with the fact that scaphoid fractures are intra-articular, may lead to non-union. Fracture may also interrupt the blood supply to the proximal pole of the scaphoid, leading to avascular necrosis.

Classification

Fractures of the scaphoid may be divided into stable and unstable injuries (Fig. 2). Stable injuries have the best prognosis. Fractures of the tubercle (A1) are never associated with avascular necrosis and non-union is not a problem. Undisplaced hair-line fractures of the waist (A2) have a relatively good prognosis although avascular necrosis of the proximal fragment may sometimes arise. The

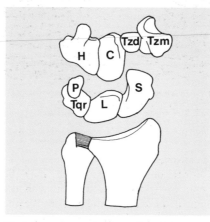

Fig. 1 **The radiocarpal and carpal row joints.**
H = hamate; C = capitate; Tzd = trapezoid; Tzm = trapezium; P = pisiform; Tqr = triquetral; L = lunate; S = scaphoid.

prognosis is poorer in unstable injuries, which have the highest incidence of non-union and avascular necrosis. The most common patterns of the injuries that are seen include oblique fractures involving the distal third of the bone (B1); displaced fractures through the waist (B2); fractures of the proximal pole (B3) where the incidence of avascular necrosis is particularly high; fractures of the scaphoid found in association with carpal dislocation (B4); and comminuted or multifragmentary fractures of the scaphoid (B5).

Treatment

Where a fracture has been suspected, but not confirmed by X-ray, it is common practice to apply a cast for 2 weeks and then carry out a further X-ray examination of the scaphoid out of plaster. If a fracture shows up in the second set of radiographs, then 2 weeks immobilisation has been gained; if no fracture is seen, then in most cases the injury may be accepted as being a sprain and the cast discarded.

Established stable fractures of the scaphoid are treated by cast fixation. There is some debate about the need to include the thumb and the best position in which the wrist should be held when the cast is being applied, but the classical scaphoid cast includes the proximal phalanx of the thumb, with the wrist in dorsiflexion and radial deviation. After a 6 week period of immobilisation union should be assessed by clinical and X-ray examination. If the fracture has united, then mobilisation may be commenced; if not, plaster fixation should be continued. Then, at 12 weeks the situation

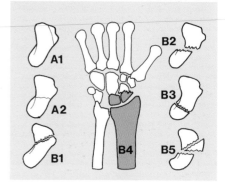

Fig. 2 **Fractures of the scaphoid.** A: stable; B: unstable.

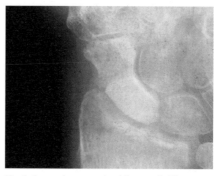

Fig. 3 **Avascular necrosis of the scaphoid.**

should be carefully reappraised. If avascular necrosis is present, surgical treatment should be considered (e.g. excision of the scaphoid with a prosthetic replacement). If there is established non-union, internal fixation (e.g. with a Herbert screw) and bone grafting are normally advised. If union is minimal, but there is no evidence of established non-union, internal fixation or a further period of fixation may be considered.

If on the initial radiographs the scaphoid is seen to be displaced, it is important to exclude the presence of a carpal dislocation. The amount of displacement should be assessed: if this exceeds 1 mm, or if the angulation of the fragments is greater than 15 degrees, then primary internal fixation should be carried out.

Complications

Sudeck's atrophy (reflex sympathetic dystrophy). This may be treated along general lines.

Avascular necrosis (Fig. 3). Excision of the scaphoid, with or without a prosthetic replacement, may be undertaken before secondary osteoarthritic changes supervene.

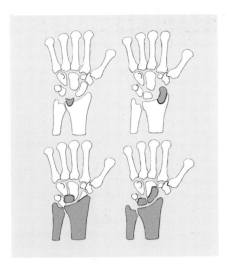

Fig. 4 **Carpal dislocations. Top**: dislocation of lunate; ...on of scaphoid. **Bottom**: perilunar dislocation ...; periscapholunar dislocation of carpus.

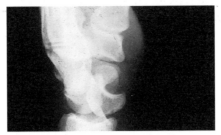

Fig. 5 **Dislocation of the lunate.** Note its halfmoon shape with the concavity facing anteriorly.

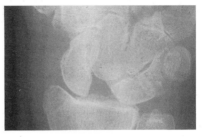

Fig. 6 **Scapholunate dissociation:** in the radiograph taken in ulnar deviation note the gap between these two bones.

...nion. Unless long established ...ught unlikely to cause symptoms, ...fixation and bone grafting ...e considered.

...rthritis of the wrist. Radio-...sion is the most reliable treat-...h the best prospects of pain ...nation and supination move-...e retained, but radiocarpal ...t is of course lost. Other treat-...metimes advocated include ...f the proximal row of the ...he use of an orthotic device to ...wrist.

CARPAL DISLOCATIONS

Carpal dislocations are comparatively uncommon, and fall into two main groups. In the most common situation the majority of the carpal bones and the hand remain in alignment with the radius, with one or more carpal bones dislocating (e.g. dislocation of the lunate, Figs 4 and 5); in the second group of injuries one or more of the carpal bones remain fast bound to the radius, while the rest of the carpus dislocates (e.g. peri-lunar dislocation of the carpus).

Dislocation of the lunate

Of all dislocations of the carpus, this is the most common. When the lunate dis-locates (which it does anteriorly), it may press on the median nerve, giving rise to paraesthesia in the thumb and index finger and sometimes weakness of the small muscles of the thumb. The diag-nosis is confirmed by the characteristic X-ray appearances; care must be taken in interpreting these, as the diagnosis is not infrequently missed (Fig. 5).

Treatment

Dislocations of the lunate may be reduced by applying traction with the hand in dorsiflexion and pressing the dis-located lunate back into position with the thumb; when the bone reduces, the hand is brought into the neutral position.

Any accompanying median nerve symptoms generally settle rapidly after prompt reduction. If there is delay in making the diagnosis, open reduction of the lunate may be required. In all cases there is a risk of avascular necrosis; if this complication ensues it may be treated along similar lines to avascular necrosis of the scaphoid.

Treatment of other carpal dislocations

The majority of other carpal dislocations may be treated by manipulative reduc-tion followed by a short period of plaster fixation. Where there is an associated unstable fracture of the scaphoid, its internal fixation is usually desirable.

CARPAL INSTABILITIES

These may follow a traumatic incident or degenerative joint disease (e.g. rheuma-toid arthritis) and are characterised by a loss of the normal alignment of the carpal bones. The main complaints are of pain and weakness of the wrist, and sometimes of clicking sensations from the joint on certain movements. In *static instabilities*, the abnormality is constant and normally shows in X-rays of the supinated wrist taken in radial and ulnar deviation. Scapholunate dissociation is the most common of these abnormalities (Fig. 6).

In *dynamic instabilities* the instability is momentary, and the patient is often able to toggle his carpal alignment from normal to abnormal and back again by moving his wrist in a certain way. The presence and nature of such abnormali-ties may be hard to confirm. Techniques available include the comparison of radi-ographs of the carpus (with lead markers over tender points) taken in the normal and subluxed positions; image intensifier screening of the wrist in motion; arthrog-raphy; and radioisotope bone scans to detect local inflammatory changes.

Treatment

The treatment of carpal instability is spe-cialised and is determined by the nature and severity of the instability, as well as the risks of secondary osteoarthritis in the carpal or radiocarpal joints. The most common and most useful procedure is the repair of the torn intercarpal ligaments responsible for the instability, the best results being obtained when such proce-dures are performed at an early stage. Some also advocate and claim good results from stabilising intercarpal fusions.

Fractures and dislocations of the carpal bones

- Fractures of the scaphoid may be difficult to detect, and special X-ray projections must be taken.
- If the initial radiographs are negative, further radiographs should be taken after 10–14 days if there is continuing local tenderness.
- Unstable fractures of the scaphoid should be treated by internal fixation.
- Avascular necrosis is a serious complication of both scaphoid fractures and dislocations of the lunate.
- Dislocations of the lunate may be accompanied by median nerve palsy requiring prompt treatment.
- Carpal instability may require extensive investigation before its presence and nature can be confirmed.

FRACTURES AND DISLOCATIONS OF THE METACARPALS

In assessing any metacarpal (or phalangeal) fracture, consider the following points:

- Is the fracture in an acceptable position? This is generally the case if there is at least 50% of bony contact, there is no rotational deformity and any angulation is less than 10 degrees (more can be accepted in the case of the fifth metacarpal neck).
- Is the fracture stable? If it is not, careful consideration must be given to what method is used to maintain its position; this is especially the case after operative reduction, and may be an indication for internal fixation. Instability is associated with badly displaced fractures, multiple fractures, comminuted fractures, many oblique and spiral fractures and displaced articular fractures.
- Are the fractures open and/or is there any major skin damage?
- Is there any accompanying vascular, nerve or tendon injury?

INJURIES OF THE THUMB

The thumb is most commonly injured as a result of being forced backwards (stave), from axially applied violence (e.g. from administering a punch) or from direct violence. At the base, the five most common patterns of injury include (Fig. 1):

(a) dislocation of the metacarpal
(b) dislocation of the first ray — that is, dislocation of thumb along with the trapezium
(c) Bennett's fracture–dislocation of the base of the thumb
(d) transverse fracture of the metacarpal
(e) Rolando fracture (T- or Y- fracture of the metacarpal involving the joint at the base of the thumb (trapezometacarpal joint)).

The clinical appearance of these injuries is often rather similar, but the diagnosis is easily established by standard radiographic projections.

Treatment

Pure dislocations at the base of the thumb are usually easy to reduce by the application of traction and, on the whole, these injuries are then comparatively stable. After reduction a few weeks' rest in a protective plaster cast is advisable; thereafter mobilisation is usually rapid and physiotherapy is seldom required.

In *Bennett's fracture–dislocation* the characteristic deformity is one of both

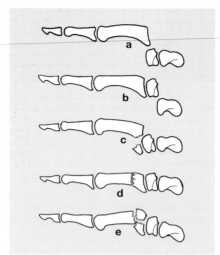

Fig. 1 **Five common injuries at the base of the thumb.**

proximal and lateral subluxation of the base of the metacarpal, with a small triangular fragment of bone from the metacarpal base remaining in an undisplaced position (Fig. 2). The principle of reduction is to realign the metacarpal with this fragment, which is generally quite easy to achieve by applying traction to the thumb and pressure over the metacarpal base. Maintaining reduction is often much more difficult, as this is an unstable injury. In a majority of cases the position may be held in a plaster cast, with the thumb in an abducted position. While the cast is setting, traction is maintained and the plaster moulded firmly round the base of the thumb which should be protected from the effects of local pressure with suitable padding. Careful follow-up is essential in case late slipping occurs. Alternatively a small screw may be used to bring the small fragment and the metacarpal into realignment or the metacarpal may be stabilised by means of two Kirschner wires, one passed through the first metacarpal into the second and the other into the trapezium.

Transverse fractures of the metacarpal seldom present any problem in management and should be treated along routine lines with a 6 week period of immobilisation in a cast. If the fracture is badly displaced, manipulation will be required.

Rolando T- or Y- fractures have a less good prognosis due to disturbance of the joint between the metacarpal and the trapezium. While a number of these may be dealt with by manipulation and cast fixation, others will require an attempt to restore the articular surface of the metacarpal base by open reduction and

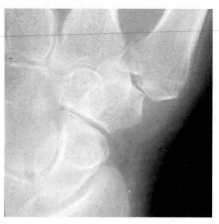

Fig. 2 **Bennett's fracture–dislocation of the thumb.**

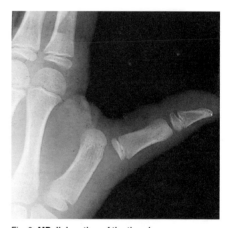

Fig. 3 **MP dislocation of the thumb.**

internal fixation with small screws or Kirschner wires.

Comminuted fractures through the shaft of the thumb metacarpal generally result from direct violence (e.g. in crushing injuries). Their treatment must be individually planned, being dependent on the accompanying deformity, the degree of comminution and whether the fractures are open or closed.

MP JOINT DISLOCATIONS AND SUBLUXATIONS

The MP joint of the thumb may be dislocated (Fig. 3) if the thumb is inadvertently forced back. This injury is particularly common in children. The metacarpal head may 'buttonhole' through the joint capsule and in some cases this may render manipulative reduction impossible. In treating these cases theatre facilities for open reduction should be available in case the dislocation cannot be corrected (under general anaesthesia) solely by traction and flexion of the thumb. After reduction a light plaster splint should be worn for 2–3 weeks.

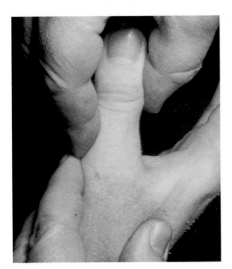

Fig. 4 **Testing the ulnar collateral ligament of the thumb.**

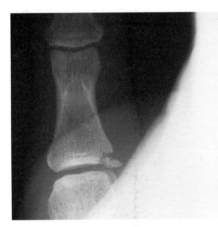

Fig. 5 **Avulsion of the bony attachment of the ulnar collateral ligament with displacement.**

ULNAR COLLATERAL LIGAMENT INJURIES

Abduction stress may sprain, tear or avulse the bony attachment of the ulnar collateral ligament of the thumb. This is an injury which is particularly common on artificial ski slopes when in a fall the thumb catches in the matting. It can be quite disabling if not recognised and treated. It may be suspected if there is complaint of pain and tenderness at the MP joint of the thumb close to the web space. The ligament should be tested by seeking laxity when an abduction stress is applied to the (extended) MP joint (Fig. 4). If laxity is slight, or if there is an undisplaced avulsion fracture, a 6 week period of immobilisation in a plaster cast of scaphoid pattern is advised, with retesting of the ligament at the end of this period. If there is an avulsion fracture which is displaced (Fig. 5) this should be reduced and fixed by open operation. Surgical repair is also advisable for very unstable or late diagnosed injuries.

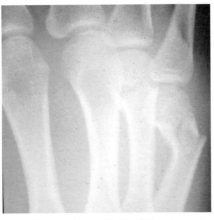

Fig. 6 **Fracture of the neck of the fifth metacarpal.**

INJURIES OF THE FIFTH METACARPAL

Fracture of the neck is the most common injury affecting the fifth metacarpal. It is most frequently acquired as a result of administering a punch. Diagnosis by clinical examination is usually easy and is confirmed by radiographs (Fig. 6). The distal fragment is often tilted anteriorly as a result of the blow, but the position may be accepted unless the tilt exceeds 45 degrees, when manipulative reduction will usually succeed in reducing the angulation to an acceptable level. The fracture may then be supported by a Colles' type plaster with an extension to support the proximal phalanx, with elevation in a sling for a few day until any swelling subsides. Transverse Kirschner wires may also be used to preserve the reduction.

Fractures near the metacarpal base, and spiral fractures of the midshaft (assuming that as is usually the case they are not significantly displaced or rotated) may be treated by rest in a Colles' type plaster cast for 3–4 weeks.

Transverse fractures of the midshaft of the metacarpal may be markedly displaced or badly angled (more than 20 degrees) and such deformities should be corrected. Various methods of internal fixation may employed, including the use of small plates, intramedullary or transverse Kirschner wires, or intra-osseous wiring.

Dislocation of the joint between the base of the fifth metacarpal and the hamate can generally be reduced by traction, but the injury is often unstable and may have to be stabilised with a Kirschner wire for 3–4 weeks.

Fractures involving a small fragment only of the head of the fifth metacarpal may be treated by strapping the ring and little fingers together; the fracture is thereby supported, while at the same time early movements are encouraged.

INJURIES TO THE OTHER METACARPALS

One or more metacarpals may be fractured as a result of direct trauma, particularly from crushing injuries. If there is significant skin damage, this must be taken into account in planning treatment, and the aim should be to establish skin cover at the earliest possible stage.

It is important to make sure that there is no rotational deformity at the fracture. When assessing this and also when applying splintage, note that under normal circumstances all the fingers when flexed strike the palm just distal to the scaphoid; where there is rotation in a metacarpal fracture the corresponding finger will fail to do so. Again, if the fingers are flexed to a right angle at the MP joints, and extended at the interphalangeal joints, the finger nails should lie in the same plane.

The most common situation is that of a stable metacarpal fracture with no significant soft tissue injury. Support in a simple cast, with initial elevation of the limb, is all that is usually required. Where unstable, displaced fractures have been sustained, reduction and internal fixation (e.g. by transversely running Kirschner wires, small plates, etc) may be called for.

Fractures and dislocations of the metacarpals

- Always assess the deformity and stability of a metacarpal fracture, and always look for any associated soft tissue injury.
- An X-ray examination is necessary to clarify the nature of any injury at the base of the thumb.
- Bennett's fracture–dislocation requires careful reduction and maintenance of the reduction.
- Metacarpophalangeal dislocations of the thumb may require open reduction.
- Rupture of the ulnar collateral ligament of the thumb may give lasting disability if not recognised and treated.
- Angulatory deformity is common in fractures of the neck of the fifth metacarpal and may be accepted unless very marked.
- In any metacarpal fracture look for the presence of rotational deformity.

PHALANGEAL INJURIES

INJURIES TO THE DISTAL PHALANX

The distal phalanx of a finger or thumb is most commonly fractured as a result of a crushing injury, e.g. from a misdirected hammer blow or from closure of a car door. The fracture may involve the terminal tuft, the neck or the base, with or without displacement (Fig. 1). The actual fracture is of much less importance than the accompanying soft tissue injury. If there is a painful subungual haematoma then some relief may be obtained if this is evacuated. If there is a skin wound making the fracture in effect open, then it should receive scrupulous attention to avoid the risks of bone infection. If there is loss of pulp skin, then an appropriate plastic surgical procedure should be carried out (e.g. full thickness skin graft, etc). As for the fracture itself, simple splinting to protect the finger from the pain of contact or stubbing should be provided (a plastic mallet-finger splint is often satisfactory). Only rarely, when the articular surface of the phalangeal base has been split without fragmentation and the bony components have separated, might reduction have to be considered.

MALLET FINGER

A mallet finger deformity occurs when function in the terminal part of the long extensor tendon (EDL) is lost or impaired. The result is that the long flexor tendon (FDP) pulls the distal phalanx into flexion and the distal interphalangeal joint cannot be actively extended (Fig. 2). Full passive movements are possible. The condition may result when an extended finger is forcibly flexed. It is commonly seen in cricketers; it also occurs in housewives when tucking sheets under a mattress. The cause is either a rupture of the distal slip of the extensor tendon close to its insertion or an actual avulsion of its bony attachment. If the bone fragment is large (more than 20% of the articular surface), the terminal phalanx may in some cases sublux (Fig. 3). If the condition has been present for some time, the proximal interphalangeal joint of the finger may hyperextend, producing a minor degree of swan neck deformity of the finger.

Treatment

Unless there is subluxation of the distal phalanx, a simple plastic splint (Stack or Abouna splint) may be used to hold the

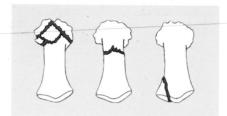

Fig. 1 **Common terminal phalangeal fractures.**

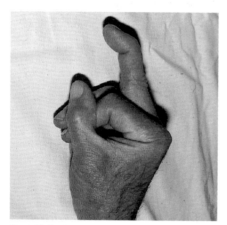

Fig. 2 **Mallet finger.**

DIP joint in extension until healing in the damaged structures is well advanced. Apart from removal for hygiene purposes (when the distal joint must be maintained in extension) the splint is worn constantly for 6 weeks and then for a further 2 weeks at night. On removal of the splintage there is often some slight recurrence of the deformity, but over the course of a year or so contraction in the fibrous tissue which forms in the torn tendon generally leads to spontaneous improvement; any residual functional impairment is generally minimal.

In those cases where there is subluxation of the distal phalanx, it is generally advisable to reattach the small bone fragment into which the extensor tendon is inserted; this is generally done with non-absorbable sutures.

FRACTURES OF THE MIDDLE AND PROXIMAL PHALANGES

These can be amongst the most difficult of injuries to treat, especially if there is accompanying skin, tendon, nerve or vascular damage. Fracture angulation from unbalanced tendon pull is common and reduction may be difficult to achieve and hard to maintain. Internal fixation may be technically challenging because of the small size of the bone fragments. If

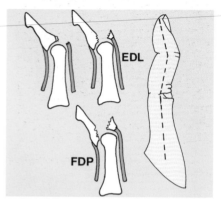

Fig. 3 **Lesions in mallet finger.** EDL = long extensor tendon; FDP = long flexor tendon.

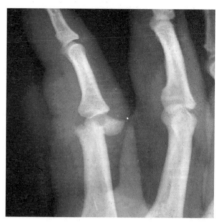

Fig. 4 **Badly displaced fracture involving a PIP joint.**

external fixation methods are employed, there is always the conflict between the need to support the finger for an adequate length of time (e.g. until union is sufficiently far advanced) and the necessity for early mobilisation before there is permanent stiffness in the related joints, with serious implications as far as hand function is concerned.

Assessment of closed injuries

Note the position of the fracture and its stability. The position of the fracture can generally be accepted if:

- any angulation is less than 10 degrees in the shaft or 20 degrees in the metaphysis
- there is more than 50% of bony contact
- there is no rotational deformity.

The fracture is likely to be unstable if:

- there is appreciable fragmentation at the fracture site
- it is of spiral pattern and rotated

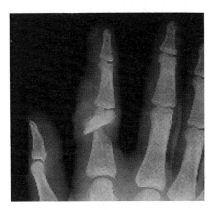

Fig. 5 **Displaced unstable fracture requiring open reduction and internal fixation.**

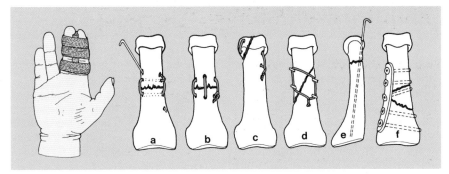

Fig. 6 **Garter strapping and some methods of internal fixation of phalangeal fractures.**

- there is considerable displacement
- it is a badly angled fracture of the neck of a proximal phalanx
- there are multiple fractures
- the fracture involves an articular surface and is displaced (Fig. 4).

If the fracture is in an acceptable position and appears to be stable, treatment is directed to relieving pain and swelling by providing elevation and local support. In practice this is usually achieved by: (i) the application of garter strapping (where adjacent fingers, with padding between, are strapped together, thereby providing support while at the same time allowing early movement) (Fig. 6), and (ii) high elevation of the limb in a broad arm sling for 2–3 days. In some badly displaced fractures it may be possible to obtain a good reduction by manipulation, after which the fracture may be sufficiently stable to be treated in a similar fashion or by a plaster cast or padded aluminium splint. In the latter case it is important to support only the injured finger, with its MP joint flexed at 90 degrees.

Many badly displaced fractures require open reduction and some form of internal fixation may have to be considered (Fig. 5). Many methods are available (Fig. 6) including:

(a) a single stainless steel wire passed through both fragments and reinforced with a percutaneous Kirschner wire
(b) two wires at right angles to one another
(c) small fragment wiring
(d) tension band wiring
(e) percutaneous intramedullary Kirschner wires
(f) the use of small plates and screws.

In some cases it may be desirable and possible to use a mini external fixator.

OPEN FRACTURES

Where the fracture is open the results become less predictable and many factors must be taken into consideration before deciding what is the best line of treatment for the particular patient and his injury. Often of great importance is the patient's work and his other interests and hobbies. If the wound is clean, primary closure is often possible, with fixation appropriate to the fracture. Treatment in ideal circumstances may also be extended to primary repair of any associated tendon or nerve injury. Where there is tissue contamination and the risks of infection are high, it may be wiser to delay nerve and tendon suture. Where there is soft tissue loss every effort should be made to obtain skin cover at the earliest opportunity, and the use of a mini external fixator may be helpful. Where the vascular supply to the finger is impaired, a decision may have to be made between making an attempt at restoring the circulation by microsurgery or amputating. With the former, treatment is likely to be prolonged and at best uncertain; a decision to embark on this will be dictated by the severity of the soft tissue injuries and the particular needs of the patient. Similar factors apply to replantation.

FINGER DISLOCATIONS AND SPRAINS

Dislocations of any of the finger joints (Fig. 7) are usually easy to reduce by traction. Thereafter, the finger should be splinted with garter strapping for 2 or 3 weeks until stability has returned (assessed by stressing the joint that was involved). In finger sprains and momentary lateral subluxations, garter strapping may also be employed until pain has settled and the joint is found to be stable on testing.

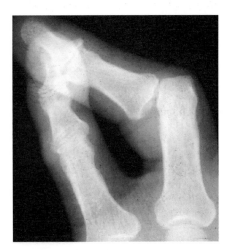

Fig. 7 **PIP joint dislocation.**

Phalangeal injuries

- Fractures of the distal phalanx seldom require any active treatment, as opposed to the soft tissue injuries which may accompany them.
- If there is no subluxation of the DIP joint, most cases of mallet finger may be treated satisfactorily by splintage.
- Fractures of the proximal and middle phalanges must be mobilised early, otherwise permanent stiffness and disability will be inevitable.
- In any fracture of a proximal or middle phalanx, make a careful assessment of the deformity and of the stability of the fracture.
- If the deformity is slight, and the fracture stable, simple methods of splintage will usually suffice.
- In unstable injuries, some form of internal fixation should be considered to allow early mobilisation.
- In the treatment of open fractures, especially with other associated soft tissue injuries, each case must be assessed on its individual merits.
- Finger dislocations should be reduced by traction and treated thereafter like sprains, supported for a period with garter strapping.

HAND INFECTIONS

Because of the good vascularity of the hand, primary infections are relatively uncommon, but they require prompt treatment to avoid prolonged disability. The majority are caused by relatively minor injuries which may be dismissed by the patient at the time. Scratches, minor grazes or rose-thorn pricks whilst gardening may be sufficient to allow the entry of pathogens. Animal or human bites are common and almost invariably become septic. While infections in major injuries are often successfully aborted by prompt administration of antibiotics, unfortunately, neglected sepsis is a cause of much disability, often leading to oedema, stiffness or tethering of the tendons within their sheaths. Once stiffness is established, it may be very difficult to eradicate even with intensive physiotherapy.

ANATOMY

A knowledge of the anatomy of the hand is helpful in understanding how infections within the fingers or hand may be contained or how they may spread.

The *fingertip pulp* is divided into a large number of tight compartments (loculi) by a series of fibrous septa which serve to tether the skin to the bone (Fig. 1). These are filled with fat and are well innervated, making them exquisitely sensitive to any rise of pressure.

The *synovial sheaths* lie within fibrous tendon sheaths in the fingers. In the case of the thumb and little finger, the synovial sheaths routinely extend proximally above the wrist (Fig. 2) and communicate in 50% of cases.

In the hand there are a number of potential spaces which can become infected. Deep to the flexor tendons (and superficial to the interossei and the metacarpals) lie the fascial lined *mid-palmar* and *thenar spaces* separated by a septum attached to the third metacarpal (Fig. 3). This septum is sometimes defective proximally, allowing infection on occasion to spread from one space to the other. The palmar spaces may also connect with *Parona's space* (which lies in the distal forearm between the flexor tendons and pronator quadratus): this communication lies deep to the flexor tendons and within the carpal tunnel. On the dorsum of the hand the extensor tendons are linked together with fascial bands which, along with the deep fascia, form an aponeurotic sheet. The *dorsal subaponeurotic space* lies deep to this (and superficial to the metacarpals and interossei, Fig. 3).

Infection may spread rapidly through any of these spaces, through the tissue planes, or by the lymphatics (causing lymphangitis, axillary lymphadenitis and usually systemic upset).

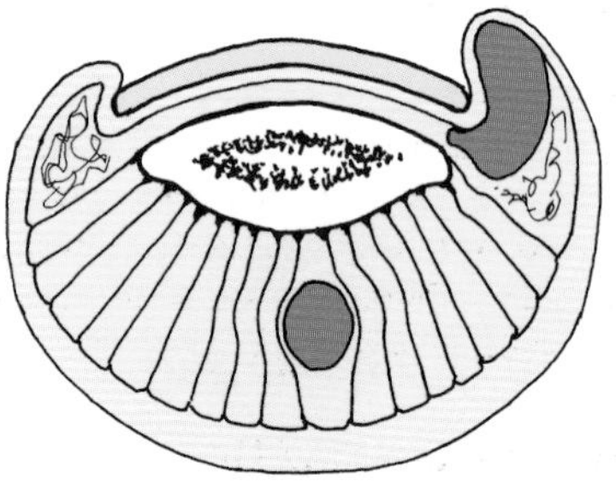

BACTERIOLOGY

The most common organism is the staphylococcus aureus. Streptococcal infections are rarer, but are responsible for rapidly spreading infections, not uncommonly seen after gardening injuries. Bite injuries often cause mixed organism contamination, including anaerobes; antibiotic treatment must cover this possibility.

DIFFERENTIAL DIAGNOSIS

Many conditions can mimic infection, but the most common is gout; inflammatory arthropathies, sarcoidosis and metastatic deposits should also be considered.

PARONYCHIA

This infection is usually initiated by rough manicuring or a hang-nail being torn off. It starts at the corner of the nail, but if left untreated can 'wrap' round the edge of the nail to its underside (Fig. 4);

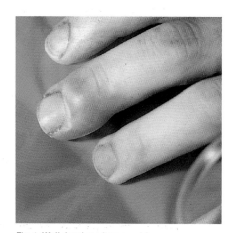

Fig. 1 **Pulp space and paronychial infections.**

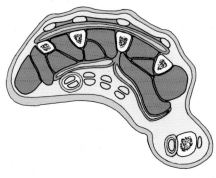

Fig. 3 **The mid-palmar and thenar spaces lie superficial to the interossei and adductor pollicis, and deep to the flexor tendons.** The dorsal subaponeurotic space lies deep to the extensor tendon mass.

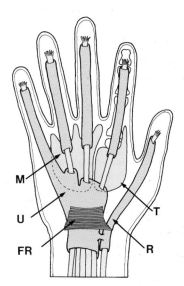

Fig. 2 **The communicating ulnar (U) and radial (R) bursae, and the synovial tendon sheaths are shown in pink.** M = mid-palmar; T = thenar spaces; FR = flexor retinaculum.

Fig. 4 **Well developed paronychia.**

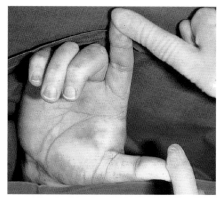

Fig. 5 **Tense (infective) swelling in the web between the thumb and index finger prior to surgical drainage.**

it may eventually cross to the opposite side, lifting the nail from the nail bed.

Treatment

The infection is treated by surgical drainage. This may be effected by an incision parallel to the edge of the nail. Depending on the extent of tissue involvement and the efficacy of drainage, part or all of the nail may require removal.

PULP SPACE INFECTION

This is usually caused by a minor injury which inoculates one or more of the pulp spaces. Pain is of rapid onset and is severe, because the spaces are small and unyielding and rapidly become tense. The finger tip becomes red, swollen and tender and the patient takes great care to protect it.

Treatment

Surgical drainage rapidly relieves the pain and generally prevents the development of an osteitis of the terminal phalanx.

WEB SPACE INFECTIONS

These form in the fat-filled spaces between the fingers at the level of the metacarpophalangeal joints. These spaces are loose, and pus can track along the fingers in the subcutaneous plane or onto the dorsum of the hand. Typically the presentation is late, by which time a large abscess has usually formed, pushing the fingers apart (Fig. 5).

Treatment

The space is drained by an incision in the web.

PALMAR SPACE INFECTIONS

These are almost always caused by penetrating injuries. They are now relatively uncommon as they are often aborted by the prompt use of antibiotics. If untreated, they result in severe swelling of the whole hand, great tenderness, stiffening of the fingers and pain on finger movements.

Treatment

Surgical drainage of the appropriate space is generally required. This usually necessitates incisions in the palm, which must be carefully planned and executed to avoid injuring important structures and to minimise scarring. Postoperatively, early mobilisation is necessary to avoid stiffness.

TENDON SHEATH INFECTIONS

Although now less common these must be recognised promptly to avoid disastrous tendon tethering or necrosis. The organisms responsible are usually inoculated through a penetrating wound in a flexor crease, and through this the synovial sheath is entered. This is a closed and tight compartment, and it soon becomes tense and painful. This leads to disruption of blood flow to the tendons within, and, although their oxygen consumption is low, necrosis will ultimately occur if the tension is not relieved. The most common organisms are the staphylococcus aureus and streptococcus pyogenes, although mixed organisms are not uncommon. Clinically, the affected finger becomes tense, swollen and motionless. Tenderness is marked, and whilst some active movement may be possible and relatively pain-free, passive motion is extremely painful. The synovial sheaths of the thumb and little finger often communicate proximally, and the wrist should be palpated carefully to assess possible spread between them.

Treatment

This is by surgical drainage and irrigation of the sheath. In late cases, the necrotic tendon may have to be excised and reconstruction attempted with tendon grafting. The results are somewhat unpredictable, and it is seldom that full function can be restored.

SEPTIC ARTHRITIS

This is uncommon in the hand and wrist and is almost exclusively secondary to traumatic puncture wounds. Typically the puncture is caused by *a bite*: this usually occurs when the patient's clenched fist strikes an opponent's tooth during a fight (Fig. 6). The metacarpophalangeal joint is most frequently penetrated and the extensor tendon damaged. Over 40 organisms have been identified in the human mouth, so the chances of inoculating the joint with virulent organisms is high.

Treatment

Very often the patient presents late with an established septic arthritis requiring urgent decompression of the joint. If seen at an early stage, as first measures a bacteriological swab should be taken, the wound debrided and left open (as in a contaminated open fracture), a broad spectrum antibiotic administered, and the hand splinted and elevated.

OSTEOMYELITIS

This is now rare, and the most common site is in the terminal phalanx following a crush injury, a partial amputation, or a pulp infection.

Treatment

This is similar to that of bone infections elsewhere, where radical excision of all infected and dead bone is generally indicated. In a digit, a terminal amputation may be the best treatment.

PYOGENIC GRANULOMA

Following a penetrating injury, and as a result of chronic infection, a tumour-like, friable granuloma is formed. Staphylococcus aureus is usually the offending organism.

Treatment

The granulomatous tissue is excised; as much of the lesion lies beneath the skin, this must be meticulously performed to avoid recurrence.

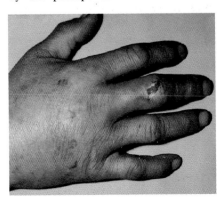

Fig. 6 **Bite injury with gross infection of the middle finger.**

Hand infections

- Most infections are caused by penetrating injuries which are often of a trivial nature.
- Staphylococcus aureus is the most common organism.
- Streptococcal infection can spread rapidly and cause systemic upset.
- Many infections can be aborted by prompt and appropriate antibiotic administration, but surgical drainage is frequently required.
- Beware the 'bite' injury which frequently causes septic arthritis.

DUPUYTREN'S DISEASE / HAND TUMOURS

DUPUYTREN'S DISEASE

The primary pathological process involves fascial tissue; it most commonly affects the palmar fascia, leading to significant finger contractures and impairment of hand function. The palmar fascia (aponeurosis) lies superficial to the flexor tendons, and extends distally to the level of the distal interphalangeal joints. Proximally, the palmaris longus is inserted into it. It has vertical, horizontal and transverse fibres through which it is attached to the skin and deep structures; these fibres serve to anchor the skin and thereby enhance its grip characteristics.

Aetiology

The cause is not known, but there is a definite genetic predisposition, with 60–70% of affected patients having a family history of the disease. Trauma has often been implicated, but this probably acts only as a precipitant in a genetically susceptible individual. Other factors such as alcoholism, epilepsy and liver disease have been said to be causative, but the evidence for this has not been satisfactorily established. The disease is extremely common in Northern Europe, with males being affected ten times more frequently than females. It is rare in the Chinese, African and Indian populations. It seldom presents before the age of 40 years, but becomes progressively more common with increasing age. In the affected young patient there is usually a strong family history, and the course is much more rapid.

Pathology

The histology shows a dense and often aggressive fibrous tissue reaction originating in the palmar fascia. The extent of infiltration is related to the activity of the disease; if severe it can involve all the fascial bands, and in extreme cases has been mistaken for fibrosarcoma. In common with fibrous tissue elsewhere, it tends to contract, and this is responsible for the deformities with which it is associated.

Clinical features

In the early phase pain-free nodules appear, usually in the palm. The skin typically becomes puckered and multiple nodules may coalesce. Eventually pretendinous bands produce contractures of the fingers, with gradual impairment of hand function. The ring and little fingers are most commonly affected,

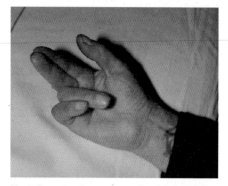

Fig. 1 **Dupuytren's contracture involving the little and ring fingers, and to a lesser extent the middle finger.** There is another prominent band at the thumb.

although all the digits can become involved (Fig. 1). The contractures may progress slowly over a number of years, although there are often periods of more rapid activity (perhaps provoked by a traumatic incident). Although the contractures are not usually painful, they can be a nuisance to the patient when trying to perform simple tasks such as grasping a cup or face washing. In extreme cases pressure of the nails of the affected fingers against the palm may cause local ulceration. Nodules and bands may also occur in the soles of the feet and rarely on the penis (Peyronie's disease). In addition, firm lesions are commonly found on the knuckle pads of the proximal interphalangeal joints; these are asymptomatic and require no treatment other than reassurance.

Treatment

Where nodules are present without contractures, reassurance about the diagnosis and a watching policy can be adopted. Once contractures have developed and are causing functional difficulties, fasciectomy is indicated (Fig. 2). In general terms, contractures of the metacarpophalangeal joints can usually be completely corrected, but in the case of the proximal interphalangeal joints only partial correction is usually possible, due to contractions of the collateral ligaments and joint capsules. Postoperative physiotherapy and splintage are essential to achieve a lasting result.

TUMOURS AND SWELLINGS

In the hand, primary tumours are relatively uncommon, and their assessment and treatment does not differ in essence from elsewhere. The following are most frequently encountered.

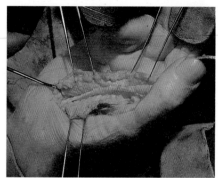

Fig. 2 **Dissection of Dupuytren band to thumb prior to excision.**

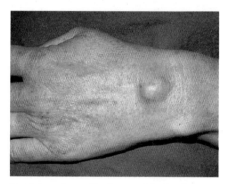

Fig. 3 **Ganglion on the dorsum of the hand.**

GANGLION

This is the most common 'tumour' in the hand. It usually presents as a tense swelling on the dorsum of the hand (Fig. 3) or the anterolateral aspect of the wrist. Ganglions are seldom painful. They typically enlarge during activity and gradually recede after rest; this is a diagnostic feature. They are usually found near joints with which they may communicate (suggesting in this instance that they may arise from a herniation of synovial tissue). This communication forms a one-way valvular mechanism which delays drainage back to the joint and may help to explain the slow fluctuations in size. Some have no joint communication and may arise from mucoid degeneration of interstitial tissue. A small group arise from the digital flexor sheaths at the base of the fingers. These ganglions are small and firm and do not move during finger flexion. Occasionally they are tender and may cause pain when hard objects are gripped. The peak incidence of ganglions is in young adults. In older patients they may be associated with degenerative changes in a joint. Nerve compression due to a ganglion is rare, but may occur in the canal of Guyon,

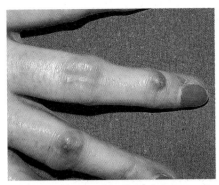

Fig. 4 **Multiple mucous cysts, with Heberden and Bouchard (osteoarthritic) nodes.**

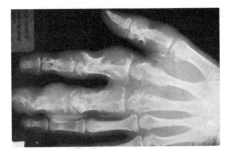

Fig. 6 **Ollier's disease.**

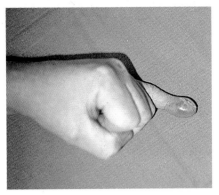

Fig. 7 **Secondary tumour involving a terminal phalanx.**

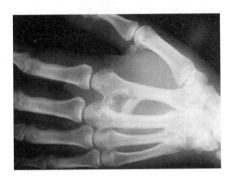

Fig. 5 **Ecchondroma of index metacarpal.**

through which the ulnar nerve runs in the hand. This tends to cause selective motor palsy, although sensory symptoms can occur. In the region of the proximal tibiofibular joint, a ganglion may cause a common peroneal nerve palsy and a drop foot.

Treatment

At least 50% disappear spontaneously, so reassurance about the diagnosis may be sufficient. Aspiration produces a clear viscous fluid and may lead to resolution. Those remaining can be removed surgically, although recurrence is common. Where there is a nerve palsy, exploration is always required.

INTRAOSSEOUS GANGLIONS

Radiographs of an affected area show one or more cystic spaces lying close to an articular surface. The joint may be otherwise normal, which distinguishes isolated intraosseous ganglions from conditions such as rheumatoid arthritis or osteoarthritis. Occasionally they present with pain or even a pathological fracture. If significantly symptomatic, it is justifiable to carry out a curettage of the ganglion with bone grafting of the defect.

MUCOUS CYST

These cysts always occur at the distal interphalangeal joints of the fingers in association with osteoarthritis. Although similar to ganglions, they are distinguished from them on the consistent basis of the site (Fig. 4) and the fact that they occur in an older age group. Excision is generally best avoided (as they are notoriously difficult to eradicate), but occasionally an attempt is justified when a synovial fistula develops following rupture of a cyst.

EPIDERMOID CYSTS (INCLUSION DERMOIDS)

These occur as a result of a penetrating injury which implants a fragment of skin into the subcutaneous layer. They are common in the hand because of its vulnerability to trauma. The cysts are generally small and tense, and filled with a creamy fluid; although painless, they are often tender on pressure, and this may impair hand function. Excision is curative.

OSTEOID OSTEOMA

This is a benign tumour which classically produces unremitting local pain relieved by aspirin. The carpal bones and the terminal phalanges are most commonly affected, although any of the bones in the hand can be involved. Diagnosis may be delayed as there may be few clinical signs. Typically the X-rays show an area of sclerosis, with a central radio-opaque nidus surrounded by a radiolucent 'halo'. Where X-ray changes are doubtful, an isotopic bone scan showing a 'hot spot' is the most reliable method of confirming the diagnosis. There is some evidence that spontaneous resolution may occur over a period of 1–2 years, but if symptoms are marked early excision is usually curative.

CHONDROMA

This is the most common benign tumour and is usually found in the metacarpals or proximal phalanges. It is generally confined within the bone (enchondroma), but occasionally can break out into the soft tissues (ecchondroma, Fig. 5). It is often solitary, although multiple tumours of a similar nature are found in Ollier's disease (Fig. 6), which has a hereditary diathesis. The condition often presents acutely after fracture. Chondromata can be treated conservatively if asymptomatic, but if troublesome because of pain or recurrent fracture, curettage and bone grafting may be necessary.

METASTATIC TUMOURS

These are uncommon and have a preference for involving the terminal phalanges (Fig. 7). Misdiagnosis is common unless care is taken. Although any tumour can metastasise to bone, the most common primary sites by far are lung and breast. Treatment is dependent on the nature of the primary tumour.

Dupuytren's disease / hand tumours

- Dupuytren's disease has a genetic predisposition and is 10 times more common in men than women.
- Surgical intervention is only necessary when contractures occur and the function of the hand is impaired.
- Ganglions are the most common tumours in the hand, and 50% resolve spontaneously.
- Chondroma and osteoid osteoma are the most common bone tumours in the hand.
- Metastatic tumours favour the terminal phalanges and can be misdiagnosed if care is not taken.

TENDON INJURIES IN THE HAND

The tendons in the hand are vulnerable to traumatic division, tenosynovitis and rupture from attrition or trauma. A careful assessment is necessary to ensure that an early diagnosis is made, and a sound knowledge of the anatomy of the tendons and their sheaths is essential.

FLEXOR TENDON INJURIES

A flexor tendon may be divided by a sharp instrument (such as a knife, chisel or saw) which comes into contact with the fingers or hand; or sometimes if an assailant's weapon (e.g. a knife, sword or bayonet) is grasped to ward it off or withdraw it. In the latter case in particular, both flexor tendons to one or more fingers may be divided. With extensive lacerations the neurovascular bundles may be damaged, with the risk of compromising the viability of the fingers (Fig. 1).

Diagnosis

It is necessary to have a clear understanding of the anatomy of the flexor tendons, especially in the fingers. The flexor digitorum profundus (FDP) is inserted into the distal phalanx, and the flexor digitorum superficialis (FDS) into the middle phalanx. One of the main differences between them is that the FDP has a mass action, whilst the FDS has single muscle units which activate each finger. To test the integrity of the FDS, begin by holding all the fingers in an extended position (to abolish the mass action of the FDP). Then free each finger in turn to see whether it can be flexed (at the proximal interphalangeal joint); if it can, then the FDS tendon to that finger is intact. The site of any division is important, as injuries within the flexor tendon sheaths of the fingers are much more troublesome than more proximally situated injuries. The hand is divided into five zones, zone 2 being the most troublesome (the so-called 'no man's land') (Fig. 2). It should also be remembered that the flexor tendons have an excursion of 5–7.5 cm from full extension to full flexion; thus the position of a skin laceration relative to the site of the tendon injury depends on the position of the finger, both at the time of the injury and the examination (this is important if exploration is being undertaken). Following division of a tendon the natural balance of the digits will be lost, and this is usually clinically obvious on inspection.

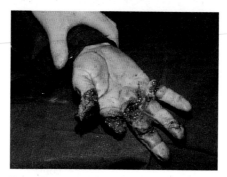

Fig. 1 **Circular saw injury.** Apart from attention to the tendons and skin wounds, injuries of this pattern may require fixation of fractures, and repair of digital nerves and vessels.

Treatment

It is generally agreed that to obtain the best results flexor tendons should be surgically repaired as soon as feasible. With improved techniques this is now also true for tendons divided in no man's land, where there is risk of adhesions occurring between the FDS and FDP tendons within the intimately confined space of the digital tendon sheath. Postoperatively, specialised splintage for 3–6 weeks is essential to protect the tendon from re-rupture, whilst at the same time allowing protected motion to minimise adhesions. If the case presents late, the only option is tendon grafting. This involves transposing an independent segment of tendon (free tendon graft) into the gap in order to restore the integrity of the divided tendon.

PROFUNDUS TENDON RUPTURE

This is an uncommon injury where the FDP tendon is avulsed from the distal phalanx, sometimes with a fragment of bone. It is caused by a forced extension injury whilst the finger is powerfully flexed (e.g. when a rugby player attempts to grasp an opponent's shirt as he pulls away). The patient cannot flex the DIP joint, and during attempted flexion the finger adopts a typical posture (Fig. 3). The treatment is usually surgical repair. As the tendon normally retracts to the level of the decussation of the FDS, this can be difficult.

DIVIDED EXTENSOR TENDONS

These do not generally cause any problems in management, although care must be taken in assessment. This is particularly true on the dorsum of the hand,

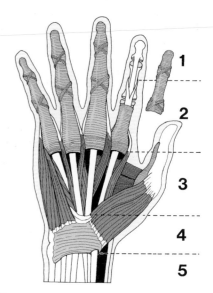

Fig. 2 **The zones of the hand.** Zone 1 = area distal to the insertion of FDS; zone 2 = 'no man's land' between zone 1 and the entrance to the flexor tendon sheaths; zone 3 = the lumbrical region in the palm; zone 4 = beneath the flexor retinaculum; zone 5 = proximal to the retinaculum.

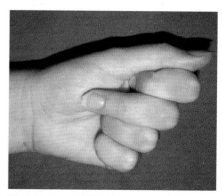

Fig. 3 **Rupture of FDP with loss of flexion in the terminal joint of the middle finger.**

as the intertendinous bands may allow metacarpophalangeal joint extension even when a tendon has been completely divided. Beware the laceration which divides an extensor tendon over the knuckle or proximal phalanx; typically both phalangeal joints can be extended by intrinsic action, but the metacarpophalangeal joint can not. Treatment is usually by surgical repair followed by 3 weeks of protective splintage.

AVULSION INJURIES

These occur at either the distal or proximal interphalangeal joints. At the distal joint an extensor tendon avulsion leads to a mallet finger (see p. 92). At the level of the proximal interphalangeal joint, a forced flexion injury may lead to the central slip of the extensor tendon being avulsed from the middle phalanx, with a resulting boutonnière deformity (Fig. 4). The initial deformity may be slight, but it often progresses as the two lateral parts of the tendon slip over the condyles of the middle phalanx. Once they come to lie anterior to the centre of rotation, they become flexors, causing the typical deformity (flexion of the proximal and hyperextension of the distal interphalangeal joints). This deformity can also occur in rheumatoid arthritis secondary to erosion of the bony insertion of the central slip.

Treatment
If the deformity is not fixed, splintage for 4–6 weeks in extension will usually suffice. If it has become fixed, surgical correction is necessary.

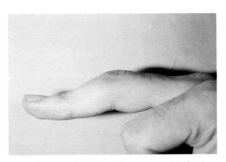
Fig. 4 **Boutonnière deformity.**

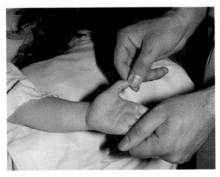
Fig. 5 **Stenosing tenosynovitis of the thumb. The IP joint has become permanently flexed.**

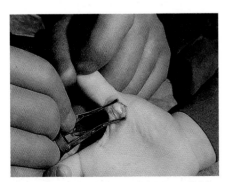
Fig. 6 **Same case as in Figure 5 just prior to division of the tendon sheath.** Note the local thickening at the level of the metacarpophalangeal joint.

EXTENSOR POLLICIS LONGUS RUPTURE

This is a comparatively uncommon problem which occurs after a distal radial fracture. Its aetiology is uncertain, although it is thought that attrition of the tendon or some disturbance in its vascularity as it passes around the dorsal tubercle of the radius may be responsible. Strangely enough it is more common after relatively undisplaced fractures. It usually presents at 4–8 weeks with sudden loss of thumb extension. Although the thumb tends to get in the way when attempting to grip objects, the disability is generally minor.

Treatment
Transfer of the extensor indicis proprius tendon to the distal part of the thumb extensor is normally advised.

'BITE' INJURIES

Beware a small laceration over the metacarpophalangeal joint found after someone is involved in a fight. It is often caused by the front teeth of the recipient of a punch. It may divide the tendon, but more importantly can inoculate the joint with bacteria, leading to a septic arthritis (p. 95).

TRIGGER FINGER (STENOSING TENOVAGINITIS)

This is a striking complaint which often has no obvious precipitating cause, although there is sometimes a history of minor trauma or a degree of local synovitis. A discrepancy arises between the size of the tendon (which sometimes has a local nodular swelling) and the entrance to the tendon sheath (which may be thickened and narrowed). The flexor tendons are able to bend the finger and draw the obstruction clear of the sheath, but when an attempt is made to straighten the finger, resistance is

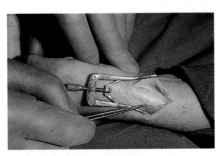
Fig. 7 **De Quervain's tenovaginitis.** The common tendon sheath of abductor pollicis longus and extensor pollicis brevis is greatly thickened and will be divided to free the tendons.

encountered which the extensor tendon is not at first able to overcome. With greater effort however the finger suddenly extends (triggering). As the condition progresses, the affected digit (usually the ring finger) may eventually have to be physically extended, and later still it may become fixed in a permanently flexed position. A variation of the condition occurs in the thumbs of infants, where there is no triggering, but the interphalangeal joint is held in a permanently flexed position. In most cases there is palpable thickening in the region of the metacarpophalangeal joint where the pathology is always situated (Figs 5 and 6).

Treatment
In adults in the early stages a steroid injection into the sheath may abort the condition, but later surgical release of the proximal part of the tendon sheath is required and gives immediate gratifying relief. In babies the condition tends to resolve spontaneously by 18 months, but if not, surgical release may also be performed.

DE QUERVAIN'S STENOSING TENOVAGINITIS

This is an inflammatory condition which involves abductor pollicis longus and extensor pollicis brevis as they pass through their common sheath on the lateral side of the distal radius. It can be intensely painful, and there is often local swelling and tenderness (Fig. 7). If the thumb is flexed across the palm and then the wrist forced into ulnar deviation, the patient complains of great pain which is virtually diagnostic of the condition.

Treatment
Steroid injections into the sheath with splintage can often produce dramatic results. In resistant cases, surgical decompression may be necessary.

Tendon injuries in the hand
- Severed flexor or extensor tendons require immediate surgical repair.
- Careful assessment of all injuries is essential to avoid missing any associated neurovascular damage.
- Triggering of a tendon can often be aborted with a steroid injection into its sheath.
- Late diagnosed tendon ruptures may require specialised treatment.

ARTHRITIS IN THE HAND AND WRIST

Degenerative changes in the hand and wrist are common. The most frequent causes are osteoarthritis and rheumatoid arthritis, although any of the inflammatory arthropathies (e.g. psoriasis) or metabolic diseases (e.g. gout) are capable of causing joint destruction. Each disease process has its own pattern of joint involvement which may help to establish the diagnosis. Rheumatoid arthritis tends to start in the metacarpophalangeal joints, whilst osteoarthritis almost uniquely affects the distal interphalangeal joints.

OSTEOARTHRITIS

As is the case in other regions, primary osteoarthritis tends to have a gradual onset. The most common joints to be affected are the distal interphalangeal joints of the fingers and the carpometacarpal joint of the thumb (trapeziometacarpal joint). Although the other joints can be affected, they tend on the whole to be spared. In the case of secondary osteoarthritis, the onset is usually more rapid. The most common precipitating factor is a fracture involving an articular surface (note that the proximal interphalangeal joints are often damaged in sporting injuries, and may be misdiagnosed as 'staves' when there may in fact be a fracture or fracture–subluxation: if left untreated, these injuries result in degenerative changes and joint stiffness).

THE THUMB

The joint at the base of the thumb (trapeziometacarpal or carpometacarpal) is one of the most common joints in the body to be affected and can lead to significant morbidity. It typically causes pain when gripping objects (such as a pen or a tool) and worsens with activity. Crepitus can be found on clinical examination. In extreme cases, the metacarpal subluxates under the influence of abductor pollicis longus (which is inserted into the base of the metacarpal). This may be obvious clinically, with the base of the thumb becoming prominent and a fixed adduction deformity developing (Fig. 1). It makes the gripping of objects progressively more difficult.

Treatment
In the early phase analgesics are used. If the condition is more troublesome, steroid injections may be tried. In the later stages, excision of the trapezium and interposition of either a segment of tendon as a 'spacer' or a silastic implant (Fig. 2) can be used with good functional results.

THE FINGERS

The distal interphalangeal joints are frequently affected, leading to pain whilst attempting to grip objects. Classically there are palpable dorsal osteophytes (Heberden's nodes, Figs 3 and 4), commonly with associated mucous cysts which are resistant to excision. Less commonly the proximal interphalangeal joints may be involved (Bouchard's nodes).

Treatment
This is aimed at relief of pain, with the use of simple analgesics as necessary. In some instances a joint may be suitable for fusion in a position of slight flexion (the position the finger adopts in gripping).

RHEUMATOID ARTHRITIS

In rheumatoid disease there are two aspects to consider, namely the synovitis and the subsequent arthropathy. Each has its part to play in the progressive deformity and ensuing disability.

TENOSYNOVITIS

This only occurs under retinacula. The retinacula prevent the tendons from bow-stringing during motion, and it is in these areas that synovium is present to aid the gliding of the tendons. The sites commonly affected are on the dorsum of the wrist, in the carpal tunnel, and in the digital sheaths. If the condition is severe it not uncommonly leads to tendon rupture, the digital extensors being most frequently affected. Probably the most frequently occurring synovitis affects the dorsum of the wrist. It has a typical

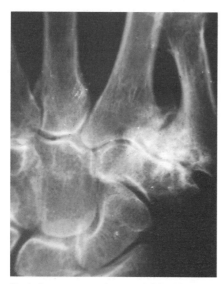
Fig. 1 **Carpometacarpal osteoarthritis of the thumb with adduction deformity.**

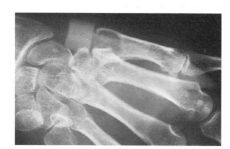
Fig. 2 **Silastic implant for carpometacarpal osteoarthritis of the thumb.**

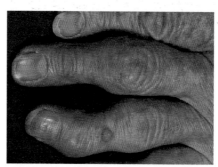
Fig. 3 **Osteoarthritis of the distal and proximal interphalangeal joints of the fingers.**

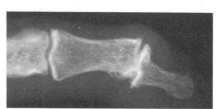
Fig. 4 **Radiograph showing osteoarthritic subluxation of a distal interphalangeal joint and the formation of a Heberden's node.**

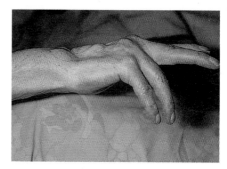
Fig. 5 **Rupture of the extensor tendons to the little and ring fingers.**

dumb-bell appearance as it bulges both proximal and distal to the retinaculum. In the carpal tunnel, a bulky synovitis can cause compression of the vulnerable median nerve as it passes through that confined space (carpal tunnel syndrome). Synovitis affecting the digital flexor tendons may in mild cases cause 'triggering' of the tendons, and in severe cases, tendon ruptures.

Treatment

This is usually medical in the first instance, with splintage and steroid injections where appropriate, but in resistant cases surgical decompression may be required.

RUPTURE OF THE EXTENSOR TENDONS

This is common (Fig. 5) and usually affects the little finger initially before progressing (if untreated) in a radial direction to involve all the fingers. Treatment is by surgical decompression of the synovitis and tendon transfer to restore tendon function.

RUPTURE OF THE FLEXOR TENDONS

While this is common, in the first instance only one digital flexor tendon may be affected (i.e. a superficial or a deep flexor); fair digital function may therefore be maintained. Once both the superficial and the deep flexor tendons

have ruptured, it is necessary to decompress the sheath surgically; a tendon transfer is the only way of restoring function.

ARTHRITIS

This occurs as a result of the synovitis which destroys the cartilaginous articular surfaces. The ligamentous insertions may become eroded as the disease progresses, leading to instability, subluxation or even dislocation. Typically the first joints to be involved are the metacarpophalangeal joints, followed by the radiocarpal and radioulnar joints (Fig. 6). However, any or all of the joints in the hand can be affected.

The most common deformity at the wrist is one of ulnar deviation, with palmar subluxation of the carpus. In addition, the ulnar head may dislocate dorsally and contribute to attritional rupture of the extensor tendons. If an attempt is made to press the ulnar head back into its proper alignment, there is complaint of severe pain (the 'piano key' sign). The ulnar deviation of the wrist tends to encourage the extensor tendons to subluxate in an ulnar direction at the level of the metacarpophalangeal joints, contributing to the typical ulnar deviation and palmar subluxation of the fingers. Secondary tightness of the intrinsic muscles may further worsen the deformity and may contribute to swan-neck deformities of the fingers (where the

proximal interphalangeal joints are extended and the distal joints flexed, Fig. 7). A boutonnière deformity can occur if the insertion of the central slip of the extensor tendon is eroded and becomes detached from the middle phalanx. It can be appreciated that all the deformities are interlinked and, once established, progression is inevitable.

Treatment

If multiple deformities are present this can be complex as several may have to be addressed if improvement is to be sustained. Stabilisation with maintenance of function is the aim, but is often difficult to achieve. Synovectomy is useful if the joint is only mildly diseased. Excision of the distal end of the ulna can relieve pain in the distal radioulnar joint and may also restore pronation and supination. If there is gross destruction of the radiocarpal joint, fusion may have to be undertaken. (Although some replacements of this particular joint are available the results are at present a little unpredictable.) Prosthetic replacement of the metacarpophalangeal joints is however often successful, allowing correction of the ulnar deviation. Release of the intrinsic muscles at the same time is usually necessary. Fusion of individual finger joints in a functional position probably gives the most satisfactory results.

Rheumatoid arthritis in the thumb has two typical deformities. The first is the Z-deformity (Fig. 8) caused by primary disease in the metacarpophalangeal joint which becomes flexed; there is secondary hyperextension of the interphalangeal joint. This may be controlled by fusion of the metacarpophalangeal joint. The second deformity starts in the carpometacarpal joint and leads to hyperextension of the metacarpophalangeal joint and flexion of the interphalangeal joint. Fixed adduction of the thumb also occurs. In this situation, excision of the trapezium and fusion of the metacarpophalangeal joint is necessary to correct the deformity.

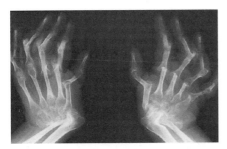

Fig. 6 **Gross deformities of the wrists and fingers in advanced rheumatoid arthritis.**

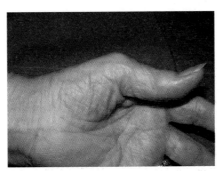

Fig. 8 **Z-deformity of the thumb.**

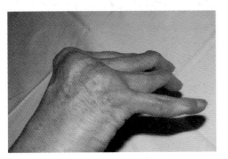

Fig. 7 **Ulnar drift at the MP joints, and swan-neck deformities of the ring and middle fingers.**

Arthritis in the hand and wrist

- Osteoarthritis usually affects the base of the thumb and interphalangeal joint. If found in the metacarpophalangeal joint it is usually the result of trauma.
- In rheumatoid arthritis, tenosynovitis only occurs under retinacula.
- If left untreated, rheumatoid tenosynovitis will eventually cause tendons to rupture.
- Rheumatoid arthritis can affect any joint in the hand, but usually starts in the metacarpophalangeal joints.
- Surgical intervention is often needed to correct deformities.

CONGENITAL DISLOCATION OF THE HIP

Pathology

Congenital dislocation of the hip (CDH) is a condition in which a child is either born with a dislocated hip, or whose hip dislocates within the first few months of life. In the latter case, the hip immediately prior to the dislocation is considered to have been unstable. There are a number of well established aetiological factors associated with this condition:

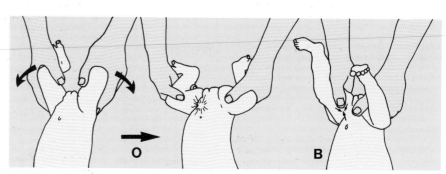

Fig. 1 **The Ortolani (O) and Barlow (B) tests (left hip).**

- It is much more common in girls than boys.
- There is a familial tendency.
- It is more common after breech presentations.
- It commonly accompanies other congenital abnormalities.
- There is a geographical variation in its incidence.

Diagnosis

The earlier the condition is diagnosed, the better the prospects of cure. Every newly born child should be examined for evidence of dislocation or hip instability. In the Ortolani test, the hips are first flexed and adducted, with the thumbs of the examiner being placed in front of the hips and the fingers behind (Fig. 1). The hips are then abducted. If either hip is dislocated, a clunking sensation will be felt near full abduction as the head of the femur slips back into the acetabulum (i.e. as the hip reduces). The Barlow test may be used to detect hip joint instability. In performing this, one hand fixes the pelvis while the thumb of the other is used to apply gentle backward pressure on the head of the femur. If the head of the femur is felt to sublux backwards, it should reduce by wider abduction of the hip or forward pressure of the examining fingers. Note that X-ray examination of suspect hips is of limited value under 3 months.

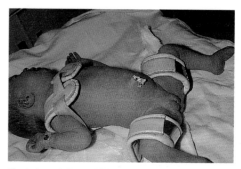

Fig. 2 **A newly born child with CDH being treated in a Barlow splint.** This allows free access to the perineum, facilitating local hygiene.

If these tests are negative, routine re-examination of the hips at 6 months is often advocated, and this is especially desirable if a child is in a high risk category (e.g. if there is a family history of the condition, or if there has been a breech delivery).

Treatment

The aim of treatment of the early diagnosed congenital dislocation of the hip is to reduce the dislocation and hold the hip in the reduced position until stability is restored (by concentric growth of the hip and the acetabulum and adaptive changes in the ligaments, capsule and acetabular labrum).

In the unstable hip, diagnosed at birth, the aim is to avoid dislocation occurring. Because it is recognised that some untreated cases of instability never progress to frank dislocation, a number of surgeons keep cases of instability under observation only, retesting the hip at frequent intervals; they reserve treatment only for those cases where instability persists. Others advocate treatment of all cases of dislocation and instability as soon as diagnosed, by supporting the hips in a position of flexion and abduction. To this end a number of splints have been devised (Fig. 2). The splint is worn until the hip is demonstrated as being stable (often in about 12 weeks) and is checked at regular intervals thereafter.

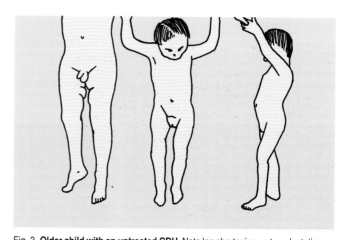

Fig. 3 **Older child with an untreated CDH.** Note leg shortening, external rotation of the limb, asymmetrical skin folds in the thighs, broadening of the perineum and increased lumbar lordosis.

CDH IN THE OLDER CHILD

The suspicion that something may be amiss may not arise until the child starts walking. At that time any hint of an abnormality in the hips should be investigated without delay (Fig. 3).

The ossification centre for the femoral head appears at about a year and radiographs of the hip may then give valuable confirmation (Figs 4 and 5); MRI scans may also show the extent of the soft tissue pathology in the hip.

Treatment of CDH in the older child

The aim of treatment is to restore the hip to as near normal as possible. Each case must be assessed on its own merits, but as a rule the same general plan is followed.

The head of the femur must be reduced into the acetabulum. A preliminary period of traction may be required to bring the proximally displaced femoral head down to the level of the acetabulum. The joint may then be reduced by manipulation, but sometimes surgery may be needed to clear

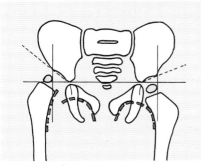

Fig. 4 **X-ray interpretation: each hip may be divided into quadrants by the construction shown.** The epiphysis (blue) should lie in the inner, lower quadrant. The radiographs may show a break in Shenton's line (red), the hyperbolic curve running between the obturator foramen and the medial side of the femur, and an increase in the slope of the acetabulum (which contributes to the instability of the hip).

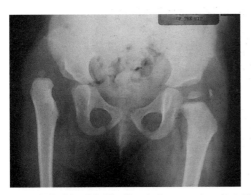

Fig. 5 **CDH of the right hip.** Note the features referred to in Fig. 4 and the relative small size of the capital epiphysis (another common finding).

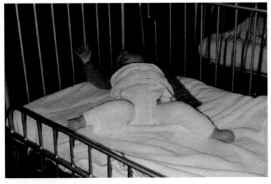

Fig. 6 **A Batchelor plaster used to support a dislocation which reduces and is stable when the hip is in internal rotation.** Note that both hips must be included even though the dislocation is unilateral.

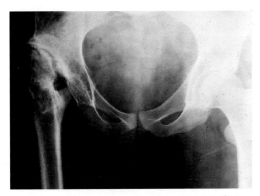

Fig. 7 **Untreated congenital dislocation of the right hip in an adult.** Note the false, arthritic joint which has developed above the original acetabulum.

Table 1 **Clinical features which might suggest the presence of CDH in the older child.**

- Delay in the child walking
- Walking with a limp (unilateral dislocation) or waddle (bilateral dislocation)
- Abnormal posture of the leg, especially external rotation of the hip (Fig. 3)
- Shortening of the leg
- Asymmetrical skin folds in the thighs
- Increased lumbar lordosis and widening of the perineum
- Limited abduction of the hip and a positive Trendelenburg's sign

the entrance to the acetabulum which may have become blocked by the thickened acetabular labrum (often referred to as the limbus).

After reduction the hip must be held in such a way that it does not redislocate; and it must be maintained in this position until it becomes stable. This is best achieved when the acetabulum and the head of the femur, by their contact and surface movement, grow in such a fashion that they become quite concentric. A common method is to apply a Batchelor plaster which is retained for about 12 weeks (Fig. 6).

Excessive anteversion must be corrected. In a large number of cases there is an abnormal degree of anteversion of the femoral neck which puts the head of the femur in adverse alignment with the acetabulum. This may be dealt with surgically by dividing the proximal part of the femur, correcting the deformity and fixing the bone with a small plate, i.e. by performing a rotational osteotomy.

Acetabular abnormalities may require correction. In some cases the acetabulum fails to develop properly so that instead of becoming deep and cup shaped it remains shallow; in addition it may not be tilted downwards in the normal manner but be inclined upwards ('sloping acetabular roof'). This leads to instability and predisposes the hip to early degenerative changes. These so-called dysplastic changes are sometimes tackled by carrying out a Salter osteotomy: in this procedure the pelvis is divided proximal to the acetabulum and the acetabular segment is rotated so that the mouth of the acetabulum is pointing downwards in a normal fashion.

CDH IN THE ADULT

If CDH has not been recognised in childhood, or if treatment has been neglected or failed, later in life secondary osteoarthritic changes will develop in the false joint that forms between the displaced femoral head and the pelvis (Fig. 7); secondary arthritic changes in the spine, due to the lurching or waddling gait, are also common. These complications are treated along general lines, but in a number of cases, in spite of a very shallow acetabulum, it is technically possible to carry out a total hip replacement procedure, often with very satisfying results.

Congenital dislocation of the hip

- Examine every new born child for the presence of CDH or hip instability.
- Repeat the examination at a later date in susceptible individuals.
- The earlier treatment is started, the better the chances of a successful outcome.
- In the older child, always suspect CDH if the child is slow to walk and the gait abnormal.
- Where dislocation persists into adult life, total hip replacement may be possible.

THE DYSPLASTIC HIP / SLIPPED UPPER FEMORAL EPIPHYSIS

THE DYSPLASTIC HIP

The principal feature of this condition is that the acetabulum does not wholly contain the femoral head, as it is often shallow and has an excessive slope (Fig. 1). The mechanical imperfection of the joint leads to secondary osteo-arthritis. At first there may be complaint of mild pain and stiffness, frequently presenting in the late teens or the twenties, but deterioration is often rapid. If seen early, surgery to improve the containment of the femoral head may be carried out: the methods available include the construction of an acetabular shelf, a femoral osteotomy or a Chiari osteotomy of the pelvis (which like the Salter osteotomy allows the acetabulum to be tilted in a more downward direction).

SLIPPED UPPER FEMORAL EPIPHYSIS

This is a disease of adolescence which affects the epiphyseal plate of the proximal femur. The epiphyseal plate is responsible for part of the growth in length of the femur, with the actively multiplying cells situated next to the capital epiphysis. The newly formed cartilage cells undergo hypertrophy in the area of the plate adjacent to the proximal femoral shaft, and this is its weakest point. During the rapid growth of adolescence, the strength of this part of the epiphyseal plate may be reduced to such a level that it is unable to resist the normal stresses to which it is subjected. As a result the head of the femur and the shaft lose their normal relationship. The capital epiphysis is well supported by the acetabulum, but the femur tends to externally rotate and move proximally under it.

Aetiology

The condition occurs in the 11–14 age group, and is much more common in boys than in girls. Many of those affected are overweight and some have the appearance of those suffering from Fröhlich syndrome, although attempts to demonstrate a hormonal disturbance have been generally unsuccessful. It has been suggested that the stresses placed on the hip by excess weight are of greater importance than any disordered hormone activity. Nevertheless some cases have been found in association with hypothyroidism.

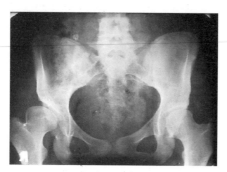

Fig. 1 **Dysplastic right hip.** Note the slope of the acetabular roof and the poor containment of the femoral head.

There is often a history of a traumatic episode and it would seem that in a number of cases at least local stress may be a factor. An important feature is that the condition is often bilateral, with the slipping of the second side often occurring when the patient is resting in bed during treatment of the first.

Diagnosis

There is often complaint of pain which may be felt in the groin or referred to the knee. There is usually a marked limp and in severe cases it may not be possible to bear weight. There is no systemic disturbance, but on clinical examination the affected hip is usually seen to be held in external rotation. There is invariably restriction of internal rotation and abduction is often also impaired. The diagnosis is confirmed by X-ray examination of the hip which shows the disturbance in the relationship between the capital epiphysis and the femoral neck and shaft.

In the early stages, where the degree of slip is small, the radiographs require careful scrutiny. Both hips should be visualised not only to allow them to be compared but also to help detect an early slip on the symptomless side. The first signs appear in the lateral projections (Fig. 2), where it is found that a line drawn up the centre of the femoral neck no longer passes through the middle of the base of the capital epiphysis. Later, the proximal movement of the femoral neck and shaft become obvious in the AP view (Fig. 3). Later still, some weeks after the onset, there is new bone formation and adaptive changes in the inferior part of the femoral neck (buttressing). Once the femoral neck has become distorted the slip is described as being chronic. The severity of the slip may be

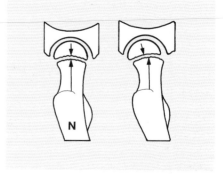

Fig 2 **The earliest radiographic signs of slipped femoral epiphysis appear in the lateral projection.** (N = normal)

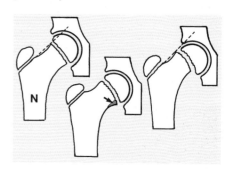

Fig. 3 **Other radiographic signs of slipped femoral epiphysis.** In the established case, in the AP projection, a line drawn along the lateral aspect of the femoral neck fails to cut the epiphysis. In a chronic slip, new bone forms below the neck. (N = normal)

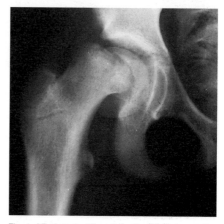

Fig. 4 **AP view showing major acute slip.**

judged by noting the percentage of the femoral epiphysis which has lost contact with the femoral neck.

The history and radiographic appearances allow any case to be assigned to one of three groups:

- **Acute slips.** Here the history is short (under three weeks) and there is no radiological evidence of buttressing (Fig. 4).
- **Acute on chronic slips.** In these cases there is often a history of

intermittent limp and discomfort in the hip for several weeks with recent, sudden deterioration. Any buttressing is slight.

- **Chronic slips.** Here the history is of many weeks' duration and buttressing is a feature (Fig. 5).

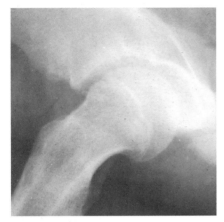

Fig. 5 **Lateral view showing chronic slip and inferior buttressing.**

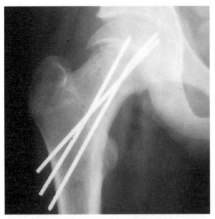

Fig. 6 **Slipped femoral epiphysis where a residual deformity has been accepted and fixed with three Knowles pins.**

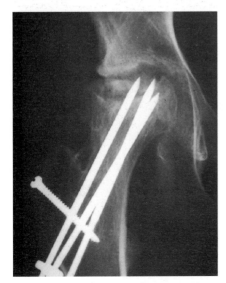

Fig. 7 **Avascular necrosis after open reduction and fixation.**

Treatment

If untreated, a minor displacement may progress and become severe. When the epiphysis comes to unite with the neck of the femur, the persisting displacement will lead to some permanent shortening of the limb, loss of internal rotation and abduction in the hip and increased susceptibility to osteoarthritis of the hip in the third and fourth decades. Treatment is itself complicated by the risks of causing avascular necrosis of the head of the femur (by disturbing its rich and somewhat delicate blood supply). For this reason forcible manipulation of the hip in an attempt to obtain a reduction must be avoided. Similarly, if operative reduction of the displacement is thought necessary and unavoidable, it must be performed with great care to avoid stretching or division of the blood vessels which are closely related to the femoral neck as they travel towards the capital epiphysis.

If the slip is less than 30%, then the displacement may be accepted and the epiphysis fixed internally with an appropriate device, e.g. with AO screws and Knowles pins (Fig. 6). If the slip is greater than this, and recent (i.e. an

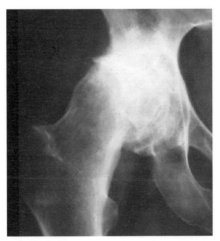

Fig. 8 **Osteoarthritis secondary to slipped femoral epiphysis.**

acute slip or an acute on chronic slip), then a gentle manipulative reduction may be tried. If this is successful in reducing the deformity to less than 30%, then it is reasonable to proceed to internal fixation, accepting this level of residual displacement. If closed reduction is unsuccessful, then operative reduction and internal fixation may be attempted, bearing in mind the risks of avascular necrosis (Fig. 7). After pinning, it is usually not long before the epiphysis unites with the diaphysis. As the condition occurs in adolescence, and as most longitudinal bone growth occurs at the distal end of the femur, little additional shortening of the limb results. During convalescence the unaffected hip must be closely observed clinically and by repeated X-rays.

Where the diagnosis is made late and the epiphysis has closed with severe deformity, there will be restriction of movement in the hip and a risk of secondary osteoarthritis (Fig. 8). The prognosis may be improved by a corrective osteotomy. This is performed at the subtrochanteric region, with removal of a wedge of bone to correct external rotation, adduction and flexion.

If avascular necrosis supervenes but symptoms are minor, analgesics may be used to control pain during revascularisation and after. In many cases, however, where there is marked deformity of the femoral head, treatment poses a difficult problem. A choice may have to be made between the following:

- **Arthrodesis.** This is often difficult to achieve, and where there are long-term risks of osteoarthritic changes in the ipsilateral knee, the spine, and the other hip
- **Osteotomy of the hip.** The results are somewhat unpredictable and not necessarily of long duration
- **Total hip replacement.** This has a degree of risk and long-term uncertainty.

The dysplastic hip / slipped upper femoral epiphysis

- In dysplasia of the hip, the risks of early onset osteoarthritis may be reduced by pelvic osteotomy.
- Slipped proximal femoral epiphysis is a condition occurring in adolescence.
- It is more common in boys than in girls.
- It may present in acute, acute on chronic and chronic forms.
- The diagnosis is best established by lateral radiographs of the hip.
- It is bilateral in 60% of cases; silent slipping of the other hip must not be missed during treatment.
- Avascular necrosis is a serious complication: forced manipulative reduction must be avoided and great care taken during any open procedures.

THE IRRITABLE HIP

The term 'irritable hip' is used to describe a syndrome which is seen in children, particularly in the 4–8 age group. The main feature is the presence of a limp. Although some vague traumatic incident may be recalled and thought to be responsible, trauma is in fact not thought to be a significant factor. In the majority of cases the onset is insidious. Often there is no pain. The most outstanding clinical feature is loss of internal rotation in the affected hip. Several quite distinct conditions may be responsible for this syndrome. The three most common causes are *transient synovitis of the hip, tuberculosis of the hip* and *Perthes' disease*. It is common practice to admit children with irritable hips for symptomatic treatment until the diagnosis has been firmly established.

TRANSIENT SYNOVITIS OF THE HIP

This is the most common cause of irritable hip syndrome. There is no accompanying systemic upset, with the sedimentation rate and the number of white cells and their distribution remaining undisturbed. The main and perhaps the only pathological feature is the presence of excess synovial fluid in the hip joint. As a result the X-ray findings are either completely normal or show some evidence of distension in the joint: there may be signs of a slight increase in the joint space compared with the other side with, for example, an increase in the gap between the head of the femur and the 'tear drop', the name given to the elongated, pear-shaped radiographic shadow cast by the anterior part of the acetabular floor (see p. 108). Aspiration of the joint is not routinely performed, but if this is carried out the synovial fluid will be found to have a clear appearance and be sterile on culture.

Treatment

The joint is rested by confining the child to bed and it is usual to apply a little light skin traction to the affected limb. The hip is kept under observation and weight bearing permitted when movement has fully recovered, usually by about 6 weeks.

TUBERCULOSIS OF THE HIP

About a quarter of all cases of bone and joint tuberculosis affect the hip. In the UK, after the introduction of routine chest screening and effective antituberculous chemotherapy it became a rarity, but recent increases in the overall incidence of tuberculosis make it clear that it can still present a problem.

Clinical features

The condition is progressive. At first there is a limp which may be painless to begin with. Later there is complaint of groin pain and pain in the hip at night becomes a feature. The limp becomes more marked as the child tries to spare the limb and muscle wasting may become quite pronounced. The hip becomes held in a permanently flexed position and the ability to extend the joint is lost (fixed flexion deformity). An

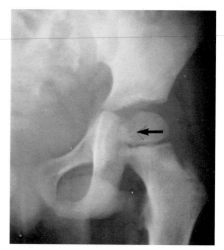

Fig. 1 **The arrow points to an early tuberculous cavity in the femoral head, before spread to the joint space has occurred.**

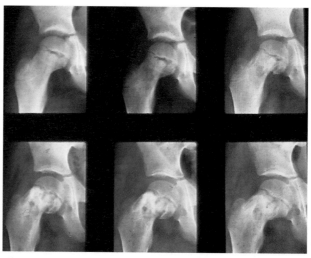

Fig. 2 **Progress over 1 year (from top left to bottom right) of a tuberculous focus in the femoral neck, without spread to the joint space.**

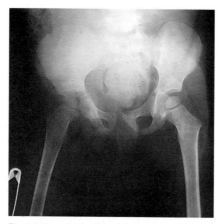

Fig. 3 **Tuberculosis of the right hip in a child with evidence of joint distension.** Note an increase in the tear drop distance, and reduction in the amount the epiphysis and metaphysis overlap the ischium.

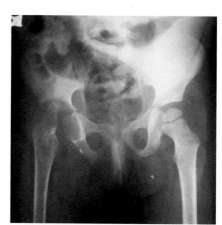

Fig. 4 **The same case as Fig. 3 seven months later.** The femoral head has been destroyed and the joint is distended with tuberculous pus.

increase in lumbar lordosis develops to compensate for the fixed hip flexion and other hip joint movements become progressively reduced. Eventually all movement may be lost, with the joint space filled with fibrous tissue (fibrous ankylosis) or, much less commonly, with bone (bony ankylosis).

Pathology

The tubercle bacillus is blood borne from elsewhere in the body, becoming first established either in the synovial membrane or in the bone of the epiphysis (Fig. 1), acetabulum or femoral neck. From these bony sites its spread to the joint space is usually rapid, although in the case of the femoral neck the infection may be locally contained (Fig. 2). Symptoms may not appear until the joint itself is involved, when an initial tuberculous synovitis is followed by destruction of the articular cartilage. The joint becomes distended with tuberculous pus, the bone of the femoral head and the acetabulum become involved and the articulation is irreparably damaged (Figs 3 and 4). The femoral head may sponta-

neously dislocate and with rupture of the joint capsule pus may track through the tissues and present in the groin or buttock, forming a so-called cold abscess (Fig. 5).

Diagnosis

In the very earliest stages it may be indistinguishable from other causes of irritable hip, but often when it is first seen it may be suspected by the extent of the muscle wasting and the flexion deformity of the hip. Radiographs of the hip may show some increase in the joint space, and a raised sedimentation rate calls for further investigation. The diagnosis is confirmed by histological and bacteriological examination of synovial biopsy specimens or by bacteriological examination of the aspirate.

Treatment

In the initial stages, before the diagnosis has been established, bed rest and traction are employed. On confirmation of the infection antituberculous therapy is commenced and this is tailored to the bacterial sensitivities as these become available. If after the initial investigative procedures there is evidence of a buildup of pressure within the joint from the formation of pus and excess synovial fluid, aspiration of the joint should be carried out to avoid further destruction of intra-articular tissues.

Prognosis

If discovered and treated early, complete resolution may be expected.

If there is delay and the joint has been extensively damaged by the infection, debridement may be called for and efforts made to obtain a joint fusion. In late diagnosed cases, where the infection is chronic and still active, an extra-articular arthrodesis may be considered.

In this procedure, to avoid dissemination of the infection, the joint is not opened: instead, it is rendered immobile by means of strut bone grafts placed like flying buttresses between the proximal part of the shaft of the femur and the pelvis.

PERTHES' DISEASE

The third of the most common causes of irritable hip is described on the following page.

ACUTE PYOGENIC ARTHRITIS OF THE HIP

Pyogenic infection of the hip is a serious condition which must be dealt with promptly and efficiently. The cause is usually a blood borne staphylococcus. The onset is rapid and is accompanied by a profound systemic disturbance. The child is unable to weight bear, is toxic with a high fever and is often delirious. There is complaint of great pain in the hip with protective muscle spasm and movement of the joint is reduced and feared. Unless promptly treated the hip becomes rapidly and irreversibly destroyed (Fig. 6).

Treatment

Traction is applied to the hip and blood cultures performed. The hip may require aspiration to reduce intra-articular pressure, relieve pain and obtain pus samples for bacteriological examination. Antibiotic therapy should be started immediately (usually a broad spectrum antibiotic is administered intravenously pending the arrival of sensitivities). With prompt treatment the infection is usually aborted, but if there is delay and much joint destruction, arthrodesis may be required.

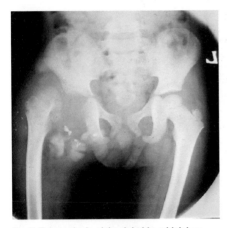

Fig. 5 **Tuberculosis of the right hip, which has dislocated.** There is calcified tuberculous pus in both sides of the thigh, with sinus formation.

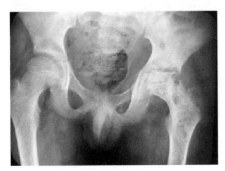

Fig. 6 **Septic arthritis of the hip.** The joint space has been destroyed and the femoral head flattened. There is an abscess cavity with a sequestrum in the metaphysis.

The irritable hip

- The most common causes of the irritable hip syndrome are transient synovitis of the hip, tuberculosis of the hip and Perthes' disease.
- The presenting feature is a limp which is generally painless and there is usually little systemic disturbance.
- In contrast, in acute pyogenic infections of the hip, there is a profound toxic illness.
- In the case of tuberculosis of the hip, as it advances fixed flexion deformity and increased lumbar lordosis develop and the leg muscles become very wasted.
- All cases of irritable hip syndrome are treated initially in the same way, by bed rest and traction.
- Later an exact diagnosis must be made, so that any additional treatment that is required may be carried out.

PERTHES' DISEASE OF THE HIP

Perthes' disease is a further cause of the irritable hip syndrome (see previous page). The child usually presents with a limp of insidious onset and there is no systemic upset. It is more common in boys than girls. It generally comes to attention in children between the ages of 2 and 6, but may sometimes appear as late as 9.

Pathology

The condition is the result of a disturbance of the blood supply to the femoral epiphysis. The cause is unknown, but it has long been suspected that it may arise from an error in the reorganisation of the blood supply to the proximal end of the femur which occurs about this time during child development. Both hips may be involved, either simultaneously or with an interval between them. In its most extreme forms its effects resemble those of avascular necrosis of the femoral head.

When the condition is in an active phase the bone involved becomes quite soft. If an appreciable portion of the femoral epiphysis is affected, the pressure of weight bearing will lead to deformity of the femoral head. The acetabulum in turn adapts to the change in the shape of the epiphysis of the femoral head, and itself becomes misshapen.

Clinical features

It frequently presents with a limp which may be painless. Often, however, there is complaint of discomfort or vague pain in the region of the hips, the thighs or the knees. (Remember, pathology in the hip quite frequently gives rise to pain which is referred to the knee!) When the condition is active, there is always some loss of internal rotation in the affected hip, and in severe cases this may be reduced to zero; its main cause is protective muscle spasm. There is usually loss of extension (mainly due to accumulation of excess synovial fluid within the joint) and of other movement to a much lesser degree.

The natural tendency is towards spontaneous resolution, which occurs by revascularisation of those areas of bone within the femoral epiphysis which have become avascular. This process is slow, usually being spread over 18 months or so. When complete, protective muscle spasm is no longer required and it disappears. As a result, movement in the hip improves and in some cases may return to normal. In others, where there is permanent deformity of the femoral head, recovery will inevitably be incomplete. With the loss of muscle spasm the child usually adapts to the residual loss of movement in the joint; the limp often disappears and former activities are resumed. Nevertheless, the altered shape of the femoral head and the acetabulum predispose the joint to the development of secondary osteoarthritis. This may often present as early as the third decade when the choice of treatment may be limited and difficult.

Diagnosis

At the very beginning, radiographs of the hip may show signs of joint effusion (as in acute synovitis and tuberculosis of the hip in their early stages) (Fig. 1). By the time the child usually presents with symptoms, specific diagnostic features are almost invariably present. Of these the most outstanding is an apparent increase in the density of the epiphysis of the femoral head, which often appears smaller than normal (Fig. 2). The radiographs may also be used to judge and grade the severity of

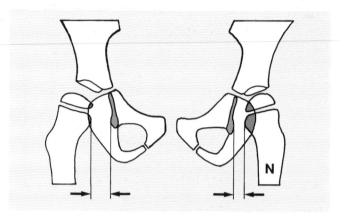

Fig. 1 **Effusion in the hip leads to an increase in the distance between the tear drop (blue) and the femoral head, and a decrease in the amount the head and neck overlap the acetabulum (red).** (N=normal side)

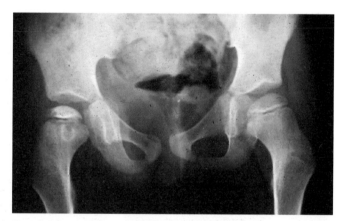

Fig. 2 **Perthes' disease of the right hip.** Although there is some rotation of the pelvis, there is still evidence of effusion on the right; the femoral head is dense and small.

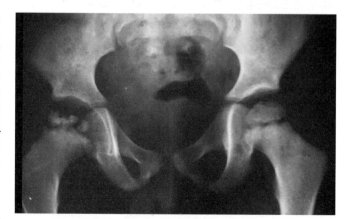

Fig. 3 **Perthes' disease, grade 1 on the left, grade 4 on the right.**

the case, to suggest a prognosis and perhaps to act as a guide to treatment. Arthrography or MRI scans may be employed to assess articular congruity; and MRI or radionuclide bone scans can unequivocally identify how much of the femoral head has become avascular.

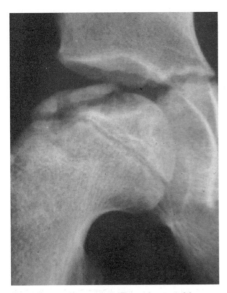

Fig. 4 **Late stage, grade 2.** The major part of the femoral head has been spared, and the bone density in the rest is almost back to normal.

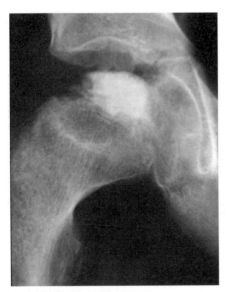

Fig. 5 **Early grade 3 Perthes' disease.** Most, but not all, the epiphysis is involved.

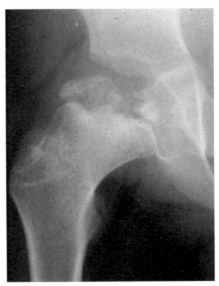

Fig. 6 **Grade 4.** All of the epiphysis has been affected, with gross fragmentation and some lateral extrusion. There is broadening of the metaphysis.

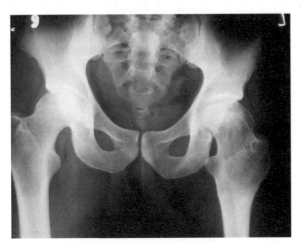

Fig. 7 **Ten years after the acute phase of a grade 3 Perthes' disease.** The degree of femoral head deformity suggests osteoarthritis of the hip is likely before the end of the fourth decade.

Catterall grading of Perthes' disease

Grade 1

Cyst formation has occurred in the anterolateral aspect of the epiphysis only (Fig. 3). The area involved may successfully revascularise without any deformity of the head occurring, and as a result the prognosis is good.

Grade 2

More of the femoral head is involved (Fig. 4), and some bony collapse will occur; recovery will be incomplete.

Grade 3

Most of the head is affected (Fig. 5).

Grade 4

All of the head is involved, and these cases naturally have the poorest prognosis (Fig. 6).

In addition to these changes in the epiphysis of the femoral head, the metaphysis may widen and the acetabulum become shallow and deformed; cystic changes may appear in both. Softening of the femoral epiphysis may lead to its flattening and extrusion beyond the lateral edge of the acetabulum. If this occurs, permanent deformity of the femoral head will be severe and secondary osteoarthritis inevitable. Other poor prognostic indicators include any tendency to lateral subluxation of the femoral head and the presence of Gage's sign — a V-shaped sequestrum in the capital epiphysis.

Treatment

In the initial stages, if there is discomfort or pain in the hip, admission for bedrest and simple skin traction is usually advised. If the severity is established as in grade 1 in the Catterall classification, then once the acute symptoms have settled, no other treatment is required, although the child should be kept under out-patient observation.

Where much or all of the femoral head is involved it is thought that progressive deformity may be minimised in a number of ways: these include (i) bedrest and splintage to avoid the pressures of weight bearing on the hip; and (ii) osteotomy of the femoral neck, which may help the acetabulum to contain the femoral head during the period when progressive revascularisation is taking place.

After revascularisation, it is usually possible to give a reasonably accurate prognosis based on the residual deformity of the femoral head (Fig. 7). This may permit the giving of advice regarding both the choice of career and athletic activities in order to help delay the onset of secondary osteoarthritis.

Perthes' disease of the hip

- Perthes' disease at its onset resembles other causes of the irritable hip syndrome.
- It is associated with avascular changes in the bone of the femoral head.
- The diagnosis is confirmed by its specific radiographic appearances.
- The radiographs may also permit the case to be graded in severity.
- The greater the proportion of the femoral head involved, the poorer the prognosis.
- Limiting deformity of the femoral head reduces the risks of secondary osteoarthritis.

FRACTURES OF THE PELVIS

When the pelvis is fractured, there is often the risk of serious internal haemorrhage, and in some cases the internal organs that the pelvis serves to protect may be damaged. If the fracture is proximally displaced or involves the sacroiliac joints or the acetabulum, lower limb function may be adversely affected and persistent pain is often a problem. These complications are often closely related to the pattern of the fracture, so that a careful assessment is required.

The first point to note is that normally the two halves of the pelvis and the sacrum form a stable cylinder of bone, the so-called pelvic ring, which protects the pelvic organs and transmits the body weight to the lower limbs. If this ring of bone is broken at its periphery or at one level, the fracture is stable; if there is disruption at two levels, then there is potential for displacement (Fig. 1).

Diagnosis

Fractures of the pelvis commonly result from falls from a height, road traffic accidents and crushing injuries. Screening films of the pelvis should always be obtained in cases of multiple trauma (especially in the presence of unexplained shock) and should be considered in blunt abdominal injuries and fractures of the femoral shaft.

In displaced fractures, the relationship between the bony components may be more clearly interpreted by CT scans; where the acetabulum is involved, oblique projections and CT scans, especially with 3-D imaging, are often helpful.

STABLE FRACTURES OF THE PELVIS NOT INVOLVING THE PELVIC RING

These are the least serious of pelvic fractures. Sudden muscle contraction may lead to an avulsion fracture of the anterior superior iliac spine (sartorius), the anterior inferior iliac spine (rectus femoris, Fig. 2), the ischial tuberosity (hamstrings) and the posterior superior iliac spine (erector spinae). Fracture of the lateral lip of the ilium or the blade

may result from direct violence. These injuries are best treated symptomatically, although severely displaced fractures of the ischium may sometimes require internal fixation.

STABLE FRACTURES OF THE PELVIC RING

Fractures of the ilium running into the sciatic notch or the sacroiliac joint (Figs 3a and 3b) will remain stable if the symphysis is undisturbed. If the pubic rami are fractured, there will be no instability provided the strong sacroiliac ligaments are unaffected; this may even apply to butterfly (or quadripartite) fractures (Fig. 3c), where although the ring is split at two levels, any displacement is usually confined to the butterfly segment. Fractures of this pattern are not infrequently complicated with urethral or bladder damage. The pelvic fractures themselves only require a few weeks bed rest until local pain, especially on attempted weight bearing, has settled.

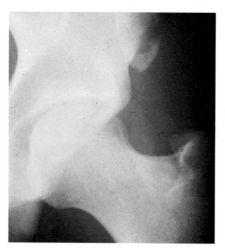

Fig. 2 **Avulsion fracture of the anterior inferior iliac spine.**

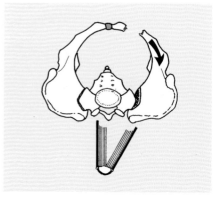

Fig. 4 **'Open book' fracture of the pelvis.**

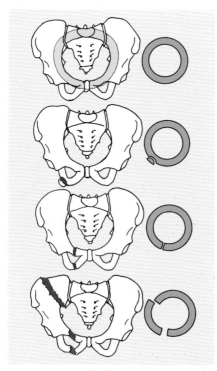

Fig. 1 **Stable and unstable fractures of the pelvic ring.**

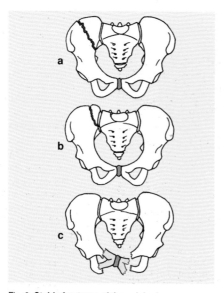

Fig. 3 **Stable fractures of the pelvic ring.**

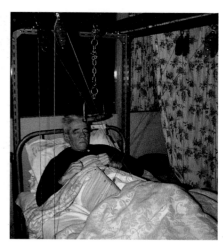

Fig. 5 **The use of a canvas sling with crossed cords and weights to reduce a displaced 'open-book' fracture of the pelvis.**

UNSTABLE FRACTURES OF THE PELVIS

Unstable fractures of the pelvis fall into two main patterns. In one, the two halves of the pelvis are free to come together or move apart, but remain stable in a vertical direction, so that shortening does not occur (rotationally unstable, vertically stable fractures). In the second, there is so much disruption that one or both halves of the pelvis may become displaced in a proximal direction (rotationally and vertically unstable fractures).

ROTATIONALLY UNSTABLE, VERTICALLY STABLE PELVIC FRACTURES

These injuries frequently result from the pelvis being crushed. When the compression occurs from front to back (anteroposterior compression fracture, e.g. in a road traffic accident when someone in the supine position is run over by the wheel of a vehicle) the pelvis

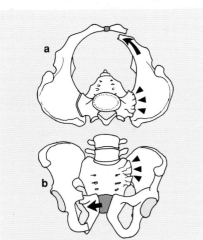

Fig. 6 **Lateral compression fractures of the pelvis.**

opens out, resulting in the so-called open book fracture (Fig. 4). In front, the pelvic ring splits at the symphysis or through the rami; behind, the ring is usually broken by disruption of sacroiliac joint ligaments. If the posterior damage is judged to be slight, and the anterior separation 2.5 cms or less, bedrest and observation will suffice. Where the separation and instability are greater, an external fixator (with pins inserted into the pelvic rims and an anterior fixator) may be used to bring the two halves of the pelvis together. These injuries may also be treated by the use of a canvas sling, with traction cords and weights adjusted to apply side-to-side compression of the pelvis (Fig. 5). (Note too that in an emergency, if other injuries will allow, lying the patient on his side may improve the position.)

Lateral compression fractures result from the pelvis being compressed from side to side. In ipsilateral injuries the sacroiliac joint and the pubic rami fail on the same side, and there may be overlap at the front (Fig. 6a). In contralateral compression fractures (Fig. 6b) the anterior and posterior lesions are on opposite sides of the pelvis. Both patterns of lateral compression injury may be treated by bed rest, unless displacement and mobility are marked, when an external fixator may be employed.

ROTATIONALLY AND VERTICALLY UNSTABLE INJURIES

The pelvic ring is broken in two or more places. In unilateral cases half of the

pelvis may become displaced in a proximal direction; in bilateral cases both sides of the pelvis may migrate proximally in relation to the sacrum. Posteriorly the sacroiliac joints may be completely disrupted (Fig. 7) or there may be fractures of the posterior part of the ilium or sacrum; anteriorly there may be involvement of the rami, symphysis or both.

These are serious injuries, potentially disabling, and often life threatening, due to the severe internal haemorrhage with which they are almost invariably accompanied. Massive blood replacement may be required. Further bleeding may be minimised by the application of a stabilising external fixator as an emergency procedure; proximal migration of the hemipelvis may be controlled by the use of leg traction applied with a Steinman pin.

Once the patient's condition has stabilised, definitive treatment may be considered. In many instances this will mean continuation of traction and the use of an external fixator. Where there is persistent dislocation of a sacroiliac joint, open reduction and internal fixation should be considered. This can be technically demanding and potentially hazardous. Methods available include plate and screw fixation of the symphysis, rami and iliac fractures; fixation of a sacroiliac joint by cancellous screws run into the body of the sacrum or by anterior plating of the sacroiliac joint; and fixation of sacral fractures and sacroiliac joint dislocations by threaded bars (studding) passed between the posterior iliac spines.

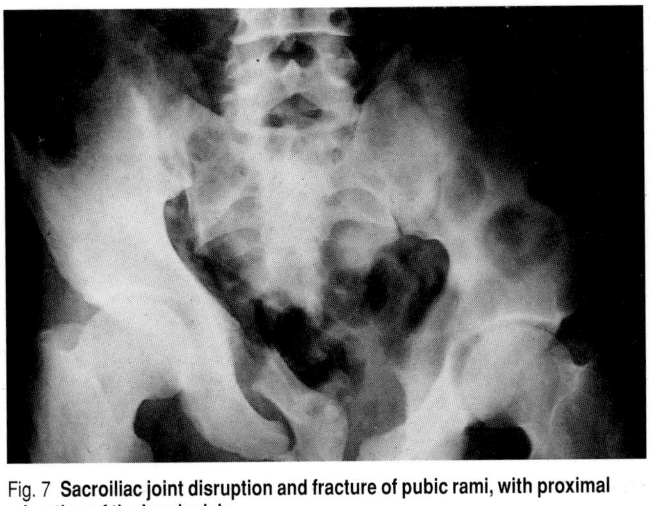

Fractures of the pelvis

- Internal haemorrhage is the most important immediate complication of pelvic fractures.
- Blood loss and the other complications of pelvic fracture are related to the pattern of injury.
- In assessing a pelvic fracture the most important consideration is to decide whether the injury is stable or unstable.
- Stable fractures either affect the pelvic ring at one point, or they do not involve it at all.
- Avulsion fractures seldom present any difficulty unless when one of the ischial tuberosities becomes markedly displaced.
- Although injuries to the rami are generally stable, the possibility of urethral or bladder complications must always be kept in mind.
- 'Open book' fractures may be treated by bed rest alone, by a canvas sling or by an external fixator, depending on their stability and displacement.
- Vertically unstable fractures are serious and potentially life threatening.
- A persistently dislocated sacroiliac joint is an indication for open reduction and internal fixation, although this is recognised as being technically difficult and potentially hazardous.

Fig. 7 **Sacroiliac joint disruption and fracture of pubic rami, with proximal migration of the hemipelvis.**

FRACTURES OF THE ACETABULUM / COMPLICATIONS OF PELVIC FRACTURES

FRACTURES OF THE ACETABULUM

The acetabulum may be involved in the more severe compression and vertically unstable fractures described on the previous page. More commonly, it is fractured as a result of force transmitted through the femoral head, for example, from a fall from a height on to the feet, from road traffic accidents in which the knees strike a car dashboard, or from a fall on the side. The head of the femur tends to be pushed medially, so that this particular class of pelvic fracture attracts the term of central dislocation of the hip.

Pathological features

In the normal pelvis, forces transmitted through the acetabulum are carried by two bony buttresses referred to as the anterior and posterior columns (Fig. 1). The anterior column includes the anterior inferior iliac spine, the anterior part of the acetabulum and the pubis. The posterior column includes the posterior part of the acetabulum, the anterior part of the sciatic notch and the ischium. One or both of these columns may be fractured and any decision regarding the necessity for surgical treatment and how this may best be carried out is dependent on a careful analysis of the extent of this involvement. In so-called Type A fractures, only one column is fractured. Type B fractures involve both columns, but part of the acetabular roof remains in continuity with the ilium (Figs 1 and 2). In Type C fractures, both columns are again fractured, but none of the acetabulum stays connected to the weight transmitting part of the ilium.

Diagnosis

The fracture is easily diagnosed on plain films and ideally in the first instance an AP view of the pelvis (to allow comparison of both sides) and a lateral of the affected side should be obtained. Thereafter the extent of the acetabular damage and displacement should be assessed, which can prove difficult. Oblique projections of the pelvis, CT scans and, best of all, 3-D pelvic imaging may be required.

Treatment

Each case must be considered on its own merits. Ideally the acetabular floor should be rendered congruous with the femoral head if the risks of secondary osteoarthritis are to be reduced. Obviously operative treatment is unnecessary if the fracture is not significantly displaced (e.g. the displacement is less than 2 mm). Under these circumstances 6 weeks' traction (with a Steinman pin inserted through the tibial tuberosity) will usually give a good result. Physiotherapy to encourage hip movements is commenced while the patient is in traction and continued during the later stages of mobilisation. Conservative treatment should also be advised if there is such a degree of comminution of the acetabulum that reduction is not feasible for technical reasons. If there is significant disturbance of the acetabulum but little comminution, and open reduction and internal fixation are thought to be possible, the surgical approach will be dependent on the fracture type and the access required. The procedure is often long and technically demanding, with attendant haemorrhage and risk of post-operative infection. The patient's fitness for surgery requires most careful assessment and precautions must be taken to minimise the risk of complications.

FRACTURES OF THE SACRUM AND COCCYX

Fractures of the ala of the sacrum may occur in compression fractures of the pelvis and transverse fractures through the body of the sacrum may occur in falls on hard surfaces. In some cases there may be some neurological disturbance. Treatment of sacral fractures is symptomatic, with 2–3 weeks' bed rest; if the neurological disturbance is severe and fails to improve spontaneously (as is the usual course) laminectomy may be advised.

The coccyx may be injured as the result of a fall on a hard surface. It may fracture, or become anteverted as a result of subluxation at the sacrococcygeal joint or fracture of the end piece of the sacrum. The initial treatment is symptomatic. In some cases pain becomes persistent (coccydynia) when local short wave diathermy or injections of long-acting local anaesthetics may be tried. Response to treatment is often poor; in severe cases where all else has failed coccygectomy is sometimes carried out.

COMPLICATIONS OF FRACTURES OF THE PELVIS

HAEMORRHAGE

Severe internal haemorrhage is a common and life-threatening complication of pelvic fractures, especially where there is disruption of the pelvic ring or where there is vertical instability. Apart from the signs of oligaemic shock, bruising

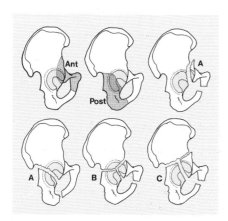

Fig. 1 **The anterior and posterior columns and the main types of acetabular fracture.**

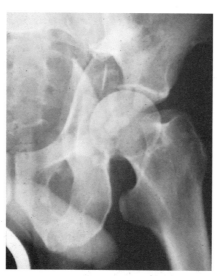

Fig. 2 **Type B fracture with disruption of the acetabulum.**

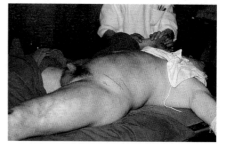

Fig. 3 **Lower limb ischaemia complicating a fracture of the pelvis from a run-over injury.** Note tyre stretch marks in groin.

appearing in a buttock, groin or scrotum or the development of a palpable retroperitoneal haematoma are evidence of substantial blood loss. In addition, intraperitoneal haemorrhage may result from the tearing of mesenteric blood vessels; this will lead to a progressive increase in abdominal girth, absent bowel sounds and a blood stained peritoneal tap. In some cases the iliac arteries may be damaged, leading to lower limb ischaemia (Fig. 3).

Treatment

Shock should be anticipated in any pelvic fracture and immediate measures taken; massive blood replacement may be required, depending on the nature of the fracture. Where the fracture is unstable, the emergency application of an external fixator may reduce the transfusion requirements. In the majority of cases the haemorrhage results from the disruption of the veins of the pelvic plexus and responds to these measures. If not, selective embolisation using image intensifier controlled angiography may be attempted; occasionally ligation of one or both internal iliac arteries has brought the bleeding under control. Where rupture of mesenteric vessels is suspected, abdominal exploration will be required.

URINARY TRACT INJURIES

Damage to the urethra occurs most frequently after butterfly fractures of the pelvis. Rupture of the bladder is seen most often after vertically unstable fractures of the pelvis where a sharp edge of a fractured superior pubic ramus causes a tear. Intraperitoneal rupture is only likely

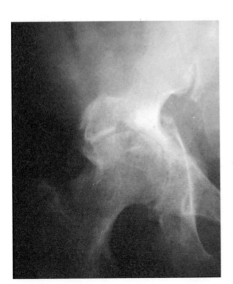

Fig. 4 **Osteoarthritis complicating an old central dislocation of the hip.**

to have occurred if the bladder was full at the time of the injury. The presence of perineal bruising is also highly suggestive of lower urinary tract injury, while blood at the tip of the penis is diagnostic (although the absence of these signs does not exclude injury).

Damage to the bladder or urethra should be suspected in all fractures of the anterior pelvis, particularly in those described, and investigated further. At the simplest, this may be to ask the patient to make an attempt to pass urine. Further investigation by a urethrogram may be required, and it is important to avoid wherever possible the dangers of a traumatic catheterisation. The treatment for injuries of the urethra and bladder is dependent on which structures are involved and the degree of continuity in the affected structures.

INJURY TO THE BOWEL

The rectum may be torn in open fractures and sometimes in closed injuries of the central dislocation type. Small bowel infarctions, perforations and mesenteric tears may be caused by crushing injuries of the pelvis. There may be abdominal rigidity, loss of liver dullness and abdominal distension. Exploration will be required.

PARALYTIC ILEUS

This complication may result from a retroperitoneal haematoma disturbing the autonomic supply to the bowel. It normally responds to intravenous fluids and nasogastric suction within 2–3 days.

RUPTURE OF THE DIAPHRAGM

Routine radiographs of the chest should be taken in all cases of major pelvic fracture in order to avoid overlooking this potential complication. If it is found, it should be formally repaired.

LIMB SHORTENING

Limb shortening may follow unreduced vertically displaced pelvic fractures and may be compensated by an appropriate shoe raise.

NEUROLOGICAL DAMAGE

The lumbosacral trunk, isolated spinal nerves or the sciatic nerve itself may be involved. Most frequently the lesion is one in continuity (neuropraxia) and exploration is seldom indicated. Impotence, which is usually permanent, complicates about a sixth of all major pelvic fractures and occurs most frequently in association with rupture of the urethra.

SACROILIAC PAIN

Chronic sacroiliac pain is a common complication, especially when there is persistent subluxation of a sacro-iliac joint, and sometimes merits sacro-iliac joint fusion.

OSTEOARTHRITIS OF THE HIP

This is a common complication of fractures of the central dislocation type (Fig. 4). In severe cases a total hip replacement may have to be considered; in these circumstances an acetabulum which has been reconstructed by an earlier procedure may facilitate this procedure, even though previously inserted metalwork may require removal.

SYMPHYSEAL INSTABILITY

Complaints of persistent pain in the region of the symphysis may merit investigation by intensifier screening, and if instability of the joint is confirmed, internal fixation may be carried out. (Note that in practice fractures of the pelvis which lead to permanent distortion of the pelvic inlet seldom give rise to any problem during parturition.)

Fractures of the acetabulum / complications of pelvic fractures

- Ideally in all cases of central dislocation of the hip the acetabular floor should be rendered congruent with the femoral head.
- In deciding to pursue this surgically, the pattern and degree of the acetabular disturbance and the operative risks must be carefully assessed.
- Symptoms following coccygeal injuries are often prolonged and a poor response to treatment is common.
- The most serious complication of pelvic fracture is haemorrhage and shock. Massive transfusion, the emergency application of a fixator and other measures may be required.
- Injuries to the urethra or bladder may complicate pelvic fractures, particularly of the butterfly or vertically unstable type.

DISLOCATION OF THE HIP / INTRACAPSULAR FRACTURES OF THE FEMORAL NECK

DISLOCATION OF THE HIP

Dislocation of the hip is comparatively uncommon, but generally results from force transmitted along the femur from the knees striking the dashboard in road traffic accidents. It may be overlooked if the same incident has resulted in a more obvious fracture of the patella or femoral shaft. It may also result from falls on the feet or heavy objects falling on the shoulders or back; posterior dislocation (Fig. 1) is much more common than anterior dislocation. Posterior dislocation is sometimes associated with a fracture of the acetabular rim and instability of the hip.

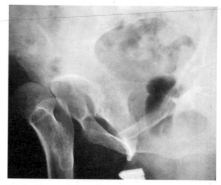

Fig. 1 **Posterior dislocation of the hip.**

Treatment

Dislocation of the hip is usually very painful and is accompanied by severe muscle spasm. To reduce a dislocated hip, general anaesthesia with complete muscle relaxation is required. The pelvis is steadied while traction is applied to the femur with the hip being held in 90 degrees flexion. After reduction it is customary to rest the hip for a period on traction. If there is a large displaced fracture of the rim, this is likely to lead to hip instability and should be reattached by screwing or plating.

Complications

Sciatic nerve palsy

This is seen in about one in ten posterior dislocations of the hip. If recovery does not occur after reduction, exploration is indicated within 24 hours of the incident especially if there is a rim fracture which may be causing local pressure on the nerve.

Avascular necrosis of the femoral head

Avascular necrosis of the femoral head due to disturbance of its blood supply is also seen in about a tenth of cases and is impervious to treatment.

Osteoarthritis of the hip inevitably develops after avascular necrosis, but is also seen where there is bony or cartilage damage to the acetabular floor. The overall incidence of this complication is 40% and it is treated along usual lines.

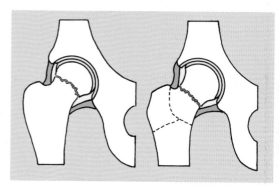

Fig. 2 **Subcapital and transcervical intracapsular fractures.** Extracapsular fractures (the dotted line shows the position of a typical extracapsular fracture) lie outwith the hip joint capsule.

INTRACAPSULAR FEMORAL NECK FRACTURES

When a fracture occurs in the femoral neck region, the fracture line may lie totally within the capsule of the hip joint (intracapsular fracture) or it may lie at or distal to the capsular attachments (extracapsular fracture, Fig. 2). Intracapsular fractures are the most common and potentially most serious of hip fractures.

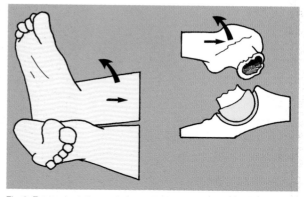

Fig. 3 **External rotation and shortening are seen most frequently in the non-impacted fracture.**

Aetiology

Intracapsular fractures of the femoral neck are much more common in women than in men. They are rarely seen before the onset of the menopause and their frequency increases with age. Osteoporosis is the most important predisposing factor; this is usually of postmenopausal origin, but in the younger patient it is sometimes secondary to chronic alcoholism.

As age advances, osteoporosis becomes more severe. The bones become increasingly fragile so that fracture may follow the most trivial injury. The most common cause is a simple fall at home. Momentary dizziness, poor muscle control and coordination and defective vision may be ancillary factors.

Diagnosis

Inability to bear weight after a fall, particularly in the case of an older woman, should alert you to the possibility of this condition. Very rarely, and generally when the fracture is impacted, weight bearing may be attempted by the patient, although there is always complaint of pain when the affected hip is rotated. If the fracture is not impacted, the leg tends to fall into

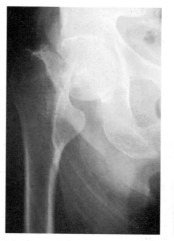
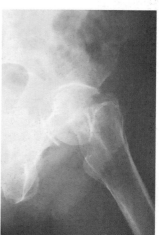

Fig. 4 **X-ray showing two views of an intracapsular fracture of the femoral neck.**

external rotation (Fig. 3). There is often a little shortening. There may be tenderness in the region of the femoral neck, but bruising is not a feature.

An X-ray examination of the hip is mandatory (Fig. 4). Occasionally, pain in the hip and difficulty in weight bearing following a fall may be due to a pubic ramus fracture rather than an intracapsular fracture of the neck of the femur. To eliminate this possibility, and to allow the injured hip to be compared with the good, it is common practice to have as the first films an AP view of the pelvis with an additional lateral projection of the injured hip. If no abnormality is found and the symptoms continue in spite of rest, further investigation will be required (e.g. repeat X-rays after a week, or radionuclide bone imaging, or a CT scan).

Complications

Avascular necrosis
Fractures in this region may disturb the blood supply to the femoral head. With the exception of a variable and unreliable supply through the ligamentum teres, all the vessels going to the head travel within the bone of the femoral neck and arise from a vascular ring at its base (Fig. 5). Disruption of the blood supply may lead to death of bone cells and to segmental or total avascular necrosis of the femoral head (Fig. 6). Radiological changes of avascular necrosis and secondary osteoarthritis may be delayed for as long as several years, although pain and restriction of movement appear much earlier.

Non-union
Because it is often difficult to hold the bone fragments in alignment for the time necessary for union to occur, non-union (Fig. 7) is the second common complication of intracapsular fractures.

Treatment
Without appropriate treatment, pain from the fracture immobilises the patient, with fatal complications ensuing in the majority of cases (e.g. hypostatic pneumonia, pulmonary embolism from deep venous thrombosis, urinary infection and renal failure, infected pressure sores, etc). Internal fixation of the fracture is the usual method of treatment. Commonly the head fragment is secured with a large diameter partially threaded screw sliding in a sleeve attached to a plate screwed to the lateral aspect of the femur (e.g. AO dynamic hip screw, Fig. 8).

In cases where the prospects are considered particularly bleak (e.g. in a very severely displaced proximally situated fracture), some form of joint replacement is often considered as a primary procedure, although there is an increased risk of complications such as dislocation and loosening. In the very frail elderly patient with a low life expectancy, a hemiarthroplasty may be carried out (this is a rapidly performed procedure where the femoral head is removed and replaced with a metal one of the same diameter, attached to a stem which passes down the femoral shaft). In the elderly but fitter patient with a good life expectancy, a total joint replacement may be considered. (A total replacement is also the usual procedure for either avascular necrosis or non-union, should these complications ensue.)

Whatever surgical treatment is carried out, the patient should be got out of bed as rapidly as possible, and it is usual to start weight bearing within a week. The patient's subsequent mobility determines after care. Ideally the patient should be able to return home, with or without back-up services and aids to daily living.

Where the fracture has been internally fixed, it should be followed up (ideally for 3 years) in case of early or late complications.

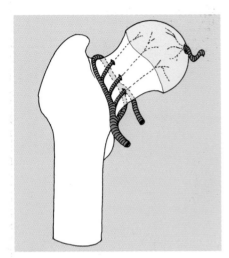

Fig. 5 **Blood supply of the femoral head.**

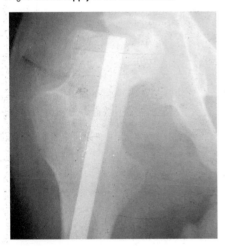

Fig. 6 **Avascular necrosis with deformity of the femoral head.**

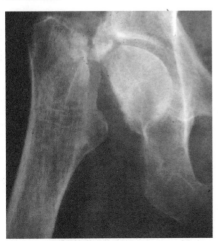

Fig. 7 **Non-union of an intracapsular fracture of the femoral neck.**

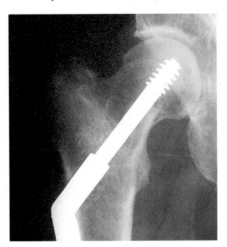

Fig. 8 **Fracture of the femoral neck held with an AO dynamic hip screw.**

Dislocation of the hip / Intracapsular fractures of the femoral neck
- Complete muscle relaxation is essential when an attempt is being made to reduce a dislocated hip.
- The two most serious complications of dislocation of the hip are avascular necrosis of the femoral head and sciatic nerve palsy.
- The more distal a femoral neck fracture is situated, the better the prognosis.
- The less an intracapsular fracture is displaced, the better the prognosis; and impacted fractures do best of all.
- Reduction and internal fixation is the most common method of treating intracapsular fractures.
- The two main complications of intracapsular fractures are non-union and avascular necrosis.
- Total hip replacement is the usual treatment for either of these complications.

EXTRACAPSULAR AND SHAFT FRACTURES OF THE FEMUR

BASAL (INTERTROCHANTERIC) FRACTURES OF THE FEMORAL NECK

Fractures at this level involve a substantial area of cancellous bone and do not interfere with the blood supply to the femoral head. They have a good prognosis as union is usually rapid and avascular necrosis is not a problem. These fractures are more common in men than in women and may result from direct violence in industrial or road traffic accidents or from falls on the side. They may be hair-line in pattern (Fig. 1) or displaced.

PERTROCHANTERIC FRACTURES

Fractures of this pattern lie distal to the intertrochanteric line and pass through or separate either of the trochanters (Fig. 2); in some cases there may be an associated spiral fracture of the proximal femoral shaft. They may pose problems with fixation, and the difficulties increase with the degree of fragmentation (comminution).

Treatment

Internal fixation is the preferred method of treatment in the majority of extracapsular fractures. In many cases, after any reduction that is required, the fracture may be held satisfactorily with a Dynamic Hip Screw, with a long plate attached to the femoral shaft. For the more unstable fracture a Gamma nail, reconstruction nail (Fig. 3) or a blade plate may be used. In all cases the patient is mobilised as soon as possible. The interval before weight bearing is permitted is dependent on the pattern of the fracture and the quality of the internal fixation; undue reliance must not be placed on the fixation device, as in fractures at this level there is an appreciable risk of its breaking and the fixation failing. As union is generally not a problem, extracapsular fractures may be treated by traction in a Thomas splint should other factors dictate that the fracture be managed conservatively.

FRACTURES OF THE FEMORAL SHAFT

Pathology

The femur is the largest bone in the body and well adapted to the severe stresses to which it is normally subjected. Considerable violence, such as may be sustained in falls from a height or road

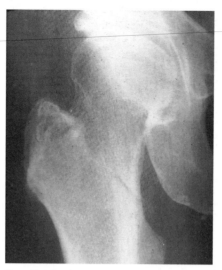

Fig. 1 **Hair-line basal fracture of the femoral neck.**

traffic accidents, is necessary before it will fracture. (If the history is of trivial violence, the possibility of pathological fracture must be considered.)

The femur is surrounded by a thick layer of muscle (the quadriceps, hamstrings and adductors of the hip) so that open fractures are relatively uncommon. Many large blood vessels run close to it (e.g. the perforating arteries); when the bone fractures, these are torn, and internal haemorrhage, with oligaemic shock, commonly accompanies femoral shaft fractures. This can be life threatening unless promptly treated, especially where the problem is aggravated by the fracture being open or bilateral. Union of this large bone takes a considerable time to reach the stage where unprotected weight bearing can be tolerated without the risks of refracture and, in conservatively treated fractures, the possibility of joint stiffness must always be kept in mind.

Diagnosis

This seldom presents any difficulty. There is usually a history of considerable violence, with severe local pain and inability to weight bear. There is often striking deformity of the leg; shortening of the affected limb may be apparent, with the foot lying in external rotation. Abduction of the proximal fragment may result in great prominence of the lateral aspect of the thigh. There is often accompanying shock. In motor vehicle accidents where a seat belt has not been worn the fracture may result from the knee striking the dashboard. It is most

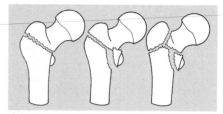

Fig. 2 **Some common patterns of per-trochanteric fracture.** These are arranged in order of increasing instability.

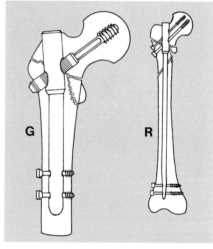

Fig. 3 **Gamma (G) and reconstruction (R) nails used to fix extracapsular fractures.**

important to note that the same forces may result in other injuries to the limb and that these are not overlooked: concurrent ipsilateral fracture of the patella, posterior dislocation of the hip and fracture of the femoral neck must always be excluded.

First aid measures

As soon as possible after the incident, and before the patient is transported to hospital, the limb should be splinted to minimise movement at the fracture site; this will reduce internal haemorrhage and shock, and help relieve pain. The simplest method is to strap the two legs together, the sound limb splinting the other. Inflatable splints may also be used, or the injured leg may be bandaged to a padded plank or similar object applied to its lateral aspect. Any open wound should be covered with a sterile dressing; this should be firmly bandaged in position if haemorrhage is brisk. In all cases the risks of oligaemic shock must be considered a priority, and particularly in the adolescent and adult an intravenous line should be set up, blood grouped and cross matched, and the pulse rate and blood pressure carefully monitored.

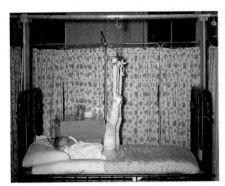

Fig. 4 **Femoral shaft fracture in a young child treated by gallows traction.**

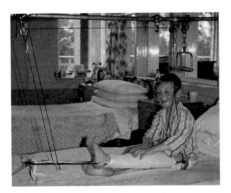

Fig. 5 **Femoral shaft fracture treated by fixed skin traction in a Thomas splint.**

Treatment of the fracture

The young child

In children up to the age of 3 (or 4 if the child is light in weight) so-called gallows traction is usually employed. Both legs are suspended with traction tapes from an overhead beam so that the buttocks are just clear of the bed. This renders nursing easy, and the child's weight provides the traction which reduces the fracture (Fig. 4). In a child of 3 this is maintained for on average about 4 weeks. This method of treatment should not be used in the older child as there is risk of vascular spasm and gangrene. Be sure to take a careful history and make a careful examination to exclude the possibility of child abuse.

The older child and adolescent

In this age group, before epiphyseal closure, surgical treatment is usually avoided and good results are generally obtained using a Thomas splint with skin traction (Fig. 5). The time taken for the fracture to unite increases with age; in a child of 11 this may be in the order of 12 weeks. Union is assessed by clinical examination and by X-ray.

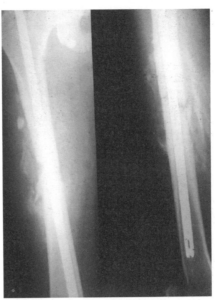

Fig. 6 **Femoral shaft fracture treated by intramedullary nailing.** Note callus formation.

The adult

Many adult fractures of the femur may also be treated successfully by immobilisation in a Thomas splint, which is especially appropriate in minimally displaced stable fractures. The skin is often unable to tolerate the amount of traction required by skin traction and skeletal traction, using a Steinman pin inserted in the region of the tibial tubercle, is usually employed. The length of time before unsupported weight bearing may be allowed is long (often 4-6 months), and as time proceeds there is increased risk of permanent knee stiffness. This becomes an even greater problem if union is delayed. In many cases it is possible to start knee movements before union is complete, either by making alterations to the traction system or by mobilising the patient with a cast brace.

To permit early mobilisation and reduce the risks of knee stiffness, many femoral shaft fractures are treated by internal fixation (Fig. 6). This is particularly important in cases of multiple injury so that the risks of prolonged recumbency (including pulmonary embolus, fat embolism, hypostatic pneumonia, etc.) are minimised. The usual method is to carry out a reduction of the fracture under image intensifier control and to insert an intramedullary nail from the trochanteric region of the femur, without direct exposure of the fracture. To counteract any tendency for the femoral fragments to rotate round the nail (torsional instability), interlocking screws may be inserted in a transverse direction across the shaft of the femur and through openings in the intramedullary nail.

OPEN FRACTURES OF THE FEMORAL SHAFT

Open fractures are uncommon and, in most cases, provided the wound is treated appropriately, the risks of infection following internal fixation are not appreciably higher than if conservative methods are employed. Where the conditions are more adverse (e.g. with extensive skin and muscle damage), careful assessment is required. Primary internal fixation may still be advocated, although reaming of the medullary cavity should probably be avoided. In other cases an external fixator may be used or the limb placed in traction in a Thomas splint until any potentially serious infection has been eliminated.

Complications

Oligaemic shock. Anticipate and treat promptly and adequately.

Fat embolism. The risks of this occurring are reduced by expert fluid replacement and by intramedullary nailing in cases of multiple injury. If it occurs, treat by appropriate measures (e.g. stabilisation of the fracture, intubation and the use of a ventilator if the blood gases are disturbed).

Non-union. This may be treated by internal fixation and bone grafting.

Limb shortening. In children this generally corrects itself spontaneously by accelerated growth; in adults, a shoe raise (or rarely, limb lengthening) may be required if the shortening exceeds 2 cm.

Knee stiffness. Prolonged physiotherapy may be necessary. Where there is permanent restriction of flexion to less than 90 degrees, a quadricepsplasty may be helpful.

Extracapsular and shaft fractures of the femur

- Union in extracapsular fractures of the femoral neck is usually rapid and avascular necrosis is not a problem.
- In fractures of the femoral shaft, be alert to the dangers of oligaemic shock.
- In any case of femoral shaft fracture, but especially in road traffic accidents, look for other injuries in the same limb.
- Treat fractures of the femoral shaft in children and adolescents by conservative methods.
- In adults, consider using internal fixation so that mobilisation may be started early and the risks of knee stiffness reduced.

FRACTURES OF THE DISTAL FEMUR AND PROXIMAL TIBIA

SUPRACONDYLAR FRACTURES OF THE FEMUR

The femur may fracture in its distal third just proximal to the femoral condyles without disturbance of the tibiofemoral articulation, although the fracture line may enter the suprapatellar pouch (Fig. 1a). Fractures of this pattern are usually the result of indirect violence (e.g. from a fall on to the feet from a height). In some cases (especially in children) the fracture is impacted without significant displacement, but in many there is a tendency to posterior angulation (pa, Fig. 1). This is due to tension in the gastrocnemius muscle whose two heads have their origin just proximal to the femoral condyles.

Treatment

An undisplaced, impacted supracondylar fracture in a child may often be treated successfully in a close fitting plaster cylinder (pipe-stem plaster) (Fig. 2). In adults, a period of traction in a Thomas splint followed by a cast brace may be employed. If the fracture is angled it must be reduced. Thereafter it may be treated conservatively or by internal fixation. With the former, for traction to be effective in maintaining the reduction, it is necessary to have an effective fulcrum behind the femur at the level of the fracture. Although this may sometimes be achieved by padding, it is often more effective to use a Thomas splint which has been bent at the level of the fracture (Fig. 3). If the fracture is being internally fixed, the internal fixation device must have a secure hold of the femoral condyles at one end and of the femoral shaft at the other. In practice this may be achieved with a blade-plate, locked intramedullary nail or a long plated dynamic compression screw (Fig. 4).

The main complication of supracondylar fractures of the femur is stiffness of the knee. In the main this is related to the length of time that the knee is immobilised after the injury, although surgical adhesions may make a signficant contribution to this problem.

FRACTURES INVOLVING THE FEMORAL CONDYLES

Fractures in this region are potentially serious as they involve the knee joint. There may be considerable disturbance of the articular surfaces, with the risk of knee joint stiffness and secondary osteoarthritis.

There are a number of methods of classifying the many different patterns of fracture in this region, but the most important points to note are the amount of deformity and whether one or both femoral condyles are involved. Unicondylar fractures (Fig. 1b) by definition involve a single condyle; bi-condylar (i.e. T- or Y-fractures) (Fig. 1c) are the most serious injuries in this region because of the disturbance that they cause to the articulation, their potential for instability and the diiffculties they may present in reduction and fixation. The latter is an especial problem when there is marked comminution (Fig. 5).

Treatment

Where displacement is slight, conservative methods similar to those employed in the treatment of supracondylar fractures of the femur may be used, although internal fixation followed by early mobilisation is usually preferred. In the case of badly displaced fractures, open reduction and internal fixation are advised unless the degree of comminution is so great that this

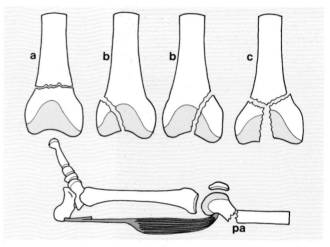

Fig. 1 **Common fracture patterns in the distal femur.**

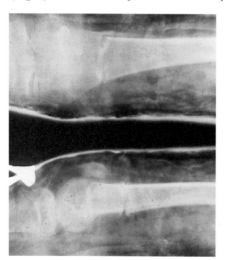

Fig. 2 **Supracondylar fracture of the femur in a child being treated in a plaster cylinder.**

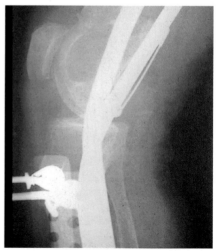

Fig. 3 **Supracondylar fracture of the femur in an adult being treated with skeletal traction in a bent Thomas splint.**

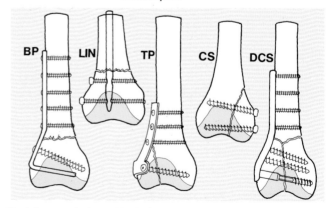

Fig. 4 **Some methods used for the internal fixation of distal femoral fractures.** BP = blade plate; LIN = locked intramedullary nail; TP = T-plate; CS = cancellous screws; DCS = dynamic condylar screw.

is technically impossible. Unicondylar fractures may be fixed with a T-plate or cancellous screws (Fig. 4). In the case of T- and Y-fractures a dynamic condylar screw, with a plate attached to the distal femoral shaft, can give good control (Fig. 4).

FRACTURES OF PROXIMAL TIBIA

Fractures of the tibial plateau (tibial tables, tibial condyles) may result from violence which forces the joint into valgus or varus. Most occur as a result of a fall or from a road traffic accident. If a medially directed force is applied to the lateral aspect of the knee (e.g. as may happen when a pedestrian is struck by a car bumper) (Fig. 6a), the medial ligament becomes taut and the lateral femoral condyle bears down forcibly on the lateral tibial plateau (lateral tibial table). This may fracture, and with greater violence all or part of the lateral tibial plateau becomes depressed below the level of the surrounding joint surfaces. If uncorrected, the disturbance of the articular surface may predispose the joint to secondary osteoarthritis and the relative slackening of the lateral ligament may lead to joint instability. Although relatively uncommon, with greater violence, the stretched medial ligament tears (Fig. 6b and Fig. 7) and the cruciate ligaments may even rupture. A similar sequence of events may follow a blow on the inside of the knee (or violence which forces the foot medially). Under those circumstances the medial tibial table may fracture and become depressed and the lateral ligament may tear. If the lateral aspect of the joint opens up, the common peroneal nerve may be stretched (Fig. 6c); this may result in a common peroneal nerve palsy, with a drop foot and loss of sensation over the side of the leg and dorsum of the foot. In many cases the nerve is completely ruptured, with extensive and irreparable damage.

Uncommonly, both the lateral and medial tibial tables may simultaneously fracture, leading to the equivalent of a T- or Y-fracture.

Treatment

More than half those patients who have a persistent depression of a tibial articular surface of 14 mm or more have a poor functional result and the chances of a poor outcome are also greater in those cases where there is malalignment or instability. Treatment is aimed at addressing these facts. Where the deformity is slight (e.g. joint surface depression of 1 cm or less) and there are no other oustanding features, a period of traction with early mobilisation of the knee usually gives good results. Where the deformity is more severe (i.e. a depression in excess of 1 cm), reduction and some form of internal fixation is usually advised. The type of fixation is dependent on the exact nature of the injury. In some cases the use of cancellous bone screws alone may suffice; in others, a combination of a T-plate and screws may be used (Figs 8a and 8b). Where the articular surface has been depressed, it may be necessary to pack this up from below with bone grafts (Figs 8a–8f). Torn ligaments may also have to be repaired to restore joint stability. A common peroneal nerve palsy should be explored.

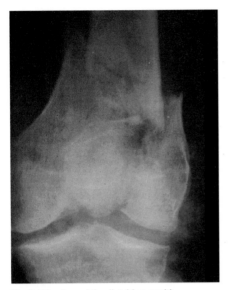

Fig. 5 **Y-fracture of the distal femur with comminution.**

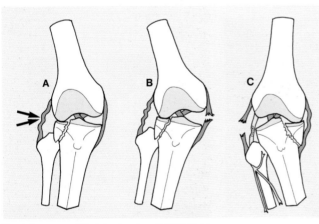

Fig. 6 **Fractures of the lateral and medial tibial tables.**

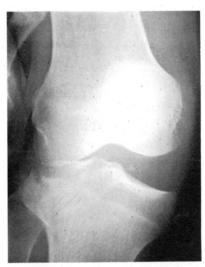

Fig. 7 **Fracture of the lateral tibial table with rupture of medial ligament of the knee.**

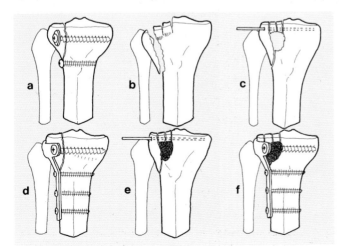

Fig. 8 **Some methods of fixing proximal tibial fractures.**

Fractures of the distal femur and proximal tibia

- Supracondylar fractures of the femur have a tendency to posterior angulation and this should be anticipated.
- Significantly displaced fractures of the femoral condyles and of the tibial tables are generally best treated by open reduction and internal fixation.
- Fractures of the medial tibial table may be complicated by common peroneal nerve palsy.

FRACTURES AND DISLOCATIONS OF THE PATELLA

FRACTURES OF THE PATELLA

The patella may fracture as the result of direct violence, e.g. if the knee strikes the edge of a step after a fall on stairs or if it hits the dashboard of a car in a road traffic accident. It may also fracture as the result of a sudden contracture of the quadriceps muscle.

Treatment

This is dependent on the site, the severity and the degree of displacement of the fracture. The aim of treatment is, if possible, to retain the patella and to restore its articular surface with a degree of accuracy that will minimise the risks of secondary patello-femoral osteoarthritis.

An undisplaced fracture (Fig. 1), particularly if it is of hair-line pattern, may be treated by a cylinder plaster for 6 weeks. Care must be taken to ensure that if late displacement occurs it is detected and dealt with promptly.

Fractures of the upper and lower poles which involve a small portion only of the articular surface may be dealt with by excision of the fragment, followed by reattachment and repair of the torn soft tissues of the quadriceps insertion, so that the ability to extend the knee is restored.

Where **two or three substantial fragments** are displaced (Fig. 2) but which can be reduced with accuracy, then internal fixation, e.g. by tension band or Pyrford wiring (Fig. 3), should be carried out.

Where there is much **comminution**, so that accurate reconstruction is not at all possible, the patella should be excised and the tendon repaired. Following patellectomy for trauma, a 6 week period in a plaster cylinder is advised before mobilisation is commenced. Initially there is usually an extension lag, but ultimately recovery of a full or excellent range of movements may be expected, although some loss of strength and occasional sensations of instability in the knee when going down slopes are not uncommon.

OTHER INJURIES OF THE EXTENSOR MECHANISM

Sudden muscle contraction, especially in the older patient, may result in loss of the ability to extend the knee due to disruption of the extensor apparatus of the knee at other levels. The quadriceps tendon above the patella (Fig. 4) or the patellar ligament below may rupture, or the tibial tuberosity at the insertion of the quadriceps may be avulsed (Fig. 5). These injuries are dealt with surgically either by tendon repair or reattachment of the tibial tubercle with a screw.

DISLOCATION OF THE PATELLA

The patella may dislocate laterally (Fig. 6) as a result of a blow on its medial edge, often during the course of contact sports. The patella may also dislocate spontaneously as a result of a number of predisposing factors. Due to the fact that the femur meets the tibia at an angle, the pull of the quadriceps always has a lateral component of force which tends

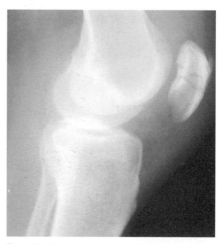
Fig. 1 **Undisplaced fracture of the patella.**

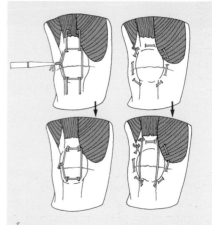
Fig. 3 **Tension band (left) and Pyrford wiring (right) of the patella.**

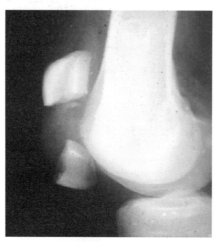
Fig. 2 **Transverse displaced fracture of the patella.**

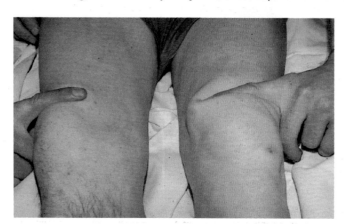
Fig. 4 **Rupture of the left quadriceps expansion with a palpable 'gap'.**

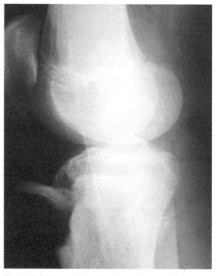
Fig. 5 **Avulsion of the tibial tuberosity with proximal displacement of the patella.**

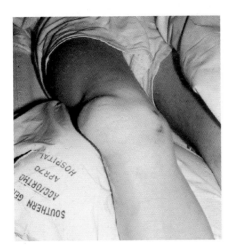

Fig. 6 **Lateral dislocation of the left patella.** Note the medial bruising.

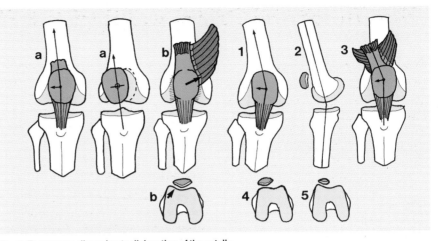

Fig. 7 **Factors pre-disposing to dislocation of the patella.**

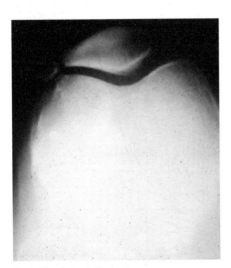

Fig. 8 **Marginal patellar fracture.**

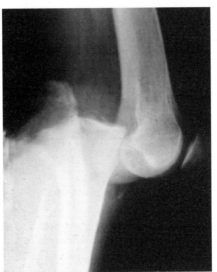

Fig. 9 **Dislocation of the knee.**

to displace the patella laterally (Fig. 7a). This is resisted by the vastus medialis and the walls of the bony gutter in which the patella lies (Fig. 7b). There is an increased tendency to dislocation (see Fig. 7) if:

1. the tibiofemoral angle is increased (as in knock knee)
2. the patella is highly placed (patella alta) so that it lies outwith the femoral gutter (this abnormality is seen most often in association with genu recurvatum (back knee))
3. the main mass of the quadriceps has an abnormally lateral insertion into the patella
4. the lateral wall of the gutter is poorly developed, offering little resistance to lateral subluxation
5. the patella is hypoplastic.

These congenital and acquired abnormalities are more common in females and account for the fact that dislocation of the patella is seen most frequently in girls, the first incident often occurring in the 14–16 age group.

The deformity is striking, but the diagnosis may be more difficult if the patella has reduced before the patient attends; nevertheless, in most cases there is no problem as a history of deformity and the age and sex of the patient should alert you to this possibility. As the patella dislocates laterally it tears its medial attachments, where there is local tenderness and where bruising may appear. Tangential views of the patella may show a marginal avulsion fracture (Fig. 8), or later, at about 3 weeks, some medial calcification in the local haematoma.

Treatment

The patella is easily reduced by pushing it medially. Thereafter the leg should be supported for 6 weeks in a plaster cylinder to allow the torn tissues time to repair. Some advocate exploration and surgical repair at the time of a first incident.

The most serious complication is recurrent dislocation of the patella, when the patella repeatedly dislocates with progressive facility, until in some cases it subluxes laterally whenever the knee is flexed. This may result in the joint giving way or secondary osteoarthritis. There are a number of surgical treatments performed for this condition (e.g. lateral release, medial reefing and medial transposition of the tibial tuberosity). Careful assessment of the causal factors is necessary in selecting the best procedure for any patient.

DISLOCATION OF THE KNEE

In this rare condition, traumatic in origin, there is loss of alignment between the femur and the tibia (Fig. 9). There is invariably major ligament disruption, and in some cases there may be damage to the popliteal vessels or the common peroneal nerve. In the uncomplicated case, reduction and conservative treatment in a plaster cast appear to give as good results as attempts at operative repair of the damaged ligaments.

Fractures and dislocations of the patella

- Displaced fractures of the patella should be reduced and internally fixed unless there is much comminution, when excision may give a better result.
- Apart from fracture of the patella, the ability to extend the knee may be lost by other disruptions of the extensor apparatus of the knee.
- Recurrent dislocation is the most common complication of patellar dislocation; it is seen most often in adolescent girls and a number of predisposing factors may be present.

MALALIGNMENT DISORDERS OF THE KNEE

The tibia and femur meet at an angle of about 7–11 degrees, and normally when the legs are adducted they touch at the knees and ankles (Fig. 1). If the tibio-femoral angle increases, the malleoli diverge, resulting in knock knee (*genu valgum*). (Some would restrict use of the term to intermalleolar gaps of 10 cm or more.) In contrast, when the knees do not touch when the malleoli come into contact, the resulting deformity is known as bow leg (*genu varum*). This may result from a decrease (or reversal) of the tibiofemoral angle, or to bowing of the tibia, femur or both. Note that normally the planes of the knee and ankle lie horizontally; a line drawn from the centre of the femoral head to the mid-point of the ankle passes through the centre of the knee; and in the erect position the inclination of that line to the vertical (normally about 3 degrees) is related to the width of the pelvis.

When the knee is fully extended and viewed from the side, the femur and tibia lie virtually in line. If the knee can extend further (i.e. hyperextend), the condition of *genu recurvatum* is present. This may result in the patella becoming highly placed (patella alta) and to lie above the intercondylar gutter.

PHYSIOLOGICAL VARIANTS

In the child, the alignment of the lower limb varies from birth until maturity. Babies are naturally bow legged at birth; this usually corrects at about 18 months, but may persist until age 4 or more. The varus is often associated with persistent anteversion of the femoral neck. This causes the child to walk awkwardly with the feet turned inwards (intoeing or hen-toed gait), so that they frequently trip and fall. In the older child, a bilateral genu valgum (knock knee) deformity often develops. This usually straightens to the adult alignment as puberty approaches.

It is common for a parent to express concern over the shape of a child's legs or gait. It is important to remember that the deformity may involve the femur, tibia and foot, and all must be carefully assessed. In most cases a malalignment disorder will be found to be responsible, and reassurance can generally be safely given. Rarely, when the deformities are much more severe, surgical correction may be required. This is usually postponed until near the end of growth.

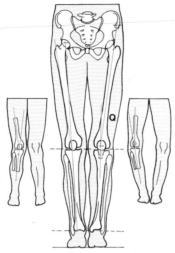

Fig. 1 **Normal joint planes and alignments (centre); disturbance of tibiofemoral angle in knock knee and bow leg (left and right).** Note the Q angle, used in assessing patellar forces, which is the angle between the patellar ligament and a line connecting the centre of the patella with the anterior superior iliac spine (ASIS).

GENERAL CAUSES OF MALALIGNMENT

When physiological growth variants are excluded, the remaining deformities are found to be due to abnormalities of growth or metabolism (Table 1).

When growth is disturbed, this is generally due to involvement of the epiphyseal plate. This may result from *fracture*, particularly of Salter and Harris Type 4 or 5 which can lead to partial fusion of the growth plate and differential bone growth. Exceptionally, a valgus greenstick fracture of the proximal tibial metaphysis, even though minimally displaced, may be followed by progressive deformity (which unlike the majority of children's fractures fails to correct spontaneously). *Sepsis*, either of the joint or periarticular bone, can affect growth. In these situations it is important to anticipate growth disturbance and keep the patient under review, although operative correction should be postponed until the infection has completely settled. Growth may also be disturbed in a number of other conditions where the cause is not local. In some there is an hereditary element, and the growth disturbances are often multifocal (the *epiphyseal dysplasias*).

Of the *metabolic causes* of deformity, rickets is by far the most common. It is caused by Vitamin D deficiency in the growing skeleton. Fresh cases are now rare in the UK, although it is seen from

Table 1 **Causes of malalignment.**

General
- Physiological
- Traumatic growth disturbance of the epiphysis and/or metaphysis
- Sepsis
- Epiphyseal dysplasia
- Metabolic, including rickets
- Soft tissue imbalance in the growing child

Specific
Genu varum
- Blount's disease
- Medial compartment osteoarthritis
- Medial tibial plateau fracture

Genu valgum
- Valgus greenstick fracture
- Rheumatoid arthritis
- Lateral tibial plateau fracture

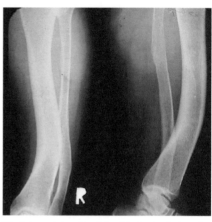

Fig. 2 **Late deformity of the tibia (in three planes) secondary to rickets.**

time to time, particularly amongst the immigrant population; it is still common, however, in many deprived countries. In the UK there remain a number of adults who have residual deformities (Fig. 2) from having had rickets as children, and they may present with secondary conditions such as osteoarthritis. In the affected child it is important to treat the rickets before contemplating any surgical correction.

GENU VARUM

The more important point is to assess whether the condition is worsening as it is this which influences the decision as to whether corrective surgery is going to be required. This generally involves observation with repeated measurements over a period. Note that with growth a constant inter-knee gap in fact indicates an improvement in the tibiofemoral angle. The diagnosis of pathological genu varum cannot be made until the child is 1–2 years old, as prior to this, deformity

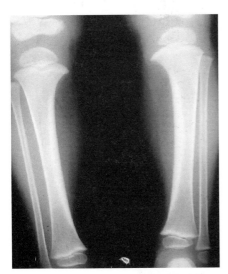

Fig. 3 **Blount's disease: note the characteristic 'beaking' of the medial tibial metaphyses.**

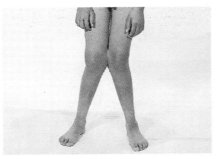

Fig. 4 **Persistent bilateral genu valgum at maturity requiring surgical correction.**

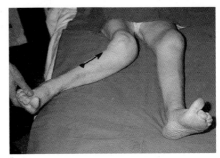

Fig. 5 **Severe genu valgum secondary to rheumatoid arthritis, about to undergo corrective surgery.**

may be physiological. Unfortunately, it is in the 2–4-year-old group that physiological varus will tend to improve and pathological varus will worsen so a watching policy is essential. After 4 years of age correction can be considered in worsening deformities, whilst continuing observation is appropriate in those which are more minor.

Blount's disease (tibia vara) is an uncommon developmental anomaly which affects the posteromedial portion of the upper tibial growth plate and tibial metaphysis (Fig. 3). This causes severe and progressive genu varum. It is more common in black Africans and Americans and in West Indians. Spontaneous resolution never occurs, and surgery, which is usually performed at about 8 years, is almost always required.

The most direct way of treating genu varum is by performing a realignment osteotomy; this involves removing a wedge of bone. Manipulative closure of the gap, which may be done immediately or after a delay (osteoclasis), then leads to correction of the deformity. Alternatively, an external fixator may be used, with fixing pins in the epiphysis and shaft to modify epiphyseal growth. While the resulting correction is slow, it can be well controlled. Finally, it is possible to slow the growth on the lateral side of the tibia by inserting staples across the growth plate; as the child grows, the deformity gradually improves.

In the adult, the main causes of genu varum are either tibial plateau fractures which cause depression of the fragments or medial compartment osteoarthritis. In displaced fractures it is important to try to minimise the deformity, and open reduction and internal fixation may be

required. In established osteoarthritis, treatment is either by realignment osteotomy or joint replacement. The latter is largely dependent on the age of the patient and the severity of the symptoms.

GENU VALGUM

As in genu varum, the progress of the deformity determines whether observation should be continued or surgery advised (Fig. 4). In children, genu valgum is much more common than genu varum and its causes are similar (although there is no equivalent to Blount's disease). It is important to assess the whole limb as it is not uncommon for genu valgum to be found in association with fixed hip deformities, rotational anomalies of the femur and tibia, or flat feet (pes planus). Treatment is much the same as in the varus deformities, with realignment osteotomies or stapling of the growth plates being most common. Correction with an external fixator is not so useful in valgus knees. Care has to be taken not to stretch the common peroneal nerve as it winds around the fibular neck, and if a traction injury does occur, recovery is always protracted.

In the adult, the deformity is most commonly seen in the rheumatoid patient, where the lateral compartment is more vulnerable than the medial (Fig. 5). It is relatively uncommon in the osteoarthritic knee. As genu valgum can

occur secondary to a fixed adduction deformity of an osteoarthritic hip, it is important to ensure that the hip is normal. If the hip pathology is not addressed first, any correction of the knee alignment is doomed to fail.

GENU RECURVATUM

In the very young child, the hyper-extension may be marked and associated with a short quadriceps tendon and generalised ligamentous laxity. The flexion range is usually restricted, but with physiotherapy and splintage the recurvatum can be controlled.

Genu recurvatum of varying degrees commonly develops in adolescent girls. This results from slowing of growth in the anterior portion of the upper tibial growth plate and frequently results from the wearing of high heeled shoes in the early teens. It also occurs in ballet dancers (where it is almost universal) as a result of point work. It may result in patella alta and may be associated with recurrent dislocation of the patella and chondromalacia patellae.

In cases of muscle imbalance, such as in cerebral palsy or poliomyelitis, genu recurvatum may gradually manifest itself over a period of years. This may not be totally disadvantageous as, if quadriceps control is lacking, a degree of recurvatum can be useful to 'lock' the knee and allow weight bearing. In these circumstances, splintage may nevertheless be helpful.

Malalignment disorders of the knee

- Tibiofemoral alignment changes from varus to valgus during normal growth.
- If significant malalignment is suspected, a period of observation will be required.
- A valgus greenstick fracture of the proximal tibia may sometimes cause a progressive deformity.
- If indicated, any malalignment may be corrected by surgery.

KNEE LIGAMENT INJURIES

Injuries to the ligaments of the knee are common and, fortunately, usually minor. In more severe injuries, where several structures may be involved, careful assessment and treatment are required to avoid permanent disability.

Anatomical features

There are four main ligaments at the knee joint, namely the anterior and posterior cruciate ligaments and the medial and lateral collateral ligaments. The cruciates are intracapsular, but extrasynovial whilst the collaterals form part of the capsular structures. The *anterior cruciate* (ACL) is attached at the front to the tibia near the spines and crosses to the medial side of the lateral femoral condyle. The *posterior cruciate* (PCL) is attached to the posterior tibia and crosses to the lateral side of the medial femoral condyle. They are under appreciable tension when the knee is in 20 degrees flexion, and it is in this position that the anterior cruciate is most vulnerable. The cruciate ligaments can be visualised on an MRI scan (Fig. 1), although injuries to them are generally diagnosed clinically. The *medial ligament*, which is strap shaped and in two layers, stretches between the medial femoral epicondyle and the anteromedial aspect of the tibia. The medial meniscus is firmly attached to the deep part by the coronary ligaments. The cord-like *lateral ligament* runs obliquely from the lateral epicondyle of the femur to the head of the fibula. Note that during the last 10 degrees of extension of the knee the femur internally rotates on the tibia, rendering the collateral ligaments taut and stabilising the joint. The ligaments also have a proprioceptive function.

ANTERIOR CRUCIATE INJURIES

This is the most common ligament to be injured and the most frequent cause of an acute haemarthrosis. Although it can be torn in isolation, other structures are often injured simultaneously. The mechanism of injury is probably one of external rotation of the tibia on the femur combined with an abduction force. In most cases of ACL rupture the patient gives a history of a significant injury, often with the sensation of something tearing or giving within the knee, sometimes with an audible 'pop'. This is invariably followed by a rapidly forming haemarthrosis. Early assessment

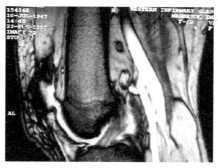

Fig. 1 **MRI scan showing a normal anterior cruciate ligament.**

(because of pain and muscle spasm) may be unreliable, but later, abnormal movement of the tibia relative to the femur may be demonstrated by the drawer and Lachman tests. Some patients present late, with a history of previous injury: they then complain of feelings of instability, and of incidents of giving way followed by effusion. There may be some difficulty in differentiating these cases from those who have meniscal tears, but it should be noted that combined injuries are not uncommon, and that a solitary ACL rupture may lead to secondary tearing of a meniscus (as result of the instability in the knee).

Treatment

This depends on prompt diagnosis which may require an examination under anaesthesia or arthroscopy. If several structures are damaged, each must be treated on its own merits. An isolated ACL injury can usually be treated conservatively (although some consider that early repair gives better long-term results). Intensive physiotherapy with a specific programme to strengthen the hamstring muscles is sufficient in most patients. Surgery is reserved for patients who during normal activities have symptoms of instability. Common reconstructive procedures use either part of the patellar ligament or woven synthetic implants. The initial results are generally very good, but later failure is not uncommon, and there remains some uncertainty about the long-term results.

Avulsion fractures generally occur in children, but are sometimes seen in adults. The anterior cruciate ligament avulses its bony attachment to the tibial intercondylar area (Fig. 2). Because of its articular cartilage covering, the fragment is always larger than it appears on X-ray. If the fracture is only slightly displaced, a 6–8 week period in a cast with

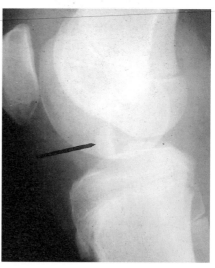

Fig. 2 **The arrow points to an avulsion fracture of the anterior attachment of the anterior cruciate ligament.**

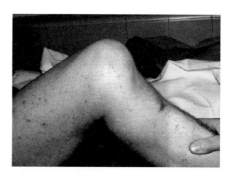

Fig. 3 **Posterior cruciate ligament tear with backward sag of the tibia.**

the knee in extension is advised (this position encourages reduction of the fragment). If badly displaced, the fragment may lie upon the medial meniscus, blocking closed reduction. Open reduction and fixation is required, taking care not to injure the growth plate of the tibia.

POSTERIOR CRUCIATE INJURIES

Rupture of the posterior cruciate ligament is much less common than anterior cruciate injury, and is often found combined with other ligament injuries. The mechanism is often one of a fall on the flexed knee or from dashboard impact in a road traffic accident. It may be overlooked unless the possibility of its occurrence is kept in mind and a careful examination is performed. When the leg is examined in the extended position, a tense haemarthrosis is usually obvious, and the joint can be hyperextended. When the knee is flexed, the tibia usually sags backwards under the femur (Fig. 3).

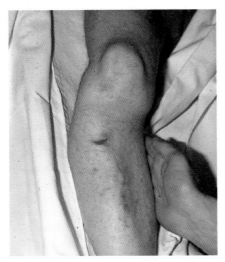

Fig. 4 **Lateral ligament tear, with opening up of the lateral side of the joint on minimal stressing with the knee extended.** In this case there was an associated common peroneal nerve palsy.

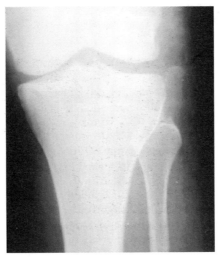

Fig. 5 **Avulsion of attachment of the lateral ligament into the head of the fibula.**

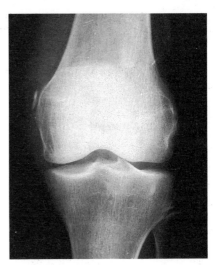

Fig. 6 **Pellegrini–Stieda disease, with calcification at the upper pole of the medial ligament.**

This can be corrected by pulling the tibia forwards (which is sometimes falsely interpreted as indicating a torn anterior cruciate ligament). If there is no backward sag, the posterior drawer test may be positive. Comparison with the opposite side is essential. In some cases an avulsion fracture of the tibia is evident on X-ray.

Treatment

In acute cases, as in isolated ACL injuries, conservative treatment is often advocated: intensive quadriceps exercises can produce good results if knee control can be maintained. With avulsion fractures, it is usual practice to stabilise them surgically. Persisting instability, however, can lead to severe and rapidly progressive osteoarthritis, and if conservative measures fail, surgical ligament reconstruction may reduce the risks of this serious complication. Again, because of this possibility, a number of surgeons advise primary ligament repair in the acute case, especially where other structures are involved.

COLLATERAL LIGAMENT INJURIES

The collateral ligaments are commonly injured, although the medial is more frequently affected. It requires significant force, such as a sporting tackle or blow on the side of the leg from a motor vehicle. Note that in a number of cases there are associated fractures of the tibial plateau (see p. 119). Three grades of ligament injury are recognised:
Grade 1. There is minor tearing of the fibres of the ligament. Although the knee is very painful and there is localised tenderness, tests for instability are negative.

Grade 2. More ligament fibres are torn, leading to some laxity of the ligament; this can usually be demonstrated (comparing one side with the other) when the knee is held in 30 degrees flexion. The knee remains stable when stress is applied to the extended joint.
Grade 3. The ligament is completely torn and the joint unstable. The instability is obvious on clinical testing in both the slightly flexed and extended positions (Fig. 4). (Some record by how much the joint surfaces open up when the joint is stressed under X-ray control.)

Diagnosis

A history of injury is always evident. Careful clinical assessment is important. A haemarthrosis or effusion may be apparent if the capsule remains intact. In more severe injuries external bruising is obvious and, strangely, a complete rupture is often less painful than a more minor tear. The lateral ligament tends to rupture at its distal end and may detach the long head of biceps or the head of the fibula (Fig. 5). In severe cases the opening up of the lateral side of the joint may damage the common peroneal nerve, with sensory loss and a drop foot. If doubt exists about the severity of any ligament injury, an examination under anaesthesia is essential.

Treatment

Grade 1 injuries usually settle rapidly over 3 or 4 weeks with conservative treatment in the form of analgesics, supportive bandaging and physiotherapy.
Grade 2 injuries need protection in a splint or plaster cast for 4 to 6 weeks.
Grade 3 injuries, where the ligament tears are complete, require surgery, with

reattachment or repair of the ligament. A period of physiotherapy to rehabilitate the muscles is essential to maintain the stability of the knee.

Note that in the middle-aged minor tearing of the upper attachment of the medial ligament may give rise to local calcification (Fig. 6), chronic pain and tenderness (Pellegrini-Stieda disease); this may usually be relieved with local hydrocortisone injections.

O'DONOGHUE'S TRIAD

While ligaments may rupture in isolation, the possible involvement of other related structures should be kept in mind. A common combination is a tear of the medial meniscus, with associated ruptures of the medial and anterior cruciate ligaments (O'Donoghue's triad). Dislocation of the patella may also occur at the same time. The treatment is related to the specific injuries.

Knee ligament injuries

- The most common cause of an acute haemarthrosis is an ACL rupture.
- If there is persistent instability following an ACL rupture, surgical reconstruction may have to be considered.
- Incomplete tears of the collateral ligaments may be treated conservatively.
- Complete collateral ligament tears generally require surgical repair.
- Intensive physiotherapy is necessary after any ligament injury to maintain muscle strength and preserve dynamic stability.

MENISCAL INJURIES

Each knee has two menisci, whose main function is to spread the loads of weight bearing on the joint surfaces. They also contribute to the stability of the joint and aid the distribution of synovial fluid; the latter is essential to articular cartilage nutrition.

Anatomy

The menisci are made up of laminated layers of tough fibrocartilage. They are semilunar in shape and conform to the surfaces on which they rest. They are attached to the tibia anteriorly and posteriorly by strong ligaments, but their peripheral attachments by means of the coronary ligaments (to bone and to the joint capsule) are relatively weak. The periphery of each meniscus has a tenuous blood supply, but the main, central part of the meniscus is nourished by diffusion only and in consequence is incapable of repair. The medial meniscus is relatively fixed, sitting in a concavity in the medial tibial plateau; the lateral meniscus rests on the flat (and indeed slightly convex) lateral tibial condyle, is comparatively mobile, and is less vulnerable to injury.

Pathology

Meniscal abnormalities can affect the stability and mechanics of the knee and in some cases may lead to secondary osteoarthritis. Apart from cysts, there are three common meniscal problems: congenital discoid meniscus, which generally presents in childhood; longitudinal meniscus tears, which occur in young adults and only exceptionally in females; and horizontal cleavage tears, which occur in both sexes in middle age.

DISCOID MENISCUS

In the early stages of development the menisci are disc shaped. Later the central portion of each meniscus is absorbed, producing the normal semilunar configuration. In some this process fails to occur and the resulting solid

meniscus tends to become detached at its periphery (Fig. 1). In infants the child may be referred as a case of flexion contracture of the knee. After weight bearing commences, whilst there is often a history of giving way and locking (see later), the striking feature is one of loud clunking sounds emanating from the joint as the detached meniscus moves in and out of alignment with the tibia: this may occur during activity or be discovered during the course of examination. If the meniscus is relatively stable, arthroscopic resection of the central portion is sometimes attempted, but in others total meniscectomy is often required.

LONGITUDINAL MENISCUS TEARS

These are by far the most common types of meniscal injury, and occur in the young adult. There is nearly always a history of a causal incident, and when this is clear three factors are generally found to have been present: the knee was weight-bearing; it was flexed; and it was twisted (i.e. subjected to rotational stress). Many result from an athletic injury, e.g. while playing football. Excessive force is not always necessary; the meniscus can be torn as a person rises from a kneeling or squatting position.

Types of tear

The meniscus, having been trapped between the femoral condyle and tibia, splits longitudinally. The *site* of the split is dependent on the degree of knee flexion and the *extent* on the amount of violence to which it is subjected. Most commonly the tear involves the mid portion of the meniscus. If the tear is extensive, the inner limb of the torn meniscus may become displaced into the centre of the joint, giving rise to the classical *bucket handle* tear. In others, further transverse tearing of the meniscus results in a *parrot beak* tear.

Posterior horn tears may allow buttonholing of the femoral condyle, and if extensive are referred to as *racquet* tears.

Tears of the anterior third are uncommon. Most tears involve the avascular substance of the meniscus; they are incapable of spontaneous healing and unlikely to respond to any attempt at surgical repair.

A further not uncommon meniscal injury is the *peripheral detachment* which results in the meniscus becoming abnormally mobile and unstable. The posterior half of the lateral meniscus is most frequently affected. Peripheral detachments are worthy of early diagnosis as they may be amenable to surgical repair.

Diagnosis

History. Although not invariably, there is usually an obvious incident which the patient can recall. A painful, twisting injury during athletic activities or whilst rising from a kneeling or crouching position are common precipitants. In the case of a football injury, unlike most of the dramatic events which seem now to be so commonplace, the player who tears a knee cartilage is unlikely to be able to finish the game.

Pain. This may be non-specific, but if confined to the joint line may indicate meniscal pathology.

Locking. In classical, true locking of a knee, the joint may be flexed, but when an attempt is made to extend it fully, a mechanical resistance is encountered, with further pressure usually causing pain. While there are other causes of a block to full extension (e.g. loose bodies in the joint, dislocation of the patella, and even osteoarthritis), this is a highly significant complaint in someone suspected of having a meniscal injury. (If the knee can be fully extended when the patient is first seen, ask him to indicate the position the joint was in when it locked. Note that the knee never locks in full extension, and if that position is indicated, some other cause — such as painful muscle spasm — must be sought. Ask the patient what caused the knee to lock, and ask how he managed to unlock it, bearing in mind that locking is a

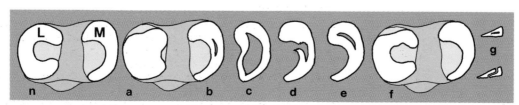

Fig. 1 **Meniscal injuries.** Normal relationship between the lateral (L) and medial (M) menisci, and the tibial plateau (**n**); discoid lateral meniscus with posterior detachment (**a**); longitudinal tear medial meniscus (**b**); bucket handle tear (**c**); parrot beak tear (**d**); racquet tear (**e**); posterior detachment of the lateral meniscus (**f**); horizontal cleavage tears (**g**).

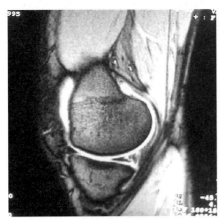

Fig. 2 MRI scan showing posterior meniscal tear.

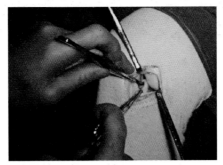

Fig. 3 **Open, total meniscectomy of a bucket handle tear.**

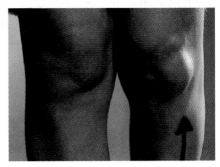

Fig. 4 **Cyst of the lateral meniscus.**

purely mechanical problem.) In the locked knee, a springy block to the last few degrees of full extension is almost pathognomonic of a displaced bucket-handle tear. Sometimes a posterior horn tear can produce painful locking with the knee acutely flexed.

Giving way. In true giving way, painful stimuli arising from the joint (i.e. from clear intra-articular pathology) lead to reflex inhibition of the quadriceps muscle, causing the knee to collapse. This term is much maligned, as a feeling of 'giving way' is common in many conditions, not least of all quadriceps weakness. More weight can be attached to this complaint if the patient is unable to save himself and gives a history of falling to the ground (sometimes sustaining additional injury).

Swelling. Rapid massive swelling of a joint after injury is indicative of a haemarthrosis and is not a normal feature of isolated meniscal injuries (less marked bleeding may occur within the joint in peripheral tears). Intermittent joint swelling is indicative of an irritative intra-articular lesion, but is non-specific. Oedema localised to the joint line is indicative of a meniscal tear.

Examination

An acutely locked knee is clinically obvious, but in many cases patients present some time later, giving a history of intermittent trouble with the joint. The presence of a slight effusion, combined with joint line tenderness and possibly quadriceps wasting should arouse suspicion. Crouching may provoke meniscal symptoms and an inability to do so comfortably or 'duck waddle' (walking in the crouched position) increases the likelihood of meniscal pathology being present. McMurray's test, part of which involves rotating the tibia on the femur with the knee fully flexed, may be helpful. Where significant energy has been

responsible for an acute injury (e.g. a sporting tackle), the ligamentous structures should be carefully assessed, particularly to exclude O'Donoghue's triad (torn medial meniscus with ruptures of the anterior cruciate and medial ligaments). This usually results in a haemarthrosis.

Investigations

Where the diagnosis is clear-cut (e.g. with a locked knee), few investigations are necessary. Radiographs are invariably negative, except in the older patient with a degenerate meniscus who may have early osteoarthritic changes. If doubt exists an MRI scan (Fig. 2) or arthroscopy may be performed.

Treatment

The acutely locked knee is an emergency and should be dealt with quickly. In all cases arthroscopic resection of the torn portion of the meniscus is now the most popular method of treatment; all types of tear can be removed and the patient can be mobilised very quickly. Open arthrotomy (Fig. 3) is mainly reserved for failed arthroscopic resections. In chronic lesions more extensive resection may be required to leave a stable remnant. Meniscal repair is controversial, but is confined to peripheral tears (often associated with concomitant ligament injuries) in the younger patient. Physiotherapy postoperatively is important where muscle wasting is

present, as muscle control is essential to the stability of the joint.

HORIZONTAL CLEAVAGE TEARS

Degenerative changes occur within the menisci as part of the ageing process and may result in tears which lie in the horizontal plane, parallel to the tibial plateau. Such tears may extend into the superior or inferior surfaces of the menisci. They are often the source of chronic pain of insidious onset. Pain may be common at night or be aggravated by prolonged standing or walking. In some cases it may resolve spontaneously after many months, but if this fails to occur, resection (preferably by arthroscopy) may ultimately be required.

MENISCAL CYSTS

These are relatively rare, but are distinctive. They are more common in the lateral meniscus (Fig. 4) and there is often a history of local trauma (such as a kick when playing football). There is frequently an associated meniscal tear which may result from local tethering of the meniscus. The cysts are in the joint line and very firm on palpation. If symptomatic, treatment is by excision which must include the meniscal root of the swelling; if there is an additional meniscal tear this may also have to be dealt with.

Meniscal injuries

- The menisci spread the high loads of weight bearing over a wider area of the joint. They contribute to the stability of the knee and help distribute the synovial fluid.
- The medial meniscus is more commonly torn than the lateral meniscus.
- True locking is almost pathognomonic of meniscal tear.
- Meniscal cysts are almost always found on the anterolateral aspect of the knee associated with meniscal pathology.
- Arthroscopic resection is the treatment of choice for symptomatic meniscal tears.

OTHER KNEE DISORDERS

RETROPATELLAR PAIN SYNDROMES

These are characterised by ill-localised patellar pain which has no specific features apart from being made worse by prolonged sitting or by walking on slopes or stairs. The pain is not usually severe, but activities may sometimes have to be modified. There is sometimes a little swelling of the joint which at times may give way. It is most common in adolescent and young adult females, and is generally self-limiting.

Pathology

There is no clear-cut pathological lesion although the deep layers of the articular cartilage of the patella may degenerate, causing 'blistering' and fasciculation of the surface (chondromalacia patellae). The lesions are thought to be capable of repair, unlike the changes seen in osteo-arthritis. On clinical examination some of the risk factors for dislocation may be present, and indeed there may be a history of patellar dislocation. The articular surface is always tender (palpated after patellar displacement). Also of diagnostic importance is pain which mimics the patient's complaint when the patella is moved under pressure against the femoral condyles, either manually or by quadriceps contraction. Investigation is by radiographs which should include a skyline (tangential) view which may reveal maltracking of the patella. Arthroscopy can be useful, although cartilaginous abnormalities of a similar nature are often observed in asymptomatic patients.

Treatment

General advice is given to avoid activities which are known to aggravate the condition, along with quadriceps building exercises. Operative treatment remains controversial.

OSGOOD–SCHLATTER'S DISEASE

This is a common problem in the young adolescent. It is a traction apophysitis, and can be bilateral. It usually causes mild pain which is worse after exercise. Typically the tibial tubercle is tender and prominent, but knee movements are unaffected. A lateral radiograph shows displacement or fragmentation of the apophysis (Fig. 1). Treatment is generally symptomatic as the condition is self-limiting. Restriction of activity may be sufficient, but in refractory cases 6 weeks immobilisation in a plaster cast, or excision of a displaced bone fragment, may be necessary. Sinding-Larsen syndrome is very similar, but affects the distal pole of the patella.

BIPARTITE PATELLA

This abnormality of ossification is often mistaken for fracture. It is usually symptomless, but if it is the source of pain the smaller superolateral fragment may be excised.

OSTEOCHONDRITIS DISSECANS

This is a condition in which a small fragment of bone just deep to the articular surface is rendered avascular. Along with the articular cartilage capping it, it becomes detached from the surrounding healthy structures (Fig. 2), and if cast into the joint, forms a loose body. The aetiology remains uncertain, but contact between the femoral condyles and the tibial spines, patella or anterior cruciate ligament may be a factor. 70% of the defects involve the lateral aspect of the medial femoral condyle. The condition tends to affect adolescents and may be bilateral. Initially it is often symptom free, but later it may cause mild aching pain in the joint and a slight effusion. A loose body may cause locking of the joint if it becomes trapped between the joint surfaces. This can occur at any angle, is painful and the patient can often 'unlock' the knee by manoeuvring the leg. Between episodes a mobile body can often be felt if it comes to lie in the suprapatellar pouch.

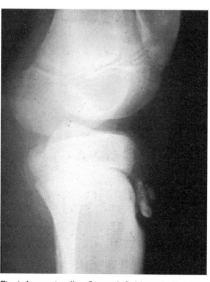

Fig. 1 **Long-standing Osgood–Schlatter's disease.**

Diagnosis

This may often be confirmed by routine radiographs of the knee, but specialised tunnel projections showing the intercondylar area are often invaluable. Arthroscopic assessment is helpful in deciding whether the fragment is becoming detached and likely to form a loose body (note that osteochondritis dissecans can occur in other joints, particularly the elbow and ankle).

Treatment

In the young patient where the fragment remains in situ, some advise observation over a prolonged period with serial radiographs in the hope that the joint will return to normal. Where a defect is evident on arthroscopic examination or is mobile, the affected area may be drilled to stimulate healing, or the fragment can occasionally be pinned back. Loose bodies should be removed, and this may often be performed arthroscopically (note that multiple loose bodies (Fig. 3) are a feature of *synovial chondromatosis* and are usually treated by synovectomy).

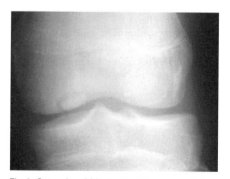

Fig. 2 **Osteochondritis dissecans of the medial femoral condyle.**

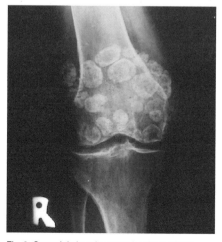

Fig. 3 **Synovial chondromatosis with multiple loose bodies.**

OSTEOARTHRITIS

The knee is a common site for degenerative change, and any or all of its three main compartments may be involved. Pain related to activity is the main symptom, and sleep may be disturbed. There may be complaint of stiffness, loss of movement, giving way, occasional swelling and perhaps locking (from the formation of osteoarthritic loose bodies). Progressive deformity, either in the form of fixed flexion or varus (secondary to medial compartment disease), is common. Clinical examination may confirm the presence of deformity, tenderness (and sometimes palpable osteophytes) in the joint line, muscle wasting, restriction of movements (in advanced cases) and crepitus on movement. When and if the disease is confined to the patellofemoral compartment the symptoms are very similar to those found in chondromalacia, except that in osteoarthritis the patients tend to be older and the symptoms are more persistent.

Diagnosis

This is confirmed by plain radiographs which will reveal loss of joint space, osteophyte formation, and often reactive sclerosis and cyst formation.

Treatment

In mild cases this is symptomatic, with analgesics, physiotherapy and modification of activities. Where there is a significant varus deformity, a corrective osteotomy may be performed, usually by dividing the tibia below the knee and removing an appropriate wedge of bone. This spreads the weight bearing loads more evenly across the joint, and may also help reduce pain by relieving intraosseous vascular congestion. It is often effective in producing relief of symptoms, at least in the short term, and is of particular value in the younger patient or where there is a history of previous bone or joint infection in the area.

In others, joint replacement has largely become the standard procedure, generally giving pain relief, retaining a good range of motion, and allowing early mobilisation. Where the arthritic process is restricted to the patellofemoral compartment, surgery is usually of little help.

RHEUMATOID ARTHRITIS

Both knees are usually involved, but unlike osteoarthritis, the lateral compartment is often more severely affected, leading to a valgus deformity. Synovitis is often the predominant feature, and pain may be severe. Treatment in the first instance is medical, but early synovectomy (which may be performed arthroscopically) can often control synovitis and prevent significant erosion of the joint surfaces. However, where major joint destruction has already taken place and disability is progressive, joint replacement is the only answer. Unlike in osteoarthritis, the procedure is not contraindicated in the young patient.

PREPATELLAR BURSITIS

Also known as housemaid's knee, this is a swelling of the bursa which develops between the patella and the overlying skin. This area is vulnerable to trauma, and the condition may follow a direct blow or the chronic irritation of prolonged kneeling. The fluctuant swelling is often tense (Fig. 4). On occasions an overlying graze or minor laceration may lead to secondary infection, with acute pain and cellulitis. The condition is common in miners, and is recognised as a prescribed disease ('beat knee'). Treatment in the first instance is conservative, with advice on the avoidance of further local trauma. For persistent swelling, excision may be required. Cellulitis may sometimes be averted by high dose antibiotics, but surgical drainage is often indicated.

INFRAPATELLAR BURSITIS

This bursa lies anterior to the patellar ligament and may become swollen (when it is known as clergyman's knee). The aetiology and treatment are the same as in prepatellar bursitis, although infection is rare.

POPLITEAL CYST

There are a number of bursae (no less than six) which lie at the back of the knee. Any one of these may become enlarged, often for no obvious reason, and the attempt to distinguish between them is academic and of no practical importance. The terms 'enlarged semimembranosus bursa' and 'Baker cyst' should be regarded as being virtually synonymous. About a third communicate with the knee joint and fluctuate in size, so that at times they may be mistaken for solid tumours. On occasion they may be associated with rheumatoid arthritis or a posterior horn tear of a meniscus, and they sometimes contain loose bodies. They may transilluminate, and on the rare occasion where there is doubt, further investigation by X-ray (which excludes any bony pathology) or ultrasound may be helpful. Beware of a pulsatile mass in the popliteal fossa as this may be an aneurysm.

Treatment

This is generally conservative, but if symptoms are troublesome, careful excision can be performed. It is important to close any communication with the joint to minimise the chances of recurrence. Note that on occasion a bursa can rupture, causing severe calf pain and swelling which may be misdiagnosed as a deep venous thrombosis, and lead to the erroneous administration of anticoagulants. It is important to warn patients and their practitioners of this possibility.

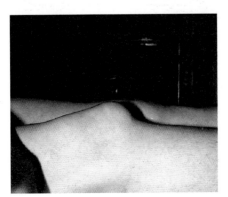

Fig. 4 **Prepatellar bursitis.**

Other knee disorders

- Osteochondritis dissecans typically involves the medial femoral condyle.
- Retropatellar pain is a common complaint, but usually responds to conservative treatment and restriction of activities.
- Traction apophysitis is common in adolescents and is usually aggravated by exercise.
- Enlargement of the bursae in the patellar region may be precipitated by trauma or excessive kneeling: if they become infected, surgical treatment may be required.
- Popliteal cysts often communicate with the joint, and may be associated with intra-articular pathology.

FRACTURES OF THE TIBIAL SHAFT

Tibial fractures commonly result from either severe twisting stresses (e.g. from skiing or other athletic activities), force transmitted through the feet in falls from a height or in road traffic accidents, or in direct violence such as a kick or a blow from falling rock or masonry.

Tibial fractures are often open because a third of the surface of the tibia is subcutaneous and unprotected. The sharp end of one of the bone fragments may penetrate the skin, rendering the fracture open from within out.

Direct violence may produce a fracture which is open from without in. The skin wounds are frequently extensive, with bruising of their margins reducing their viability. There may be skin loss, and foreign bodies such as fragments of clothing, road grit and, inevitably, bacteria may contaminate the wound. Damage to the neurovascular structures in the limb is more common in open than in closed fractures of the tibia and may threaten the survival of the limb or impair recovery of function.

First line treatment

- Any open wound should be covered with a sterile dressing to reduce the risk of further contamination.
- Significant haemorrhage may usually be controlled by local pressure, e.g. by bandaging the limb firmly while applying gentle traction. Only rarely is a properly applied and supervised tourniquet required.
- While maintaining light traction, the limb should be splinted to reduce pain, further haemorrhage and soft tissue damage. At its simplest, the leg may be bandaged to a board or to the other leg, with ties both at the knee and the foot to control rotation. An inflatable splint, if available, gives excellent support (Fig. 1).
- There should be no delay in hospitalisation and the commencement of treatment, particularly if arterial damage is suspected.

CLOSED FRACTURES

Treatment in children

An undisplaced fracture may be treated in a long leg plaster which should include the knee and ankle joints. In the anticipation of swelling, apply generous padding, (split the cast), elevate the limb and, ideally, admit for 2–3 days' observation. Depending on the child's age and the type of fracture, a walking heel may be substituted for crutches after some weeks. The cast is retained until union has occurred (e.g. at about 8 weeks in a child of 8).

If the fracture is angled or displaced, it will require preliminary reduction by traction and manipulation under anaesthesia. In all cases the position must be checked by X-rays taken after application of the cast and at regular intervals subsequently. Residual angulation may be corrected by wedging. In this procedure the plaster is cut circumferentially, but incompletely, at the level of the fracture and the angulation corrected. The gap in the cast is held with a cork wedge (Fig. 2) and locally reinforced with plaster.

Treatment in adults

If the fracture is undisplaced, or if a stable reduction can be obtained, it

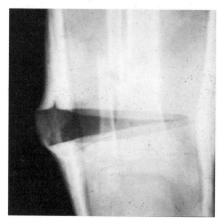

Fig. 2 **Medial angulation (lateral tilting) of a tibial fracture corrected by wedging.**

may be treated successfully along the conservative lines described. As the average time to union in an adult tibial fracture is 16 weeks, prolonged immobilisation may lead to stiffness of the knee, foot and ankle. To minimise this, in many cases it may be possible to replace the long leg cast at a fairly early stage, either with a Sarmiento below-knee cast or a cast brace.

If the fracture is unstable (e.g. many oblique, spiral and comminuted fractures), it may be difficult to achieve and maintain a good reduction using closed methods. For these fractures, primary internal fixation (by plating or intramedullary nailing) or an external fixator are the preferred methods of treatment.

Plating. A long incision over the fracture is needed to permit reduction under vision and the application of a plate of adequate size (Fig. 3). Commonly a dynamic compression plate is used so that the fracture surfaces can be brought closely together under a degree of compression to encourage stability and bone union. The plate is attached to the bone with three or more cortical bone screws both above and below the level of the fracture (Fig. 4). The screws are driven into holes drilled and tapped in the tibia. The quality of the fixation is generally such that the knee and ankle may be mobilised at a very early stage, but the commencement of unsupported weight bearing is dependent on the nature of the fracture and other factors. (If reliance is placed entirely on the plate, it is likely to fail mechanically.) If the fixation is rigid, there is little bridging callus and

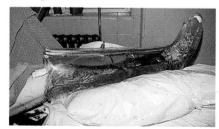

Fig. 1 **Open fracture of the tibia supported by an inflatable splint.**

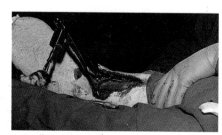

Fig. 3 **Open reduction of a fractured tibia, clamped prior to plating.**

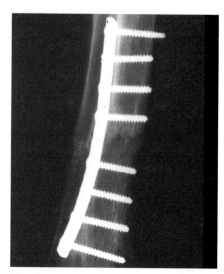

Fig. 4 **Tibial fracture held with a contoured dynamic compression plate and eight screws.**

endosteal callus may take 18 months to become established; the fixation devices should not be removed before then.

Intramedullary nailing. In most cases this may be performed without exposure of the fracture itself. The fracture is reduced under image intensifier control, with the patient set up on the operating table in such a way that there is good access to the knee and tibia and so that strong (usually skeletal traction) may be applied (Fig. 5). A guide wire is inserted through an opening made on the anteromedial surface of the tibia just below the knee joint and after reaming of the cavity an appropriately sized nail is inserted. Rotation is controlled by transversely running locking screws. Exposure of the fracture may be required if it cannot be reduced by closed manipulation.

External fixation. An external fixator may be employed as a substitute for cast fixation so that early movement of the knee and ankle may be undertaken. It may be used to hold unstable fractures and is of great value in the treatment of open fractures, especially in the presence of gross contamination where the risks of spreading infection (e.g. from wide exposure of the bone for plating or reaming of the tibia for intramedullary nailing) are great. Minimally two pins above and two below the fracture, linked with a connecting bar, are used. For the most rigid fixation, two sets of pins and connectors, at right angles to one another, may be employed.

OPEN FRACTURES

The wound
As a first measure a bacteriological swab should be taken, the wound covered with a sterile dressing to prevent further

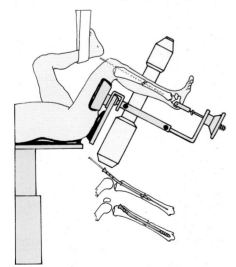

Fig. 5 **Insertion of an intramedullary nail.**

contamination and a short course of appropriate antibiotic started.

In Type I and II open fractures, the wound should be thoroughly cleaned and dressed before making a decision as to the best method of holding the fracture.

Where the wound is small, it should be extended to allow a more complete inspection. After any suspect tissue has been dealt with, a thorough lavage of the wound should be carried out. Thereafter, it is common practice to leave the wound open and apply a local dressing. It is inspected at 2–3 days, and then secondary closure, split skin grafting, or a repeat debridement may be carried out.

In Type III injuries, after a thorough debridement, it is highly desirable to obtain cover of the fracture as soon as possible (certainly in under 2 weeks from the injury and preferably as part of the initial management) to avoid antibiotic-resistant secondary infection. This may be achieved using a variety of plastic surgical techniques (e.g. a soleus flap). (Note that in a small number of cases where the soft tissue damage is profound, often with sensory and circulatory loss, primary amputation may have to be considered.)

Fixation
After the wound has been dealt with the fracture must be supported. An external fixator will give best access for later wound dressing and will allow alternative methods of fixation (should these be thought desirable) once the wounds have healed. Internal fixation by plating is probably reasonably safe in Type I open fractures. Intramedullary nailing has also been recommended as being safe for the majority of open fractures, although reaming is contraindicated in those of Type III b.

COMPLICATIONS

Joint stiffness. Stiffness of the knee and ankle are related to the duration and method of treatment. Where closed

methods of treatment are employed, it may be possible after some weeks to replace a long leg cast with a Sarmiento plaster or a plastic or plaster cast brace. Use of internal fixation or an external fixator generally reduces the risks of this complication.

Delayed union/non-union. Union of tibial fractures is normally slow with the chances of delay (and joint stiffness) increased in high energy injuries where there is bone loss, comminution of the fracture or poor peripheral circulation. If union has not occurred within the normal time, radiographs should be carefully studied at monthly intervals. If progress is noted, treatment should be continued. If not, then the diagnosis of non-union is likely and the appropriate measures should be undertaken.

In either case it may be possible to mobilise the knee while the fracture is still being supported by using a plastic tibial brace or a Sarmiento plaster. It may also be possible to encourage union by the use of pulsed electromagnetic fields applied by means of coils placed round the limb. Where non-union is established, bone grafting, with or without revision of the method of fixation, will have to be considered.

Neurovascular injury. In closed fractures the posterior tibial artery may be damaged at the level of the soleal arch in proximal third fractures, leading to distal ischaemia and Volkmann's contracture of the foot. In open fractures there may be arrest of the distal circulation from arterial compression or rupture; if this does not respond to reduction, immediate exploration, fixation of the fracture and formal arterial repair will be required.

Disturbance of the lymphatic drainage of the limb. Especially in open fractures, this may lead to chronic oedema of the limb distal to the fracture. Disturbance of the venous circulation may lead to phlebitis and varicose ulceration of the limb.

Fractures of the tibial shaft

- The majority of tibial fractures in children, and many tibial fractures in adults, may be treated successfully by closed methods.
- Unstable tibial fractures in the adult are usually best treated by plating or intramedullary nailing.
- An external fixator is often the best method of holding a severely contaminated open fracture.
- The possibility of the patient developing a stiff knee during the course of treatment should always be borne in mind and the joint should be mobilised at the earliest opportunity.
- Be on the look out for non-union and do not delay in carrying out appropriate treatment.

INJURIES ABOUT THE ANKLE

LATERAL LIGAMENT TEARS

If the hind foot is suddenly inverted (e.g. if the ankle 'goes over'), the lateral ligament is stressed as it resists the talus tilting in the ankle mortice. If the forces are great, then some of its fibres may be torn, causing a *sprain* of the ankle. Although the joint may be painful, bruised and swollen, all that is usually required is a few days' symptomatic treatment, e.g. elevation of the limb along with firm bandaging or strapping to limit swelling and the use of sticks or crutches.

If, however, the external ligament is completely torn, or if it avulses the tip of the lateral malleolus to which it is attached (Fig. 1), then the ankle becomes unstable, and if untreated may remain so. A 6 week period in a below knee walking plaster is usually advised, although some prefer to repair or reattach the lateral ligament.

A *complete tear* as opposed to a simple sprain may be suspected from the severity of the symptoms and the situation of the swelling and tenderness about the ankle. The diagnosis is confirmed by X-ray examination. If the plain films do not show an avulsion fracture, then inversion and other radiographs, taken when stress is applied to the joint, may demonstrate abnormal talar tilting (Fig. 2). In cases of *chronic ankle instability* confirmed by X-ray examination, late surgical reconstruction of the defective ligament has a high success rate.

ANKLE FRACTURES (POTT'S FRACTURES)

That part of the talus which articulates with the tibia and fibula does not readily fracture. When force is transmitted through it from the foot or heel, it may break off the malleoli or fracture other parts of the tibia and fibula. If the talus moves beyond its normal limits it may tear or avulse ligament attachments. The number of structures that may be involved and their possible combinations is large, so that any comprehensive classification is of necessity complex. For simplicity, however, most ankle injuries can be classified as being of external rotation, abduction, adduction and vertical compression pattern (Fig. 3).

External rotation injuries

These are by far the most common types of ankle injury, with the number of structures involved increasing with the violence. The talus may be externally rotated from force applied to the inside of the foot, e.g. if it strikes a piece of furniture, or more commonly from sudden inversion of the foot, e.g. if the ankle 'goes over' when walking on an uneven surface. (The talus tends to rotate in the ankle mortice with inversion because of the obliquity of the plane of the subtalar joint.) The rotating talus carries the lateral malleolus with it, at first rupturing or avulsing the anterior (inferior) tibiofibular ligament (Fig. 4) and then fracturing the lateral malleolus in spiral fashion (Fig. 5). Where the displacement is greater, the posterior part of the articular surface of the tibia (the so-called posterior malleolus) is pulled off (or the posterior tibiofibular ligament is torn). With greater violence still, the medial (deltoid) ligament is torn or the medial malleolus is avulsed.

In the majority of cases the malleoli remain aligned with the talus. In a number of cases (external rotation with diastasis) this relationship is lost, with the fibula shifting laterally away from the tibia and a gap opening up between the medial side of the talus and the medial malleolus (Fig. 6). The fibula may fracture quite proximally, even in the region of its neck, and unless anticipated this

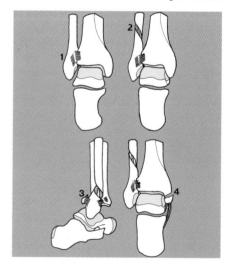

Fig. 4 **External rotation injuries of increasing severity. (1)** Rupture of the anterior inferior tibiofibular ligament; **(2)** fracture of the lateral malleolus; **(3)** fracture of the posterior malleolus; **(4)** avulsion of the medial malleolus.

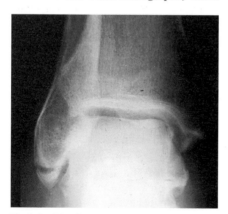

Fig. 1 **Avulsion fracture of the lateral ligament attachment.**

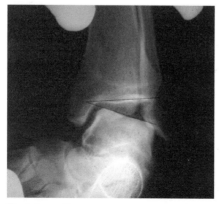

Fig. 2 **Stress films demonstrating a complete tear of the lateral ligament.**

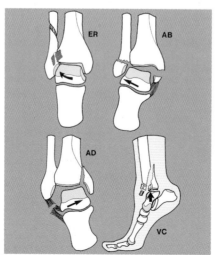

Fig. 3 **Common ankle injuries.** ER = *external rotation* with fracture of the lateral malleolus; AB = *abduction* with fracture of the lateral malleolus and avulsion of the medial malleolus; AD = *adduction* with fracture of the medial malleolus; VC = *vertical compression.*

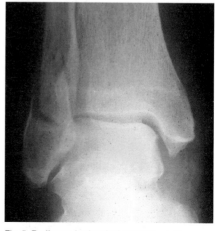

Fig. 5 **Radiograph of typical external rotation injury involving the lateral malleolus only.**

may go undetected as the proximal fibula is not included in routine radiographs of the ankle.

Abduction injuries

When the primary movement of the talus is one of abduction rather than rotation, the medial structures are the first to give; either the deltoid ligament is torn or there is an avulsion fracture of the medial malleolus. With increasing violence both inferior tibiofibular ligaments are torn and the fibula fractures at the level of the upper surface of the talus. There may also be an avulsion fracture of the posterior malleolus.

Adduction injuries

When the talus is adducted (as distinct from being rotated) the first structure to suffer is the lateral ligament and its attachments, producing sprains, complete ligament tears or avulsion fractures of the lateral malleolus as already described. With greater violence, the sharp edge at the junction of the upper and medial articular surfaces of the talus may impinge in the corner between the medial malleolus and the inferior articular surface of the tibia; this may cause a local compression fracture or split off the medial malleolus.

Vertical compression or pilon fractures

If the forces applied to the talus are mainly in a vertical direction, e.g. from falls from a height or from foot pedal pressure in road traffic accidents, there may be considerable damage to the inferior articular surface of the tibia. If at the time of injury the foot is *plantar flexed*, a large segment may shear off the posterior articular surface, with proximal subluxation of the foot. If the foot is forcibly *dorsiflexed*, the anterior tibial margin of the tibia may suffer. As the articular surface of the talus is wider anteriorly than

posteriorly, if the ankle is forcibly dorsiflexed the widening talus may push against the malleoli, causing horizontal shearing fractures. In many cases there is severe comminution of the inferior articular surface of the tibia.

DIAGNOSIS OF ANKLE FRACTURES

Suspect an ankle joint fracture if there is a history of difficulty in weight bearing after an appropriate injury and obtain relevant radiographs. If there is tenderness over the proximal fibula or the fifth metatarsal base, then additional films will be required. If a malleolar fracture is confirmed, look for tenderness elsewhere (e.g. over the deltoid ligament if the lateral malleolus is fractured) in order to confirm or eliminate an accompanying ligament tear with potential instability.

Treatment

1. By far the most common ankle fracture is a stable, undisplaced spiral fracture of the lateral malleolus with no damage to the medial ligament or medial malleolus and with no medial tenderness. This injury may be treated in a below-knee plaster with elevation of the limb for a few days. After the initial swelling has subsided, a walking heel may be applied.

2. Displacement of an isolated fracture of the lateral malleolus indicates that there is additional ligament damage and the injury is unstable. While injuries of this pattern (and in fact most ankle fractures) may be treated conservatively by manipulative reduction and the application of a below-knee plaster cast, most careful supervision is essential to detect any slipping of the fracture. To avoid delays in mobilisation, internal fixation is often preferred. Stability can generally be restored by plating the lateral malleolus;

formal repair of the medial ligament is not usually needed provided it is protected for 6 weeks with a below-knee cast.

3. If the medial malleolus is fractured, there is a tendency to non-union, particularly if the fragments are kept apart by infolding of torn periosteum. For this reason it is usual to treat all displaced fractures of the medial malleolus by internal fixation. If the lateral malleolus is also fractured, ankle stability may be restored when the medial malleolus is fixed; but if not it may also be fixed.

4. If the posterior malleolus is fractured and displaced, and if the fragment is substantial (e.g. involving a third of the articular surface or more) it should be reduced and fixed.

5. Where a vertical compression fracture has severely disrupted the inferior articular surface of the tibia, the risks of secondary osteoarthritis are high. If a reconstruction procedure is not technically possible, the patient should be admitted for traction (applied with a pin through the heel) and early mobilisation of the ankle as soon as pain will permit. Alternatively, an articulated external fixator may be used.

COMPLICATIONS OF ANKLE FRACTURE

Stiffness of the foot and ankle are common, especially if the ankle has been immobilised in a position of plantar flexion. Physiotherapy is often necessary.

Persistent **swelling and oedema** of the foot and ankle, and **Sudeck's atrophy** (reflex sympathetic dystrophy) are common complications of ankle fractures.

Secondary osteoarthritis of the ankle is most common after vertical compression fractures. In severe cases fusion of the ankle joint may be required (at present the results of ankle joint replacement are disappointing).

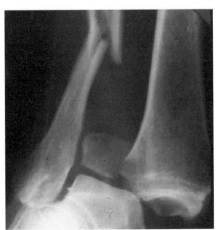

Fig. 6 **External rotation injury with diastasis.** The fibula has fractured proximally, the posterior malleolus has been avulsed and can be seen lying above the talus and the deltoid ligament has been torn.

Injuries about the ankle

- A complete lateral ligament tear can lead to permanent disability and may be easily overlooked if the plain radiographs of the ankle are normal.
- Be aware that ankle injuries may be associated with proximal fractures of the fibula and that these will only show on appropriate films.
- The most common ankle fracture is an external rotation fracture of the lateral malleolus. Provided no other major structure is involved, it is a relatively stable injury and may be treated conservatively.
- If the ankle is being held in a cast for any length of time, it is essential to position the foot at right angles to the leg, otherwise there may be permanent loss of dorsiflexion of the ankle.
- Vertical compression fractures are more likely than any other ankle fractures to be complicated by secondary osteoarthritis.
- Sudeck's atrophy is a common complication of ankle joint injuries, even when these are confined to the soft tissues.

THE TALUS AND CALCANEUS

FRACTURES OF THE TALUS

The talus is a tough structure and not easily fractured. Its weakest area is in the region of the neck. If the foot is violently dorsiflexed, the talus may crack when it contacts the sharp edge of the distal part of the tibia. In a number of cases the fracture is hair-line, but if it is displaced the proximal fragment adapts a position of plantarflexion (Fig. 1) or in severe cases is extruded from the ankle mortice.

The main problem with fractures of the talus is that the blood supply to the bone may be disrupted, leading to avascular necrosis. If this occurs it can cause much difficulty, as the talus holds a key position in no less than three joints (the ankle, the subtalar and the midtarsal). The incidence of this complication increases with displacement, ranging from 10% in undisplaced fractures to 85% where there is talar extrusion.

Treatment

The fracture should be immobilised in a below-knee cast until it has united. If the proximal fragment is displaced, reduction can generally be achieved by placing the foot in plantarflexion before application of the cast. After 3-4 weeks it is usually safe to bring the foot up to the neutral position to reduce the risks of a fixed plantarflexion deformity.

If a reduction cannot be obtained by manipulation, then it may be necessary to expose the fracture through a dorsal incision. After reduction, the fracture may be held with a Kirschner wire or cannulated screw passed through the head and into the body of the talus.

Where a large portion of the talus has been extruded backwards (Fig. 2), manipulative reduction may also be attempted. If this fails, then open reduction is demanded; the fracture may be fixed using a long cancellous screw passed from behind over a guide wire which has been previously passed through the body of the talus into its head.

AVASCULAR NECROSIS OF THE TALUS

If this is going to occur it usually declares itself in the radiographs at 6–12 weeks by an increase in the density of the talar shadow. If it occurs, weight bearing should be deferred until the bone has revascularised (usually within 8–12 months), otherwise the soft avascular bone will become greatly deformed with the forces of weight bearing. Thereafter the patient should be reviewed at regular intervals. Subsequent treatment will depend on the site and extent of secondary osteoarthritis. In minor cases restriction of activities and the prescription of analgesics may suffice; in the most severe cases, where all the talar articulations are involved, a pantalar fusion may be required (fusion of the ankle, subtalar and midtarsal joints).

CALCANEAL FRACTURES INVOLVING THE SUBTALAR JOINT

These are the most serious and potentially disabling fractures of the calcaneus (Fig. 3a). They most commonly result from a fall from a height on to the heels. It is important in such circumstances that both sides are carefully examined in case one is overlooked. In some cases the fracture is undisplaced, but in others the weight bearing part of the heel is pulled proximally and laterally by the tendo calcaneus. There is often much comminution (Fig. 4), rendering any attempt at operative reconstruction difficult or impossible. Involvement of the subtalar joint often leads to restriction in its movements, secondary osteoarthritis, chronic pain and impaired walking ability; lateral displacement makes the heel broader and squatter; and proximal displacement leads to relative lengthening of the tendo calcaneus and weakness and inefficiency of the calf muscles. To diagnose and assess the extent of a calcaneal fracture, investigation by lateral, oblique and tangential (axial) X-ray projections may be required, and a CT scan is often invaluable.

Treatment

Gross swelling, extensive bruising and pressure blistering tend to occur rapidly after any calcaneal fracture (Fig. 5). As a first measure the patient should be admitted, the limb elevated and a regime of firm bandaging over wool (to act as a temporary splint and to limit swelling) should be commenced. Thereafter an early decision should be made as to whether any attempt at reduction is undertaken. Where the displacement is marked, it may be possible to improve this by levering the heel distally using a spike

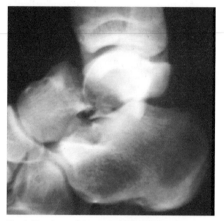

Fig. 1 **Fracture of the neck of the talus with plantarflexion of the proximal fragment.**

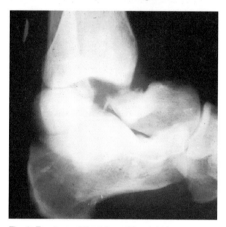

Fig. 2 **Fracture of the talus with posterior extrusion of the proximal fragment.**

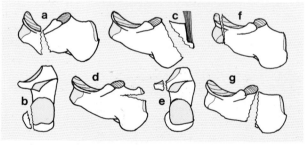

Fig. 3 **Patterns of calcaneal fracture.**

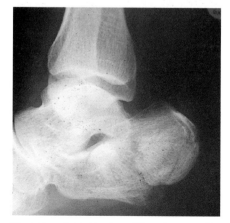

Fig. 4 **Comminuted fracture of the calcaneus with proximal displacement of the posterior fragment.**

or Steinman pin which may subsequently be incorporated into a plaster sabot. Where the fragments are large and comminution does not appear to be severe, internal fixation with the use of plates and screws may sometimes be considered; depressed articular surfaces may be elevated and supported from below with bone grafts.

In all other cases the aim is to mobilise the foot and ankle as soon as possible, while at the same time preventing any further displacement and flattening of the heel. This is best achieved by physiotherapy, and crutches should be used until the fracture has united (usually in about 6 weeks as the fracture involves cancellous bone).

CALCANEAL FRACTURES NOT INVOLVING THE SUBTALAR JOINT

Vertical fractures of the tuberosity (Fig. 3b) generally have a good prognosis and may be treated symptomatically. *Horizontal, avulsion fractures* of the calcaneus (Fig. 3c) caused by sudden calf muscle contraction should be internally fixed with a screw. *Displaced horizontal fractures* proximal to the insertion of the tendo calcaneus (Fig. 3d) may be treated by manipulative or open reduction followed by a 6 week period in a below-knee cast. *Fractures of the sustentaculum tali* (Fig. 3e) may result from eversion injuries, but as there is seldom any significant displacement, most may be treated in a below-knee cast for 6 weeks. *Fractures of the anterior process of the calcaneus* (Fig. 3f) usually involve the calcaneocuboid joint. Where the displacement of the bone fragments is minor, treatment

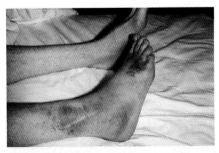

Fig. 5 **Calcaneal bruising, swelling and pressure blistering limited by firm bandaging.**

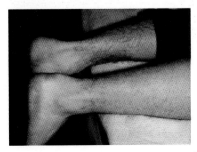

Fig. 6 **Rupture of the right tendo calcaneus with visible gap.**

may be symptomatic. Gross displacements will seriously disturb the function of the midtarsal joint (i.e. the joint between the calcaneus and the cuboid on the lateral side of the foot and between the talus and the navicular on the medial side). When this is the case, an attempt may be made to reduce and fix the calcaneal fracture; this often entails packing up depressed articular fragments using bone grafts. *Fractures of the body of the calcaneus* (Fig. 3g) may also be treated by a 6 week period of non-weight bearing in a below-knee plaster.

COMPLICATIONS OF CALCANEAL FRACTURE

Persistent pain, often with restriction of activities and a limp, is the most common complication. Treatment depends on the cause and, ultimately, the severity and duration of the pain.

Pain arising from the weight bearing portion of the heel may sometimes be relieved by the use of a Sorbo rubber heel insert to act as a cushion during heel strike.

Pain situated below the lateral malleolus often arises from the peroneal tendons being compressed between the distal end of the fibula and the distal, displaced calcaneal fragment. This may be relieved by excision of any local bony prominence and freeing the tendons.

Pain may arise from joint disturbance and secondary osteoarthritic changes. If this fails to respond to prolonged physiotherapy and is severe and disabling, then a fusion may have to be considered. If only the subtalar joint is involved, then a subtalar fusion may suffice. If the calcaneocuboid joint is also affected, then a triple fusion (i.e. a fusion of the subtalar, calcaneocuboid and talonavicular joints) will be required. Such procedures are generally successful in relieving pain, but the inevitable loss of inversion and eversion movement of the foot impair foot function so that, for example, those who are accustomed to working on roofs (e.g. roofers, plumbers) will be unable to resume these activities in safety.

In some fractures the broadening of the heel is so great that surgical shoes may be required.

RUPTURE OF THE TENDO CALCANEUS (ACHILLES TENDON)

The tendon may rupture as a result of sudden muscle contraction. In the young this generally follows some violent athletic activity. In middle age, when the injury is especially common, degenerative changes in the tendon may render it more susceptible to rupture, so that the causal force may be less severe. It is often seen after a sudden jump (e.g. when playing squash or badminton) or a sudden sprint.

There is sudden local pain, followed by difficulty in walking and standing on the toes. The tendon ruptures 4–8 cms above its insertion (although the plantaris is spared) and the gap in continuity may be obvious on inspection (Fig. 6), palpation or MRI scan.

Treatment

Calcaneal tendon ruptures may be treated conservatively, but surgical repair is often preferred in the younger patient or where there has been a delay in diagnosis. The torn ends of the tendon are exposed through a posterior incision under a tourniquet and approximated using absorbable, non-absorbable or pull-out sutures. If there is much fraying of the tendon, strips of fascia lata may be used for the repair. Afterwards the leg is supported in a long leg plaster for about 3 weeks, with the knee in 45 degrees flexion and the ankle in plantarflexion (to relieve any tension on the repair). This type of cast is then replaced with a standard below-knee cast for a further 3 weeks before mobilisation is commenced.

Conservative treatment is especially advocated for the frail or elderly patient, but may be employed for any case seen within 2 days from the time of injury. Support in plaster for 8 weeks is advised, employing the same cast regime as for surgical repair.

Complications include rerupture, weakness of plantar flexion, stiffness of the ankle, poor wound healing and deep vein thrombosis.

The talus and calcaneus

- The most serious complication of talar neck fractures is avascular necrosis. If it occurs, weight bearing should be deferred until the bone revascularises.
- In assessing any calcaneal fracture, it is important to note whether the subtalar joint is involved, as in such fractures there is risk of loss of inversion and eversion movements and secondary osteoarthritis.
- Persistent pain from subtalar joint involvement may merit surgical fusion.
- Ruptures of the tendo calcaneus may be treated either surgically or conservatively.

DISLOCATIONS AND FRACTURES IN THE FOOT

Dislocations within the foot may affect either a single bone or a major part of the foot. All are rather uncommon.

DISLOCATION OF THE TALUS

This is a rare but severe injury in which the talus not only dislocates out of the ankle mortice but loses all connection with the navicular and calcaneus. It comes to lie on the lateral side of the foot in front of the ankle with its axis lying transversely. Closed reduction can usually be achieved but avascular necrosis is almost inevitable.

PERITALAR DISLOCATION

In this more common injury, which results from severe inversion stress, the talus remains firm in the ankle mortice while the rest of the foot swings medially beneath it (Figs 1 and 2). The major portion of the blood supply to the talus remains undisturbed so that avascular necrosis does not result; but late subtalar osteoarthritis is a common complication. Closed reduction may fail due to the head of the talus buttonholing the capsule of the talonavicular joint; open reduction is then necessary. After reduction the foot should be immobilised in a plaster cast for 6 weeks before mobilisation is commenced.

MIDTARSAL DISLOCATION

If an abduction or adduction force is applied to the forefoot, the midtarsal joint may dislocate (i.e. the forefoot, at the level of the navicular and cuboid, loses its alignment with the talus and the calcaneus (Fig. 3)). In some cases there may be associated fractures of the navicular or cuboid which may render the dislocation less stable after reduction (Fig. 4). If this is the case, plaster fixation should be reinforced by the insertion of percutaneous Kirschner wires. If any accompanying fracture involves a large segment of bone, then this may be fixed with screws. Injuries of this pattern are often complicated by foot stiffness, mild chronic pain and late secondary osteoarthritis.

TARSO-METATARSAL DISLOCATIONS

If the forefoot is forcibly plantar flexed (e.g. if it is run over while the metatarsals are projecting over a pavement edge), the

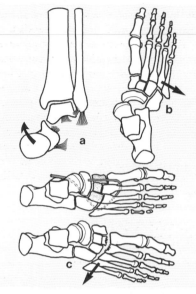

Fig. 1 **The most common patterns of foot dislocations.** Peritalar (**a**); midtarsal (**b**); tarso-metatarsal (**c**).

bases of all the metatarsals may be driven plantarwards away from the cuneiforms and the cuboid; this can occur without fracture.

If on the other hand the forefoot is violently rotated or abducted, the metatarsals may dislocate laterally. The second metatarsal is very securely keyed into the cuneiforms in this plane, so that it usually fractures close to its base (Fig. 5). In some cases, depending on the exact nature of the forces involved, the first ray (the first metatarsal and the medial cuneiform) or the first metatarsal itself may become medially displaced. These injuries are often unstable and accompanied by much swelling. The anastomotic links between the dorsalis pedis and the plantar arteries, which lie near the metatarsal bases, may be disrupted, jeopardising the distal circulation. Reduction should not be delayed. An open procedure, with the insertion of Kirschner wires for stability, is usually the best treatment.

MP DISLOCATIONS OF THE TOES

Toe dislocations may be single or multiple and generally occur at the MP joints; in the great toe, dislocation of the IP joint is not uncommon. Treatment is straightforward: the toe is reduced by traction and splinted by means of garter strapping to an adjacent toe. Instability is seldom a problem, but if it occurs, it may be dealt with by Kirschner wire fixation for 3 weeks.

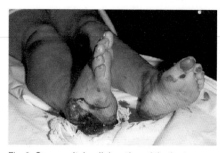

Fig. 2 **Open peritalar dislocation of the foot.**

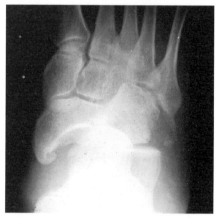

Fig. 3 **Midtarsal dislocation without significant fracture.**

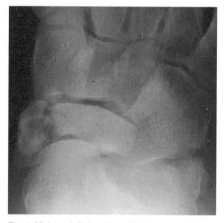

Fig. 4 **Midtarsal dislocation with fracture of the navicular.**

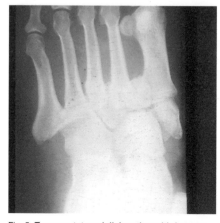

Fig. 5 **Tarso-metatarsal dislocation with fracture of the base of the second metatarsal.**

FRACTURES OF THE FIFTH METATARSAL BASE

The styloid process of the fifth metatarsal may be avulsed (Fig. 6) by the peroneus brevis which has its distal attachment here. This may happen when the foot is suddenly inverted (e.g. when walking on uneven ground) and the muscle contracts violently in an attempt to correct the position of the foot. It is an extremely common injury. It is often missed as it may be mistaken for an ankle sprain, and the fifth metatarsal base is

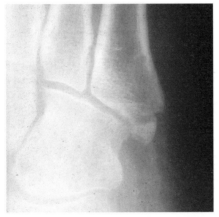

Fig. 6 **Avulsion fracture of the base of the styloid process of the fifth metatarsal.**

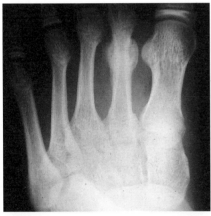

Fig. 7 **March fracture, 6 weeks old, with abundant callus.**

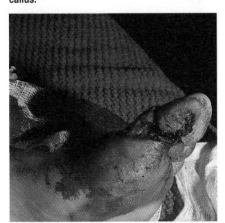

Fig. 8 **Open fractures of the proximal and distal phalanges of the great toe.**

not visualised in routine radiographs of the ankle. Treatment is symptomatic: in some cases a pressure bandage with or without crutches for 2–4 weeks may suffice, but usually a below-knee walking plaster for 5–7 weeks is recommended.

The fifth metatarsal may also fracture just distal to the joint between it and the fourth metatarsal (Jones fracture). This is often a stress fracture, but can be caused by direct violence. It is common in athletes and is often associated with delayed or non-union. It may be treated by a 7 week period of plaster fixation or by internal fixation with a cancellous bone screw. Non-union occasionally requires bone grafting.

METATARSAL SHAFT AND NECK FRACTURES

These fractures generally result from crushing injuries and, if so, any soft tissue injury takes precedence in treatment.

If displacement is minimal, then conservative measures are appropriate; if the fractures are off-ended, then open reduction and internal fixation (usually by means of Kirschner wires) is generally indicated.

MARCH FRACTURE

This is the name given to a metatarsal stress fracture (usually of the second metatarsal) which occurs most commonly in army recruits or nurses when their duties start to involve much walking. There is complaint of foot pain and the fracture may not be visible in early radiographs. Later it is rendered conspicuous by the appearance of abundant callus (Fig. 7). Treatment is symptomatic and it is usually the case that by the time it has been diagnosed the symptoms are resolving. Full recovery is the rule.

PHALANGEAL FRACTURES

Fractures of the distal phalanx of the great toe usually result from heavy weights being dropped on the foot; less commonly, the other toes may be similarly affected. Again the soft tissue injury takes precedence and, if there is an open wound (Fig. 8), debridement will be necessary. Careful assessment of the circulation, with or without admission for observation, is necessary. The toe itself may be supported by being strapped to the adjacent toe. A stout shoe, or a walking plaster with a toe platform, may also be used.

SOFT TISSUE INJURIES OF THE FOOT

The foot, having so many bony components which are small, may sustain serious injury without there being any significant accompanying fracture. This is particularly the case in run over injuries where perhaps a normal radiograph may wrongly suggest that the injury has been trivial.

Soft tissue injuries of the foot must be treated with great respect, especially in the diabetic or older patient with poor peripheral circulation. In all but the most minor cases the patient should be admitted for observation of the circulation: the foot should be elevated and lightly splinted and subsequent swelling and pressure blistering minimised by appropriate bandaging.

Particular care must be taken where the continuity of the skin has been broken. In the serious case where there has been degloving of skin, prompt plastic surgical treatment is essential. Where there has been loss or major involvement of the thick specialised skin of the sole, especially with associated neurovascular damage, amputation may have to be considered.

Dislocations and fractures in the foot

- Dislocation of the talus is a serious injury which is always followed by avascular necrosis.
- Peritalar dislocation may lead to subtalar osteoarthritis.
- Dislocations of the midtalar joint are often accompanied by fractures of the navicular or cuboid.
- Tarso-metatarsal dislocations may affect the blood supply to the distal part of the foot and the toes.
- Fracture of the fifth metatarsal base is the most common injury in the lower limb and is often missed as it may be mistaken for an ankle sprain.
- Jones and March fractures are among the most common stress fractures, and they both occur in the foot.
- Crush injuries of the foot can potentially be the most serious injuries and may not be appreciated as such, especially when they have no accompanying fracture.

FOOT DISORDERS IN CHILDREN

Perceived problems with a child's feet are a common reason for referral to an orthopaedic surgeon. Fortunately, many are minor and will resolve with growth, requiring no treatment other than parental reassurance. It is always necessary however to make a thorough general examination to exclude conditions such as cerebral palsy, and to examine the whole of the lower limb in particular to eliminate contributory conditions such as femoral neck anteversion and tibial torsion.

CONGENITAL TALIPES EQUINOVARUS (CLUB FOOT)

This occurs in about 1.2 per 1000 live births in the UK, with the incidence varying in other parts of the world. The aetiology remains obscure, although there seems to be a definite genetic component which acts in combination with predisposing environmental factors. It is 2–3 times more common in males than females. True talipes equinovarus (CTEV) is the result of an intrinsic structural anomaly, and there is no muscle imbalance. (Note that at birth some children have a mild equinovarus deformity — but not true CTEV — which resolves spontaneously; this may be secondary to intrauterine postural pressure.)

Assessment

In assessing a case it is important to decide whether the deformity is primary or secondary to another congenital anomaly (such as spina bifida, Fig. 1), tracheo-oesophageal fistula, anorectal atresia, cleft lip or a cardiac defect. In arthrogryposis multiplex congenita (a rare condition of obscure aetiology in which at birth there are multiple joint contractures due to muscle imbalance and fibrosis), the associated CTEV is particularly resistant to treatment.

Pathogenesis

There remains much controversy about the pathological process responsible for the deformity. In true CTEV, the muscles of the calf are atrophied and contracted (the triceps surae, toe flexors and the tibialis posterior are particularly affected). In addition, the tarsal bones are smaller and misshapen. Some of this may be secondary to the deformity itself.

Clinical features

In the typical deformity, the hindfoot is in equinus (i.e. fixed plantar-flexion) and in varus; and the forefoot is adducted and supinated (Fig. 2). There is always wasting of the calf muscles, and growth of both the foot and leg may be impaired. It is important to assess whether the deformity can be passively corrected. If it can, it is likely that the condition can be resolved with the use of corrective strapping applied over the course of a few weeks ('resolving' clubfoot). In those feet which cannot be passively corrected ('resistant' clubfoot), surgery is usually necessary. (Radiographs of the foot are difficult to interpret and are best reserved for the postoperative foot where a number of specialised geometric constructions may be used to assess the success of a correction.)

Treatment

The prognosis for treatment of this condition is directly related to the severity. In mild cases, resolution may be spontaneous or require corrective splintage for a few weeks only. In the more severe cases, conservative treatment is always pursued in the first instance. Although this is unlikely to lead to an improvement, it controls the deformity until the child is old enough for surgery. This is generally performed some time after 6 weeks, and within the first year; the optimal timing is dependent on the judgement of both the surgeon and anaesthetist. The types of surgical release that may be carried out remain a little controversial, but the aim is to lengthen the tight Achilles tendon (responsible for the major deforming forces) and all other tight muscular structures. In addition it is usually necessary to release other contracted structures (such as the plantar fascia and joint capsules) to allow bony realignment and maintain the correction. Tendon transfers may be necessary to restore muscle balance after release procedures. A period of splintage is necessary for a minimum of 2–3 months following surgery. It is also essential to keep each case under careful review for a prolonged period so that any tendency to relapse (Fig. 3) is promptly discovered and dealt with.

A more recent, less invasive method of correction, not yet fully evaluated, employs a sophisticated external fixator (Ilizarov); this allows gradual correction of the deformity without the need for extensive surgical release. Once the child is walking the tendency to recurrence lessens.

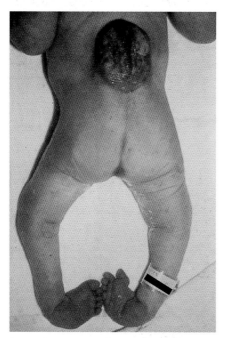

Fig. 1 **Bilateral club feet in association with spina bifida.**

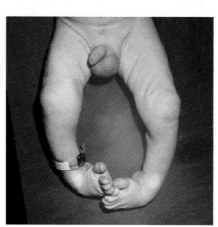

Fig. 2 **Talipes equinovarus in a newborn child.**

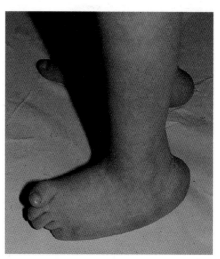

Fig. 3 **Relapsed (L) club foot.**

CONGENITAL TALIPES CALCANEOVALGUS

Here the deformity is the opposite from that found in CTEV: the hindfoot is in calcaneus (i.e. it adopts the position it has in the dorsiflexed foot) and the forefoot is dorsiflexed and twisted into eversion. While in the newborn baby it is normal for the foot to dorsiflex until its dorsal surface rests against the leg, in calcaneovalgus it is not possible to plantarflex the foot. It is common in breech births and as a consequence of intrauterine moulding (usually the result of a reduction in the volume of amniotic fluid (oligohydramnios) common in first pregnancies). It is important to look for other anomalies as it can be associated with hyperextension of the knee and, more importantly, congenital dislocation of the hip.

Treatment

Unlike CTEV this usually responds to passive stretching which the baby's mother is taught to perform. In some cases a period of splintage may be required, although surgery is rarely necessary.

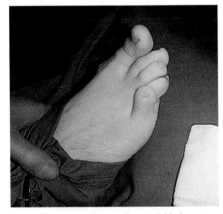

Fig. 4 **Overlapping fifth toe (in an adult) about to undergo surgical correction.**

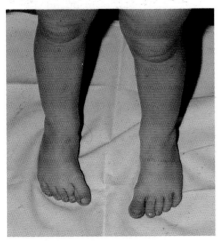

Fig. 5 **Right metatarsus adductus.**

CURLY TOES

This is a common deformity in children under a year, and is often a source of much worry to the parents, even though they themselves may have or have had the same anomaly. They seek advice about whether difficulties will develop with walking ability or shoe wear. The toes are invariably asymptomatic, but typically adopt a flexed and medially rotated posture, sometimes lying on top of each other. Despite their appearance they can usually be corrected passively.

Treatment

Reassurance is usually all that is required as the condition tends to resolve or remain static. In occasional cases surgical correction may be necessary.

OVERRIDING 5TH TOE (QUINTI VARUS)

This is similar to the above except that it invariably becomes a nuisance to the child because of difficulties with footwear. The toe is often underdeveloped and lies over the fourth toe, thus increasing the depth of the foot. A callosity can occur on the dorsum of the toe as it rubs uncomfortably against the upper of the shoe.

Treatment

Conservative treatment with splintage of the toe can be successful if the technique is religiously adhered to, but usually the deformity is resistant and surgical correction is required (Fig. 4). The parents should be warned about the surgical risk to the vascularity of the toe and the possibility of recurrence.

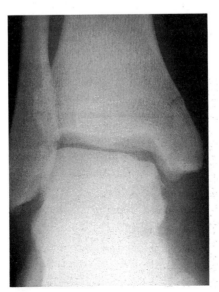

Fig. 6 **Osteochondritis of the superomedial aspect of the talus.**

METATARSUS ADDUCTUS

This is characterised by a forefoot which is adducted (Fig. 5). The hindfoot is normal, and this distinguishes it from CTEV, with which it can be confused. Parental anxiety about the intoeing and the worry that it may be causing the child to trip repeatedly is a common presentation. There may be associated neurological disease and this should be excluded during clinical assessment, as should other more common causes of intoeing (e.g. anteversion of the femoral neck, tibial torsion). The pathology is either due to a tibialis posterior which is attached more anteriorly than normal, or a tight abductor hallucis muscle.

Treatment

Most cases resolve spontaneously by the age of 3, and therefore a watching policy should be adopted. In resistant feet surgical release of the abnormal structures may be necessary. In rare cases a corrective osteotomy is required.

OSTEOCHONDRITIS DISSECANS OF THE TALUS

This is usually found in the skeletally mature. The pathology of osteochondritis dissecans of the talus is similar to that found in other sites (e.g. the medial femoral condyle): there is a localised area of ischaemia in the subarticular bone, probably of traumatic origin. The patients present with pain in the ankle, or locking if the fragment breaks loose. Typically the radiographic lesion is on the superomedial surface of the talus (Fig. 6).

Treatment

Many cases will settle with a period of immobilisation in plaster and simple analgesics. If a loose body is present, removal by arthroscopy or open arthrotomy is necessary.

Foot disorders in children

- Most deformities seen in children's feet are mild: the parents require reassurance that they will resolve with growth.
- In true congenital talipes equinovarus there is no intrinsic muscle imbalance, and surgery is required in severe cases.
- Follow up until maturity may be necessary to detect and deal with possible recurrences.

PES PLANUS / ANTERIOR FOOT PAIN / PES CAVUS

THE ARCHES OF THE FOOT

These have an important role to play in shock absorption and energy conservation during walking, running and jumping. They are not present at birth, but develop after weight bearing has become well established. Abnormalities of the arches may give rise to pain, gait disturbances and other problems.

When the feet are together they enclose a dome-like space, forming in the main a medial longitudinal and a transverse arch. The *medial longitudinal arch* is of greatest importance. At the ends of the arch lie the heel and the medial three metatarsal heads; the rest of the arch is formed by the talus, navicular and cuneiform bones. The highest point of the arch and its weakest point is at the talonavicular joint.

The *transverse arch* in each foot is in fact a half arch formed by the cuneiforms and cuboid and is of little practical importance.

There is also a *lateral longitudinal arch* which is formed by the calcaneus, cuboid and the fourth and fifth metatarsals. It is normally very shallow and during weight bearing flattens out completely (as the normal footprint reveals).

In a mobile foot there is play between the metatarsal heads which, when the foot is bare, allow it to conform to irregularities in the contours of the ground. When weight bearing, all the metatarsal heads take their share in the distribution of forefoot loads so that in practice, in the weight bearing foot, there is no real arch at the level of the metatarsal heads (the so-called anterior arch).

Factors influencing the arches

Heel posture. If the heel tilts into valgus (eversion), the medial side of the foot is lowered, leading to flattening of the arch (pes planus, pronated flat foot). Similarly, if the heel is tilted in varus (inversion), the first metatarsal must drop to maintain the contact of the forefoot with the ground (supinated foot); accentuation of the medial longitudinal arch (pes cavus) results.

Podiatrists set great store on heel alignment, which can affect the whole posture of the foot both passively and dynamically. If investigation reveals a significant disturbance they commonly advise built up insoles and other measures in an attempt to obtain correction or compensation.

Genu valgum. One of the most common causes of flattening of the medial longitudinal arches is knock knee, where the deformity leads to excessive pressure along the medial border of the foot.

Tibial torsion. During growth the shaft of the tibia may twist, disturbing the axes of rotation of the ankle and the knee in the coronal plane. Medial tibial torsion, which may be caused by congenital or other factors (e.g. rickets) is often associated with flat foot.

Hip posture. Excessive internal rotation of the hips, which is the most common cause of an intoeing, may also be associated with flat foot.

Calcaneonavicular bar (or synostosis). This is associated with the clinical condition of peroneal spastic flat foot, which occurs in adolescents. The foot is held in a fully everted position and there is often pain and severe disturbance of gait. If untreated, serial radiographs show progressive ossification in a bar of cartilage running between the calcaneus and navicular. When this process is complete (Fig. 1) it effectively obliterates movements in the subtalar and midtarsal joints and the foot is permanently flat. The condition may be treated by excision of the anomaly.

Talar tilting. This occurs in the rare (congenital) condition of vertical talus. The severe associated flat foot may require corrective surgery.

Muscle and soft tissue problems. The soft tissues which passively support the arches (e.g. the spring ligament and the plantar fascia) fail unless they receive assistance from the intrinsic muscles of the foot and from tibialis anterior, peroneus longus and tibialis posterior. Severe degrees of flat foot may be seen in poliomyelitis and muscular dystrophy; less serious forms are common in middle age where inactivity may lead to a loss of muscle bulk, the effects of which may be aggravated by an increase in body weight.

PES PLANUS

In the majority of cases the foot retains its mobility (mobile flat foot) and is symptom free (although the gait may be awkward, and shoe wear abnormal in pattern and rate). Symptoms may occur during the course of flattening of a previously normal arch, when there may be disturbance of gait and pain along the medial border of the foot (or under the metatarsal heads when there is an associated anterior metatarsalgia — see later). If secondary arthritic changes appear, or if there is a bony anomaly present, there is loss of mobility in the foot (rigid flat foot) and pain is a more common feature.

Diagnosis

This is made by clinical examination of the weight bearing foot where the contact between the medial side of the foot and the ground reveals the loss of the medial longitudinal arch (Fig. 2). The examination should include an assessment of the overall mobility of the foot, the posture of the heels, knees and hips and of tibial rotation; a search should be made for abnormal callus formation and for other deformities. If necessary, study of the footprint, a lateral X-ray projection of the weight bearing foot or gait analysis measurements may be helpful.

Treatment

In the adult, weight reduction, physiotherapy to build up the relevant intrinsic and other muscles and longitudinal arch supports may be employed. Where the heel posture has been found to be abnormal, or where breakdown of a particular part of the arch complex has been found, specialised individually tailored supports may be used.

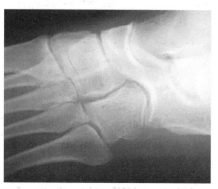

Fig. 1 **Calcaneonavicular synostosis.**

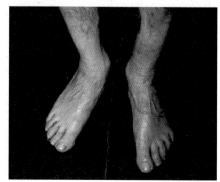

Fig. 2 **Right flat foot.**

Where there is a progressing, severe deformity (e.g. in association with poliomyelitis), in children or adolescents surgery may sometimes be indicated. The Grice sub-talar joint fusion allows correction of any valgus deformity of the heel without disturbing the growth of the foot.

FOREFOOT PAIN

The most common condition producing this complaint is anterior metatarsalgia, a well-defined entity unsatisfactorily named. It occurs in middle age, often after some weight increase, and is associated with failure of the structures which bind the metatarsal heads together (especially the transverse head of adductor hallucis and the intermetatarsal ligaments). The metatarsals tend to drift apart, leading to splaying or broadening of the forefoot; the metatarsal heads become more prominent under the skin which becomes thickened, often with much local tenderness. The broadening of the forefoot may be accompanied by other deformities, to some of which it may contribute (e.g. hallux valgus, clawing of the toes and flat foot). Anterior metatarsalgia may be relieved by podiatric measures such as trimming of local callus and the provision of dome supports. Weight reduction is advisable, and physiotherapy may help.

March fracture. See page 137.

Freiberg's disease. This is an osteochondritis of the second metatarsal head which becomes progressively deformed. There is local tenderness and often swelling of the second toe. The diagnosis is confirmed by X-ray examination (Fig. 3) and in severe cases, where pain is persistent, excision of the metatarsal head may be advised.

Verrucae pedis (plantar warts). These are a common occurrence in the forefoot (and also on the medial side of the heel and under the great toe). They are considered to be of viral origin and must be carefully distinguished from calluses: unlike calluses, they are very sensitive to side to side pressure (Fig. 4). They do not occur in areas of direct pressure, and in the forefoot they lie between the metatarsal heads. They may be treated in a number of ways, including the application of caustics (e.g. salicylic acid, acetic acid), freezing (with carbon dioxide snow) and laser light.

Plantar neuroma (Morton's metatarsalgia). This condition is seen most commonly in women in the 25–50 age group. A neuroma forms on a plantar digital nerve close to where it bifurcates; there is some controversy about the aetiology of the condition, but it may be that it results from the nerve becoming intermittently trapped between the metatarsal heads. The nerve between metatarsals 3 and 4 is most often affected. Pain is often acute and there is sometimes sensory disturbance in the distribution of the nerve. It is treated by excision of the neuroma.

PES CAVUS

Here the medial side of the foot becomes abnormally highly arched. In severe cases the lateral arch is affected as well so that it loses all contact with the ground. On weight bearing the body weight is taken by the heel and metatarsal heads alone and thick callus usually builds up in these areas. Overall the foot may be short and the forefoot broad (Fig. 5).

The condition is produced as a result of an imbalance in the muscles which are associated with the formation and maintenance of the longitudinal arches and a search for a neurological abnormality should always be made. In some cases this may be obvious (e.g. spastic diplegia). Many cases are associated with spina bifida occulta which may be suspected on clinical grounds and confirmed by X-ray.

In many cases there is an increase in the angle between the first metatarsal and the talus; the heel may be in varus, and subtalar movement may be decreased or absent. There is usually marked clawing of the toes. With the abnormal distribution of weight in the forefoot, the skin under the metatarsal head may break down, leading to chronic infection which may be difficult to heal; trophic change may contribute to the problem.

Minor cases of pes cavus may be treated by regular chiropody and supports which can help to spread the distribution of weight in the foot. Where the deformity is more severe, and there is an obvious varus deformity of the heel, a corrective calcaneal osteotomy may help avert long-term problems. In other cases weight distribution may be helped by direct correction of the abnormally high arch by a wedge osteotomy through the distal tarsus or metatarsal bases. Often surgical correction of the toes becomes necessary either by proximal interphalangeal joint fusions or transfer of the long flexor tendons into the extensor tendons.

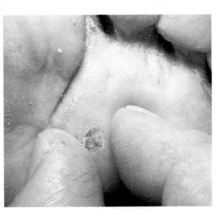
Fig. 4 **Verruca pedis.**

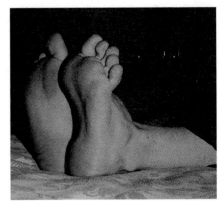
Fig. 5 **Pes cavus.**

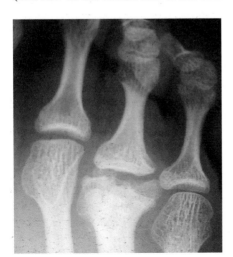
Fig. 3 **Freiberg's disease.**

Pes planus / anterior foot pain / pes cavus

- The arches of the foot are not present in the infant.
- The medial longitudinal arch is the only one of any significance and many factors influence it.
- Flat foot is commonly associated with valgus heel and/or knock knee.
- Peroneal spastic flat foot occurs in adolescents and is associated with a tarsal anomaly.
- Pes cavus is frequently seen in those who have spina bifida occulta.
- The most common forefoot problem is anterior metatarsalgia.

DEFORMITIES OF THE TOES

HALLUX VALGUS

In hallux valgus the great toe is deviated laterally in relation to the axis of the second metatarsal. The condition occurs predominantly in women, and the most important causal factor is the wearing of unsuitable footwear, particularly during growth. If the shoes have high heels, the foot tends to slide forwards so that the toes are squeezed together in the toe box. If this is wedgeshaped the great toe is deviated laterally and, depending on the duration of the constraint and continuing growth, tends to become permanently adapted to the new position. Sometimes the little toe may be similarly affected becoming medially inclined (quinti varus deformity).

The condition is also seen in children of both sexes and the wearing of socks and shoes which are too tight are important contributory factors. The patient in many cases may also be found to have a short and medially inclined first metatarsal (metatarsus primus varus) (Fig. 1).

As the toe moves further and further into valgus, the first metatarsal head is rendered more prominent (so-called *first metatarsal exostosis*) and a protective bursa may develop over it (*bunion*) (Fig. 2); friction against the shoe may give rise to inflammatory changes within it (*bursitis*), sometimes with an added bacterial infection, and the nail of the great toe may become deformed. The uncovering of the first metatarsal head and other mechanical effects may cause *secondary osteoarthritic changes* in the MP joint.

As the great toe moves laterally it crowds the other toes; it may come to lie above or, more commonly, below the other toes. The second toe is first affected (*overriding second toe*), and it may press against the shoe (Fig. 3), causing pain and difficulty in getting shoes to fit. Its IP joints may become flexed (*hammer or claw toe*), and it may rotate or dislocate at its MP joint.

The sesamoid bones under the metatarsal head of the great toe are often displaced, leading to sharply localised pain (*sesamoiditis*). The mechanics of the forefoot are disturbed, and commonly a middle-aged patient may present with spreading of the forefoot, callus formation under the metatarsal heads and complaint of *anterior metatarsalgia*.

Treatment

This potentially disabling condition is largely preventable, the key measures being:

- the dissemination of information so that parents in particular are well informed regarding the risks and how they may be avoided;
- the expert fitting, at frequent intervals, of suitable shoes, with toe boxes free from constraints and with allowance for growth (shoe shops stocking half sizes and four width fittings, with trained fitting staff, and included in the Children's Foot Register should be patronised);
- the careful choice of socks and stockings;
- support for the screening of children's feet at school by the local chiropodial/podiatric services.

In the established case treatment is dependent on the nature of the complaints and the severity of the condition.

Conservative measures

These are advised if: (i) the symptoms are minor; (ii) surgery is considered inadvisable because of the presence of diabetes, poor peripheral circulation or general frailty, etc; (iii) where the outcome of any proposed surgery is uncertain or the risks of recurrence unacceptably high. Measures which may be employed include the careful selection of suitable footwear or the provision of surgical shoes to accommodate the deformity of the great and other toes and the forefoot. Podiatric procedures include the provision of prostheses to protect a bunion or second toe and to help prevent deterioration.

Surgical treatment

More than a hundred surgical procedures have been described for the treatment of hallux valgus, a figure which points to the uncertainty of the success of any. Nevertheless good results can be expected, provided that each case is carefully assessed, and the most appropriate

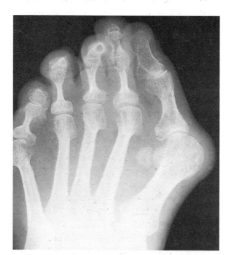

Fig. 1 **Hallux valgus; metatarsus primus varus, first metatarsal exostosis; displaced sesamoids; spreading of forefoot.**

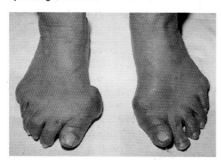

Fig. 2 **Bilateral hallux valgus with bunion on right.**

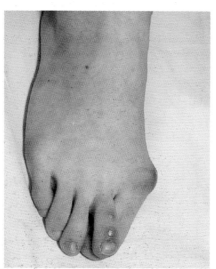

Fig. 3 **Hallux valgus with inflamed overriding second toe.**

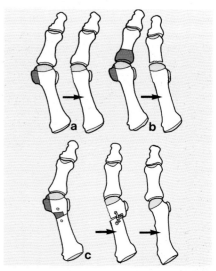

Fig. 4 **Surgical treatments for hallux valgus.**
Exostosectomy (**a**); Keller's arthroplasty (**b**); Mitchell operation (**c**).

procedure selected. (Note however that corrective surgery for hallux valgus before bone maturity is generally unrewarding.) The most popular operations include the following (Fig. 4):

Exostosectomy ('trimming of the exostosis'). The prominence on the medial side of the first metatarsal head is removed. This 'streamlines' the medial side of the foot and removes the effects of local pressure. It is a simple procedure from which recovery is rapid. It is not suitable for gross deformities, and it does not lead to any improvement in the valgus deformity itself. (Some believe that it may adversely affect it.)

Keller's arthroplasty. Here the prominence of the first metatarsal head is also removed and in addition the base of the proximal phalanx of the great toes is excised. This allows the toe to be splinted in a corrected position for a few weeks, during which time a fibrous joint forms between the phalanx and the metatarsal. Although the success rate in terms of symptomatic relief is good, the great toe is permanently shortened and its function is impaired.

Mitchell operation. This includes a displacement osteotomy through the neck of the first metatarsal. It addresses several (but not all) of the main components of the deformity. Recovery is, however, slow as fixation is best maintained until the osteotomy has soundly united.

Osteotomy of the first metatarsal base. Good results have been claimed in cases of metatarsus primus varus when this is combined with trimming of the metatarsal head and release of adductor hallucis.

Prosthetic replacement. Replacement of the first MP joint is being evaluated.

HALLUX RIGIDUS

This occurs predominantly in males and presents as pain and restriction of movement in the MP joint of the great toes. On X-ray the joint space is seen to be narrowed and there is often lipping of the metatarsal head and proximal phalanx, typical of osteoarthritis of the first MP joint (Fig. 5). The age of onset is not, however, typical of primary osteoarthritis, as hallux rigidus often presents in the late teens. If symptoms are minor, it may be treated conservatively by measures to reduce stress and movement at the MP joint (e.g. wearing boots with rigid soles). Surgically, MP joint fusion or Keller's arthroplasty both have their advocates.

DEFORMITIES OF THE LESSER TOES

In a *mallet toe* deformity, the distal interphalangeal joint is flexed and there may be complaint of pain due to pressure of the nail against the sole of the shoe. The deformity may be corrected surgically by a distal interphalangeal joint fusion or excision of the terminal phalanx.

In a *hammer toe* there is a flexion deformity of the interphalangeal joint (Fig. 6); the distal IP and the MP joints are usually dorsiflexed. The 'knuckle' of the proximal IP joint becomes prominent and often rubs against the shoe causing pain and the formation of a local hard corn. Relief may be obtained by trimming the callus and providing pressure relieving padding. In children an attempt may be made to obtain permanent correction by using restraining strapping or other measures. In the adult a permanent cure may be effected by means of a proximal IP joint fusion.

The cause of the above two conditions is not always obvious, but childhood factors, especially unsuitable socks and shoes, are common factors.

In a *claw toe* deformity, the proximal and distal IP joints are flexed and the MP joint is dorsiflexed; one or all of the toes may be affected. In the latter case, the cause is generally one of weakness of the intrinsic muscles of the foot (which normally flex the MP joint and extend the distal joints of the toes). Although it is a feature of many neurological disorders, it is particularly commonly in pes cavus.

Where a single toe is affected, the second is most frequently involved in association with hallux valgus and may be treated by fusion of the interphalangeal joint, with tenotomy of the extensor tendon. It is only reasonable to carry this out if there is sufficient space between the great and third toes to allow the displaced second toe to be brought down to lie in normal alignment. In practice, this generally means that correction of the great toe deformity must precede that of the second toe.

Multiple claw toe deformities such as occur in pes cavus may be dealt with by multiple IP joint fusions (tackling the proximal joints only) or by multiple transfers of the long flexor tendons into the extensors, thereby reinforcing intrinsic muscle action.

In *quinti varus* the little toe is deviated medially and it is often also clawed. It may be seen in isolation or in association with hallux valgus where crowding of the toes may be a common factor. There are a number of plastic surgical procedures available for the correction of this deformity.

Deformities of the toes

- Great care must be taken over the choice of well-fitting children's shoes and socks and their timely replacement during growth.
- Hallux valgus is largely acquired, but metatarsus primus varus is a commonly associated condition.
- Corrective surgery for hallux valgus (and indeed for most foot conditions) is contraindicated where there is evidence of vascular impairment.
- The results of surgery for hallux valgus can be excellent, but as there is always a degree of unpredictability, it is reasonable to treat minor cases conservatively.
- Good results are the rule following surgery for hammer toe deformity, but if there is an associated hallux valgus, this may also require treatment.
- Multiple toe clawing is seen most frequently in association with pes cavus.

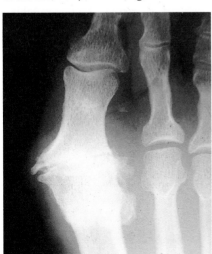

Fig. 5 **Hallux rigidus.**

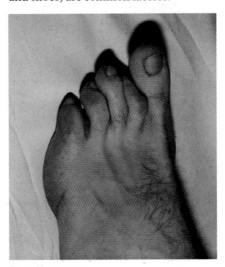

Fig. 6 **Hammer toe.**

OTHER CONDITIONS OF THE TOES AND FOOT

TINEA UNGUIUM

The toe nails may become thickened, friable and discoloured as a result of fungal infections (Fig. 1), this often occurring in those suffering from tinea pedis. Prolonged treatment with topical powders and creams (e.g. Tolnaftate), or systemic antifungals (e.g. Griseofulvin, Allylamine) may be successful, but recurrence is not uncommon. In resistant cases, avulsion of the toe nails may permit control of the situation. In extreme cases, especially in the face of sensitivity to local applications and secondary infection, ablation of the nail beds may be considered.

PSORIASIS

This may lead to pitting and softening of the nails which may thicken and become detached. Sometimes there is an associated psoriatic arthritis. The treatment is that of the underlying condition.

ONYCHOGRYPHOSIS

Growth of the nails may be disturbed (e.g. by local trauma), so that they become greatly thickened and discoloured (Fig. 2). They may be treated radically by avulsion of the nails and ablation of the nail beds; or conservatively by cutting the nails and shaping the remnants (using diamond or other abrasive cutting discs).

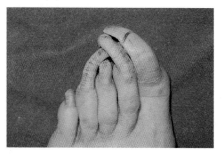

Fig. 1 **Fungal infection of the great toe nail.**

INGROWING TOE NAIL (ONYCHOCRYPTOSIS)

Here the edge of the nail (or a spur arising from it) digs into and penetrates the skin of the nail sulcus. This results in pain and local infection (paronychia, Fig. 3) which may become chronic. The many aetiological factors include pressure from tight shoes and socks, forefoot pronation, disturbance of nail growth (involution) and cutting of the nails too short at the sides. Most cases respond to conservative podiatric measures including the establishment of drainage and the removal of the causal nail splinter (or edge of the nail) under local anaesthesia. If the nail is involuted (i.e. its edges are incurved) slow correction may be obtained by using a nail brace of stainless steel wire (in the manner of the orthodontist realigning teeth). Where infection is resistant, often with the formation of much local granulation tissue, control may be obtained by avulsion of the nail. Frequent recurrences are an indication for ablation of the nail bed, either surgically (e.g. by Zadik's operation) or preferably by phenolisation (using the carefully controlled local application of phenol and alcohol).

SUBUNGUAL EXOSTOSIS

Here an exostosis arising from the tip of the distal phalanx (generally of the great toe) grows under the nail leading to local pain. The nail may become distorted and the pink, skin-covered growth is usually visible under the leading edge of the nail. The diagnosis may be confirmed by X-ray and a cure obtained by excision of the exostosis.

GANGLIONS

These cystic swellings, filled with clear gelatinous fluid, usually develop in relation to one of the dorsal tendon sheaths or one of the tarsal joints and are generally treated by excision.

BURSAE

These fluid filled sacs develop at sites of friction, frequently in relation to a bony prominence. The most common sites are at the side of the MP joint of the great toe and over an exostosis at the first cuneiform–metatarsal joint. Treatment is best reserved for the underlying bony prominence which should be excised.

PLANTAR FASCIITIS

This painful condition is most common in middle-aged men and may be associated with weight gain. There is usually marked and well localised tenderness on the medial aspect of the heel towards its plantar surface. In some cases there may be some local detachment of the plantar fascia, with ossification and the formation of a calcaneal exostosis or 'spur' (Fig. 4). (Calcaneal exostoses may however be symptom free.) It is self-limiting, although local injections of hydrocortisone, a soft rubber pad in the heel of the shoe and physiotherapy in the form of ultrasound are often advocated. (Note that in children pain in the heel may result from an osteochondritis of the calcaneal epiphysis (Sever's disease), although there is some controversy regarding this. Radiographs may show fragmentation and sclerosis (Fig. 5) of the epiphysis. Local pain usually resolves spontaneously over the course of 6 months and may be helped by the use of soft rubber heel pads.

DUPUYTREN'S DISEASE

This produces a firm swelling in the plantar fascia and may be bilateral. It is often associated with classical Dupuytren's contractures of the palmar fascia. There may be complaint of local discomfort and the unusual nature and site of the swelling may cause concern. Growth is slow and there is seldom any contraction of the toes. Treatment is by

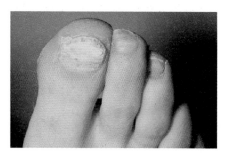

Fig. 2 **Onychogryphosis of all the toes.**

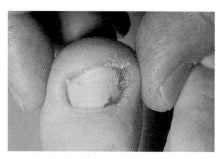

Fig. 3 **Paronychia, with pain on side-to-side pressure.** In sub-ungual exostosis there is pain on downward pressure on the nail.

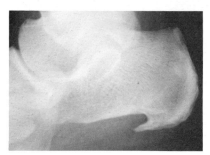

Fig. 4 **Calcaneal spur.**

excision. (Note that the histology specimens of this condition must be reviewed with the greatest of care, as the appearances are often similar to those of fibrosarcoma; confusion in the past has led to serious errors in management.)

RHEUMATOID ARTHRITIS IN THE FOOT

Although any or all of the joints in the foot may be involved, the MP joints of the toes are most commonly affected. They become inflamed and tender, rendering walking difficult. With the concurrent intrinsic muscle weakness these joints become progressively more dorsiflexed, often dislocating (Fig. 6). The toes may then cause problems by pressing against the toe caps of the shoes. The thick, specialised skin under the metatarsal heads becomes distally displaced so that the tender metatarsal heads are poorly protected. Hallux valgus and overriding of the second and often the other toes is common. Acute flat foot may be precipitated by rupture of the tibialis posterior tendon. Subcutaneous granulomatous rheumatoid nodules may develop under the metatarsal heads, over the dorsal surfaces of the toes or under the heels and they may ulcerate. Involvement of the subtalar joint may lead to pain on heel strike and a progressive deviation into valgus which

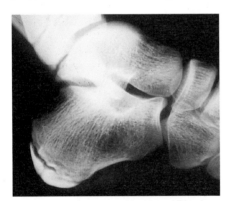

Fig. 5 **Sever's disease with sclerosis of the calcaneal epiphysis.**

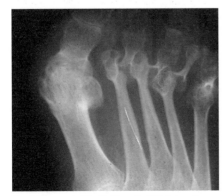

Fig. 6 **Rheumatoid arthritis, with MP dislocations of all the toes.**

contributes to further flattening of the medial longitudinal arch.

General treatment measures include drug therapy. Locally, conservative treatment may draw on the resources of the podiatrist and consists of procedures to reduce pressure on sensitive areas and spread weight bearing loads by the use of padding, insoles and foot and toe prostheses. When there is appreciable broadening of the forefoot and dorsal displacement of the toes, bespoke footwear will be required. Minor surgery may be required to excise painful bony prominences and amputate dislocated, functionless toes which are causing problems with pressure against the shoes or from intractable infections. Radical surgery is particularly indicated in those cases where the pain from prominent metatarsal heads is so great that walking has become almost impossible. In Fowler's procedure the prominent metatarsal heads are excised, along with a large ellipse of skin proximal to the forefoot pad; when the wound is closed, the pad is repositioned under the distal ends of the metatarsals, which it is then able to protect. Other measures include multiple toe corrections (e.g. of hallux valgus and claw toes) and fusions of the subtalar and midtarsal joints.

THE 'HIGH RISK' FOOT

The survival of the foot and indeed of the lower limb may become at risk in those suffering from diabetes, peripheral vascular disease or a peripheral neuropathy which carries the risks of trophic ulceration. Problems usually arise when the skin breaks down and an infection becomes established. It is imperative that every measure is taken to prevent this happening. The patient must receive guidance on the importance of foot hygiene and care of the nails, the selection of footwear and socks and how any abrasions or cuts should be cared for. 'Care of the feet' leaflets, giving good

advice in this area, are widely available from podiatrists and others dealing with these problems. Measures should be taken to minimise areas of local pressure and preserve foot hygiene (e.g. by appropriate padding or supports and avoiding adhesive dressings and prostheses retained by constricting loops or bands). Any problem which arises must be attended to without delay.

Of particular significance is the development of cellulitis; prompt treatment can reduce the ever present risk of rapid spread of infection, gangrene and the need for amputation. General treatment measures include those aimed at stabilising poorly controlled diabetes and improving the peripheral circulation. (Where there is time these might include procedures such as arterial bypass or endarterectomy.) As far as the infection is concerned, the causal organism should be isolated and its antibiotic sensitivity obtained; because of the dangers of delay a broad spectrum antibiotic should be administered until these results are to hand.

The lesion itself should be debrided, either by surgical excision of all necrotic material or the use of agents such as topical sodium hypochlorite solutions; sinuses should be loosely packed to encourage drainage and granulation from the base upwards; and in a few cases, topical antibiotics or other agents may be applied. If gangrene supervenes, amputation may be required.

GOUT

The MP joint of the great toe is affected in over 90% of cases of acute gout. The joint becomes painful, tender and red, with the acute symptoms usually lasting for several days. Repeated attacks lead to progressive destruction of the articular surfaces. Elevation, rest and anti-inflammatory drugs are helpful during the acute attacks; thereafter uricosuric therapy should be employed.

Other conditions of the toes and foot

- Psoriasis and fungal infections are the most common causes of disturbances of nail texture.
- Phenolisation of the nail bed is an effective method of nail ablation for recurrent infected ingrowing toe nail.
- The most common cause of heel pain in children is Sever's disease and, in adults, plantar fasciitis.
- Dupuytren's disease can occur in the feet as well as the hands.
- Some of the most severely deformed feet in rheumatoid arthritis may be greatly benefited by radical surgery.
- In the 'high risk' foot patient education is vital.

INDEX